MEDICAL NUTRITION THERAPY

A CASE STUDY APPROACH

FIFTH EDITION

MARCIA NAHIKIAN NELMS, PhD, RD, LD, CNSC, FAND
OHIO STATE UNIVERSITY

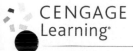

CENGAGE
Learning·

Australia • Brazil • Mexico • Singapore • United Kingdom • United States

Medical Nutrition Therapy: A Case Study Approach,
Fifth Edition
Marcia Nahikian Nelms

Product Director: Mary Finch

Product Manager: Krista Mastroianni

Content Developer: Theodore Knight

Marketing Manager: Anastasia Albinson

Art and Cover Direction, Production
    Management, and Composition: MPS Limited

Manufacturing Planner: Karen Hunt

Intellectual Property Analyst: Christine Myaskovsky

Cover Image: Dimitris Stephanides/Getty images

For product information and technology assistance, contact us at
Cengage Learning Customer & Sales Support, 1-800-354-9706

For permission to use material from this text or product,
submit all requests online at **www.cengage.com/permissions**
Further permissions questions can be e-mailed to
permissionrequest@cengage.com

Library of Congress Control Number: 2015948209
ISBN: 978-1-305-62866-3

Cengage Learning
20 Channel Center Street
Boston, MA 02210
USA

Cengage Learning is a leading provider of customized learning solutions
with employees residing in nearly 40 different countries and sales in more
than 125 countries around the world. Find your local representative at
www.cengage.com

Cengage Learning products are represented in Canada by Nelson Education, Ltd.

To learn more about Cengage Learning Solutions, visit **www.cengage.com**

Purchase any of our products at your local college store or at our preferred
online store **www.cengagebrain.com**

Printed in the United States of America
Print Number: 01   Print Year: 2015

DEDICATION

Dedicated to Sara Long Roth, PhD, RDN, LD who was my original co-author for this text and is now happily enjoying retirement!

To my students—past and present—who continue to challenge me, teach me, and guide me as I strive to enhance dietetic education.

CONTENTS

Unit One

ENERGY BALANCE AND BODY WEIGHT 1

Unit Two

NUTRITION THERAPY FOR CARDIOVASCULAR DISORDERS 35

Unit Three

NUTRITION THERAPY FOR UPPER GASTROINTESTINAL DISORDERS 73

Unit Four

NUTRITION THERAPY FOR LOWER GASTROINTESTINAL DISORDERS 105

Unit Five

NUTRITION THERAPY FOR HEPATOBILIARY AND PANCREATIC DISORDERS 151

Unit Six

NUTRITION THERAPY FOR ENDOCRINE DISORDERS 175

Unit Seven

NUTRITION THERAPY FOR RENAL DISORDERS 215

Unit Eight

NUTRITION THERAPY FOR NEUROLOGICAL DISORDERS 249

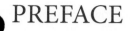

PREFACE

In teaching, I seek to promote the fundamental values of humanism, democracy, and the sciences—that is, a curiosity about new ideas and enthusiasm for learning, a tolerance for the unfamiliar, and the ability to critically evaluate new ideas.

I wish to provide the environment that will support students in their quest for integration of knowledge and support the development of critical thinking skills. Thus, I strive to develop these "laboratories" and "real-world" situations that mimic the professional community to build that bridge to clinical practice.

The idea for this book actually began more than fifteen years ago as I began teaching medical nutrition therapy to dietetic students, and now, as this fifth edition publishes, I hope that these cases reflect the most recent nutrition therapy practice. Entering the classroom after being a clinician for many years, I knew I wanted my students to experience nutritional care as realistically as possible. I wanted the classroom to actually be the bridge between the textbook and the clinical setting. In fashioning one of the tools used to build that bridge, I relied heavily on my clinical experience to develop what I hoped would be realistic clinical applications. Use of a clinical application or case study is not a new concept; the use of case studies in nutrition, medicine, nursing, and many other allied health fields is commonplace. The case study places the student in a situation that forces integration of knowledge from many sources; supports use of previously learned information; puts the student in a decision-making role; and nurtures critical thinking.

What makes this text different, then, from a simple collection of case studies? The pedagogy we have developed over the years with each case takes the student one step closer as he or she moves from the classroom to the real world. The cases represent the most common diagnoses that rely on nutrition therapy as an essential component of the medical care. Therefore, I believe these cases represent the type of patient with which the student will most likely be involved. The concepts presented in these cases can apply to many other medical conditions that may not be presented here. Furthermore, the instructor can choose a variety of questions from each case, even if he or she chooses not to have the student complete the entire case. The cases represent both introductory and advanced-level practice and, therefore, use of this text allows faculty to choose among many cases and questions that fit students' varying skill levels.

The cases cross the life span, allowing the student to see the practice of nutrition therapy during childhood, adolescence, and adulthood through the elder years. I have tried to represent the diversity of individual patients the Registered Dietitian encounters today. Placing nutrition therapy and nutrition education within the appropriate cultural context is crucial.

The electronic medical record provides the structure for each case. The student will seek information to solve the case by using the exact tools he or she will need to use in the clinical setting. As the student moves from the admission or outpatient visit record to the physician's history and physical, to laboratory data, and to documentation of daily care, the student will need to discern the relevant information from the medical record.

Questions for each case are organized using the nutrition care process, beginning with items introducing the pathophysiology and principles of nutrition therapy for the case and then proceeding through each component of the process. Questions prompt the student to identify nutrition problems and then synthesize a PES statement. It will be helpful to begin by orienting the student to the components of a case. I have provided an outline of this introduction below (see "Introducing Case Studies"). Teaching needs to be purposeful. If the instructor takes the responsibility of teaching students how to use this book seriously, it is much more likely that student autonomy will be the end result.

To be consistent with the philosophy of the text, each case requires that the student seek information from multiple resources to complete the case. Many of the articles and online sites provide essential data regarding diagnosis and treatment within that case. I have found that when students learn how to research the case, their expertise grows exponentially.

The cases lend themselves to be used in several different teaching situations. They fit easily into a problem-based learning curriculum, and also can be used as a summary for classroom teaching of the pathophysiology and nutrition therapy for each diagnosis. The cases can be integrated into the appropriate rotation for a dietetic internship, medical school, or nursing school curricula. Furthermore, these cases can be successfully used to develop standardized patient and simulation experiences.

Objectives for student learning within each case are built around the nutrition care process and competencies for dietetic education. This allows an additional path for nutrition and dietetic faculty to document student performance as part of program assessment.

New to the Fifth Edition

Several important factors have prompted the changes to this fifth edition. As we introduced in the fourth edition, the template for the cases is a typical electronic medical record (EMR). Though the EMRs used in clinics, physician's offices, and hospitals vary, these cases capture the primary sources of information that the clinician will access to provide a thorough nutrition assessment for her or his patient. The setting for some of the cases has also been changed to reflect outpatient care within the patient-centered medical home.

Secondly, our reviewers requested that the cases be shortened in length. I have streamlined all of the cases so that questions are more precise. Finally, even within a two- to three-year period, medical and nutritional care can change dramatically. These cases reflect the most recent research and evidenced-based literature so that the student moves toward higher levels of practice.

The fifth edition introduces the following new cases:

Case 8 Gastroparesis
Case 13 Gastrointestinal surgery with ostomy
Case 14 Nonalcoholic Steatohepatitis (NASH)
Case 24 Adult Traumatic Brain Injury (TBI)
Case 25 Pediatric Cerebral Palsy
Case 31 Breast Cancer
Case 32 Tongue Cancer treated with surgery and radiation

For the additional cases you will find in this edition—although the diagnosis may have been included in previous editions—the cases have also been significantly changed to reflect current medical care with appropriate changes in drugs, procedures, and nutrition interventions. For example, the presenting signs and symptoms in the celiac disease case have been changed so they are not the classic gastrointestinal complaints traditionally associated with this disorder. Case 4, on hypertension and cardiovascular disease, incorporates questions and a discussion of the Mediterranean dietary pattern. The heart failure case includes discussion of malnutrition risk. Within the open abdomen surgical case, morbid obesity with sepsis case, and acute pancreatitis case, we have incorporated the most recent literature about assessment of these critically ill patients, and the use of nutrition support has been altered to reflect current practice. Incorporation of evidence-based guidelines is encouraged throughout each of the cases, and the questions are designed to not only follow the nutrition care process but also require the student to evaluate the most current literature.

TEACHING STRATEGIES

You can find cases to emphasize specific topics that are part of the curriculum for pathophysiology and medical nutrition therapy (a list of cases by topic is provided below). I have found that when specific questions are selected for each case, they can be modified to assist in the pedagogy for other classes as well.

Nutrition Assessment: Case 1 Pediatric Weight Management; Case 3 Malnutrition associated with chronic disease; Case 4 Hypertension and Cardiovascular Disease

Fluid Balance/Acid-Base Balance: Case 13 GI surgery with ostomy; Case 27 COPD with Respiratory Failure; Case 29 Metabolic Stress and Trauma: Open Abdomen

Genetics/Immunology/Infectious Process: Case 10 Celiac Disease; Case 12 Inflammatory Bowel Disease; Case 16 Pediatric Type 1 Diabetes Mellitus; Case 17 Type 1 Diabetes Mellitus in the Adult; Case 31 Breast Cancer

Hypermetabolism/Metabolic Stress: Case 15 Acute Pancreatitis; Case 21 Acute Kidney Injury (AKI); Case 24 Adult Traumatic Brain Injury: Metabolic Stress with Nutrition Support; Case 28 Metabolic Stress and Trauma: Open Abdomen; Case 28 Burn Injury; Case 30 Nutrition Support in Sepsis and Morbid Obesity

Dysphagia: Case 22 Ischemic Stroke; Case 23 Progressive Neurological Disease: Parkinson's Disease; Case 25 Pediatric Cerebral Palsy; Case 32 Tongue Cancer Treated with Surgery and Radiation

Nutritional Needs of the Elderly: Case 3 Malnutrition associated with chronic disease; Case 6 Heart Failure; Case 22 Ischemic Stroke; Case 27 COPD with Respiratory Failure

Malnutrition: Case 3 Malnutrition associated with chronic disease; Case 6 Heart Failure; Case 26 COPD; Case 28 Metabolic Stress and Trauma: Open Abdomen; Case 29 Nutrition Support for Burn Injury; Case 30 Nutrition Support in Sepsis and Morbid Obesity; Case 32 Tongue Cancer treated with surgery and radiation

Pediatrics: Case 1 Pediatric Weight Management; Case 14 Pediatric Type 1 Diabetes Mellitus; Case 25 Pediatric Cerebral Palsy

Nutrition Support: Case 12 Inflammatory Bowel Disease: Crohn's Disease; Case 15 Acute Pancreatitis; Case 21 Acute Kidney Injury; Case 23 Progressive Neurological Disease: Parkinson's Disease; Case 24 Adult Traumatic Brain Injury; Case 28 Metabolic Stress and Trauma: Open Abdomen; Case 29 Burn Injury; Case 30 Nutrition Support in Sepsis and Morbid Obesity; Case 32 Tongue Cancer treated with surgery and radiation

ACKNOWLEDGMENTS

I first need to thank my previous developmental editor—Elesha Hyde—who has provided expert guidance for this book since its inception. I would like to thank the following Ohio State University graduate students in medical dietetics who provided input to the cases and the answer guide: Kathleen Crockett and Garrett Davidson. I also have several contributors to new cases and I am fortunate to benefit from the expertise of these outstanding clinicians:

Dena Champion, MS, RD, CSO
Deborah Cohen, DCN, RD
Holly Estes Doetsch, MS, RDN, LD, CNSC
Georgiana Sergakis, PhD, RRT, RCP
Dawn Scheiderer, RD, LD
Colleen Spees, PhD, RDN, LD, FAND
Sheela Thomas, MS, RD, CNSC

ABOUT THE AUTHOR

Marcia Nahikian-Nelms, PhD, RDN, LD, CNSC, FAND

Dr. Nahikian-Nelms is currently a professor of clinical health and rehabilitation sciences and director of the coordinated dietetic programs in the Division of Medical Dietetics. She is also nutrition faculty for the Division of Gastroenterology, Hepatology, and Nutrition, and for the Leadership Education in Neurodevelopmental Disabilities (LEND) in the College of Medicine at The Ohio State University. She has practiced as a dietitian and public health nutritionist for over thirty years. She is the lead author for the textbooks *Nutrition Therapy and Pathophysiology*; *Medical Nutrition Therapy: A Case Study Approach*; and a contributing author for *Food and Culture*. Additionally, she has contributed to the Academy of Nutrition and Dietetics *Nutrition Care Manual* sections on gastrointestinal disorders and is the author of numerous peer-reviewed journal articles and chapters for other texts. The focus of her clinical expertise is the development and practice of evidence-based nutrition therapy for a variety of conditions, including diabetes, gastrointestinal disease, and hematology/oncology for both pediatric and adult populations, as well as the development of alternative teaching environments for students receiving their clinical training. Dr. Nahikian-Nelms has received the Outstanding Teaching Award in the School of Health and Rehabilitation Sciences at Ohio State; Governor's Award for Outstanding Teaching for the State of Missouri, Outstanding Dietetic Educator in Missouri and Ohio, and the PRIDE award from Southeast Missouri State University in recognition of her teaching.

INTRODUCING CASE STUDIES, OR FINDING YOUR WAY THROUGH A CASE STUDY

Have you ever put together a jigsaw puzzle or taught a young child how to complete a puzzle?

Almost everyone has at one time or another. Recall the steps that are necessary to build a puzzle. You gather together the straight edges, identify the corner pieces, and match the like colors. There is a method and a procedure to follow that, when used persistently, leads to the completion of the puzzle.

Finding your way through a case study is much like assembling a jigsaw puzzle. Each piece of the case study tells a portion of the story. As a student, your job is to put together the pieces of the puzzle to learn about a particular diagnosis, its pathophysiology, and the subsequent medical and nutritional treatment. Although each case in the text is different, the approach to working with the cases remains the same, and with practice, each case study and each medical record becomes easier to manage. The following steps provide guidance for working with each case study.

1. Identify the major parts of the case study.
   - Admitting history and physical
   - Documentation of MD orders, nursing assessment, and results from other care providers
   - Laboratory data
   - Bibliography

2. Read the case carefully.
   - Get a general sense of why the person has been admitted to the hospital.
   - Use a medical dictionary to become acquainted with unfamiliar terms.
   - Use the list of medical abbreviations provided in Appendix A to define any that are unfamiliar to you.

3. Examine the admitting history and physical for clues.
   - Height, Weight
   - Vital signs (compare to normal values for physical examination in Appendix B)

- Chief complaint
- Patient and family history
- Lifestyle risk factors

4. Review the medical record.
   - Examine the patient's vital statistics and demographic information (e.g., age, education, marital status, religion, ethnicity).
   - Read the patient history (remember, this is the patient's subjective information).

5. Use the information provided in the physical examination.
   - Familiarize yourself with the normal values found in Appendix B.
   - Make a list of those things that are abnormal.
   - Now compare abnormal values to the pathophysiology of the admitting diagnosis. Which are consistent? Which are inconsistent?

6. Evaluate the nutrition history.
   - Note appetite and general descriptions.
   - Evaluate the patient's dietary history: calculate average kcal and protein intakes and compare to population standards and recommendations such as the USDA Food Patterns.
   - Is there any information regarding physical activity?
   - Find anthropometric information.
   - Is the patient responsible for food preparation?
   - Is the patient taking a vitamin or mineral supplement?

7. Review the laboratory values.
   - Hematology
   - Chemistry
   - What other reports are present?
   - Compare the values to the normal values listed. Which are abnormal? Highlight those and then compare to the pathophysiology. Are they consistent with the diagnosis? Do they support the diagnosis? Why?

8. Use your resources.
   - Use the bibliography provided for each case.
   - Review your nutrition textbooks.
   - Use any books on reserve.
   - Access information on the Internet but choose your sources wisely: stick to government, not-for-profit organizations, and other legitimate sites. A list of reliable Internet resources is provided for each case.

Mindmap

A mindmap is a graphic representation of the elements of the case study and the steps in its analysis. This organization can assist in connecting bodies of information and allow for further development of critical thinking skills.

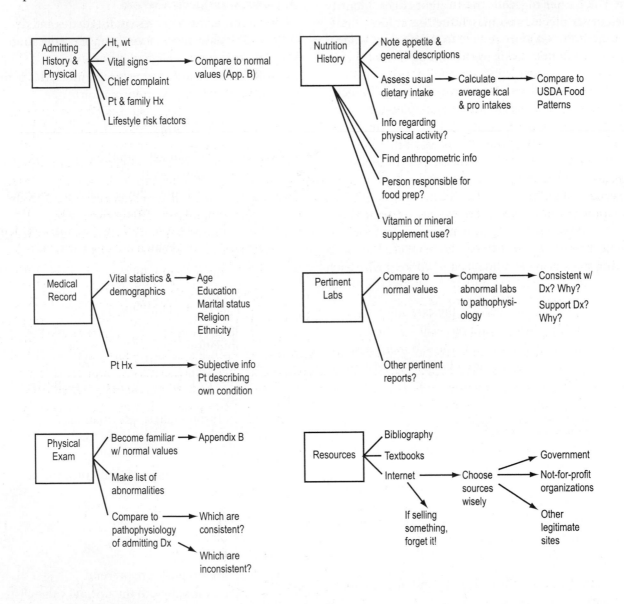

ENERGY BALANCE AND BODY WEIGHT

Unit One introduces nutrition therapy for treatment of disorders of weight balance and draws our attention to these major public health concerns in the United States. The first case uses pediatric obesity as a springboard for a discussion of the implications of the rapidly rising rate of childhood obesity. The incidence of childhood obesity has more than tripled over the past three decades with an estimated 12.5 million children and adolescents in the United States meeting the criteria for overweight and obesity. The child featured in Case 1 is representative of children ages 6–11. Pediatric obesity treatment requires complex interventions to address family, environmental, and economic concerns. This case allows the student to explore the current research and the use of evidence-based guidelines to determine appropriate nutrition therapy.

Case 2 uses the record of a bariatric surgery patient as an opportunity to learn about morbid obesity. More than 3 million individuals in the United States are considered to be morbidly obese—this is also referred to as Class III obesity or a body mass index (BMI) >40.0. Health consequences of untreated morbid obesity include type 2 diabetes mellitus, coronary heart disease and hypertension, cancer, sleep apnea, and even premature death. According to the 2013 American Heart Association and American College of Cardiology guideline for management of overweight and obesity in adults, those individuals who have failed to lose weight by less invasive means, and who meet the medical criteria, may consider bariatric surgery as a treatment method for weight control. This case allows the student to research the surgical options used for bariatric surgery and to begin to understand the progression of nutrition therapy used postoperatively.

Case 3 explores the diagnosis of malnutrition. As early as 1979, Charles Butterworth attempted to raise awareness of the increasing incidence of malnutrition in the U.S. health care system with his classic article, "The Skeleton in the Hospital Closet." Unfortunately, the rate of malnutrition is still considered to be significant today—and is associated with increased hospital costs, increased morbidity and mortality, and decreased quality of life for these individuals. Recently, new definitions of malnutrition have been proposed by the Academy of Nutrition and Dietetics (AND) and the Association for Parenteral and Enteral Nutrition (ASPEN) in an effort to more consistently identify those individuals who are at risk for malnutrition and who are malnourished, so that expedient interventions may occur. This case uses the most recent literature to provide the opportunity to recognize and apply the newly proposed diagnostic criteria for malnutrition.

Pediatric Weight Management

Objectives

After completing this case, the student will be able to:

1. Describe the physiological effects of over-weight/obesity in the pediatric population.
2. Interpret laboratory parameters for nutritional implications and significance.
3. Analyze nutrition assessment data to evaluate nutritional status and identify specific nutrition problems.
4. Determine nutrition diagnoses and write appropriate PES statements.
5. Prescribe appropriate nutrition therapy.

6. Develop a nutrition care plan with appropriate measurable goals, interventions, and strategies for monitoring and evaluation consistent with the nutrition diagnoses of this case.

Jamey Whitmer is taken to see her pediatrician by her parents, who have noticed she appears to stop breathing while sleeping. She is diagnosed with sleep apnea related to her weight and referred to the registered dietitian for nutrition counseling.

Whitmer, Jamey, Female, 10 y.o.
Allergies: No known allergies
Pt. Location: University Clinic

Code: FULL
Physician: Lambert, S. David

Isolation: None
Appointment Date: 9/22

Patient Summary: 10-year-old female is here with parents who describe concerns that their daughter appears to stop breathing while she is sleeping.

History:
Onset of disease: Parents describe sleep disturbance in their daughter for the past several years, including: sleeping with her mouth open, cessation of breathing for at least 10 seconds (per episode), snoring, restlessness during sleep, enuresis, and morning headaches. They also mention that Jamey's teacher reports difficulty concentrating in school and a change in her classroom performance. She is the second child born to these parents—full-term infant with birthweight of 10 lbs 5 oz; 23" length. Actual date of onset for current medical problems is unclear, but parents first noticed onset of the above-mentioned symptoms about one year ago.
Medical history: None
Surgical history: None
Family history: What? Possible gestational diabetes; type 2 DM; Who? Mother and grandmother

Demographics:
Years education: Third grade
Language: English only
Occupation: Student
Household members: Father age 36, mother age 35, sister age 5
Ethnicity: Caucasian
Religious affiliation: Presbyterian

MD Progress Note:
Review of Systems
Constitutional: Negative
Skin: Negative
Cardiovascular: Negative
Respiratory: Negative
Gastrointestinal: Negative
Neurological: Negative
Psychiatric: Negative

Physical Exam
Constitutional: Somewhat tired and irritable 10-year-old female
Cardiovascular: Regular rate and rhythm, heart sounds normal
HEENT: Eyes: Clear
          Ears: Clear
          Nose: Normal mucous membranes
          Throat: Dry mucous membranes, no inflammation, tonsillar hypertrophy
Genitalia: SMR (Tanner) pubic hair stage 3, genital stage 3

Whitmer, Jamey, Female, 10 y.o.
Allergies: No known allergies   **Code:** FULL   **Isolation:** None
Pt. Location: University Clinic   **Physician:** Lambert, S. David   **Appointment Date:** 9/22

Neurologic: Alert, oriented × 3
Extremities: No joint deformity or muscle tenderness, but patient complains of occasional knee pain. No edema, strength 5/5.
Skin: Warm, dry; reduced capillary refill (approximately 2 seconds); slight rash in skin folds
Chest/lungs: Clear
Abdomen: Obese

Vital Signs: Temp: 98.5   Pulse: 85   Resp rate: 27
                   BP: 123/80   Height: 57"   Weight: 115 lbs   BMI: 24.9

Assessment and Plan:

10-year-old female here with parents c/o of breathing difficulty at night. Child has steadily gained weight over previous several years— >10 lbs per year.

Dx: R/O obstructive sleep apnea (OSA) secondary to obesity and physical inactivity

Medical Tx plan: Polysomnography to diagnose OSA, FBG, HbA_{1c}, lipid panel (total cholesterol, HDL-C, LDL-C, triglycerides), psychological evaluation, nutrition assessment

.... SD Lambert, MD

Nutrition:

General: Very good appetite with consumption of a wide variety of foods. Jamey's physical activity level appears to be minimal. Her elementary school discontinued physical education, art, and music classes due to budget cuts five years ago. She likes playing video games and reading. Mother is 5'2" and weighs 225# lbs. Father is 5'10" and weighs 185 lbs. Sister has a weight/height at 85%tile with BMI at 75%tile.

24-hour recall:

AM:	2 breakfast burritos, 8 oz whole milk, 4 oz apple juice, 6 oz coffee with ¼ c cream and 2 tsp sugar
Lunch:	2 bologna and cheese sandwiches with 1 tbsp mayonnaise each, 1-oz pkg Fritos corn chips, 2 Twinkies, 8 oz whole milk
After-school snack:	Peanut butter and jelly sandwich (2 slices enriched bread with 2 tbsp crunchy peanut butter and 2 tbsp grape jelly), 12 oz whole milk
Dinner:	Fried chicken (2 legs and 1 thigh), 1 c mashed potatoes (made with whole milk and butter), 1 c fried okra, 20 oz sweet tea
Snack:	3 c microwave popcorn, 12 oz Coca-Cola

Food allergies/intolerances/aversions: NKA
Previous nutrition therapy? No
Food purchase/preparation: Parent(s)
Vitamin intake: Flintstones vitamin daily

Whitmer, Jamey, Female, 10 y.o.
Allergies: No known allergies
Pt. Location: University Clinic

Code: FULL
Physician: Lambert, S. David

Isolation: None
Appointment Date: 9/22

Laboratory Results (Pediatric)

	Ref. Range	9/22
Chemistry		
Sodium, 10–14 yo (mEq/L)	136–145	142
Potassium, 10–14 yo (mEq/L)	3.5–5.0	4.3
Chloride, 10–14 yo (mEq/L)	98–108	101
Carbon dioxide, 10–14 yo (CO_2, mEq/L)	22–30	25
Bicarbonate, 10–14 yo (mEq/L)	22–26	25
BUN, 10–14 yo (mg/dL)	5–18	8
Creatinine serum, 10–14 yo (mg/dL)	≤1.2	0.6
Uric acid, 10–14 yo (mg/dL)	2.5–5.5	3.1
Glucose, 10–14 yo (mg/dL)	70–99	112 !↑
Phosphate, inorganic, 10–14 yo (mg/dL)	2.2–4.6	3.1
Magnesium, 10–14 yo (mg/dL)	1.6–2.6	1.7
Calcium, 10–14 yo (mg/dL)	8.6–10.5	9.1
Osmolality, 10–14 yo (mmol/kg/H_2O)	275–295	302 !↑
Bilirubin total, 10–14 yo (mg/dL)	≤1.2	0.9
Bilirubin, direct, 10–14 yo (mg/dL)	<0.3	0.2
Protein, total, 10–14 yo (g/dL)	6–7.8	6.5
Albumin, 10–14 yo (g/dL)	3.5–5	4.8
Prealbumin, 10–14 yo (mg/dL)	17–39	33
Cholesterol, 10–14 yo (mg/dL)	124–201 F 119–202 M	165
HDL-C, 10–14 yo (mg/dL)	37–74	34 !↓
VLDL, 10–14 yo (mg/dL)	calculated	13
LDL, 10–14 yo (mg/dL)	64–133	118
LDL/HDL ratio, 10–14 yo	<3	9.07
Triglycerides, 10–14 yo (mg/dL)	10–121 F 10–103 M	65
T_4, 10–14 yo (µg/dL)	5.6–11.7	6.1
T_3, 10–14 yo (µg/dL)	83–213	79 !↓
HbA_{1c}, 10–14 yo (%)	3.9–5.2	4.5
Hematology		
WBC, 10–14 yo ($\times 10^3/mm^3$)	4.0–13.5	4.1
Hemoglobin, 10–14 yo (Hgb, g/dL)	11–16	13.1
Hematocrit, 10–14 yo (Hct, %)	31–43	38

Case Questions

I. Understanding the Disease and Pathophysiology

1. Current research indicates that the cause of childhood obesity is multifactorial. Briefly outline how genetics, environment, and nutritional intake might contribute to the development of obesity in children. Include at least three specific factors in each of the previously mentioned categories.

2. Describe one health consequence for obese children affecting each of the following physiological systems: cardiovascular, orthopedic, pulmonary, gastrointestinal, and endocrine.

3. How does Jamey's current weight status affect her risk of developing adulthood obesity?

4. Jamey has been diagnosed with obstructive sleep apnea. What is *obstructive sleep apnea*? Explain the relationship between sleep apnea and obesity.

II. Understanding the Nutrition Therapy

5. In general, what are the goals for weight loss in the pediatric population? Are there concerns to consider when developing recommendations for an overweight child who is still growing?

6. List four recommendations that might serve as goals for the nutritional treatment of Jamey's obesity.

III. Nutrition Assessment

7. Assess Jamey's weight using the CDC growth charts provided (p. 8): What is Jamey's BMI percentile? How is her weight status classified? Use the growth chart to determine Jamey's optimal weight for her height and age.

8. Identify two methods for determining Jamey's energy requirements other than indirect calorimetry, and then use them to calculate Jamey's energy requirements. What calorie goal would you use to facilitate weight loss?

Stature-for-Age and Weight-for-Age Percentiles: Girls, 2 to 20 Years

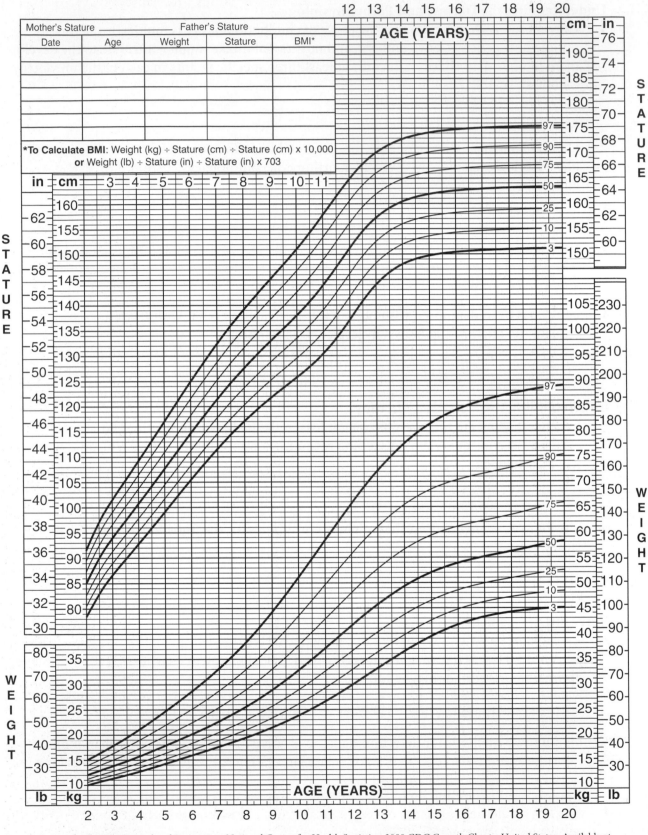

Source: Centers for Disease Control and Prevention. National Center for Health Statistics. 2000 CDC Growth Charts: United States. Available at http://www.cdc.gov/growthcharts. Accessed April 10, 2008.

9. Dietary factors associated with increased risk of overweight include increased dietary fat intake and increased calorie-dense beverages. Identify foods from Jamey's diet recall that fit these criteria.

10. Calculate the percent of kcal from each macronutrient and the percent of kcal provided by fluids for Jamey's 24-hour recall.

11. Increased fruit and vegetable intake is associated with decreased risk of overweight. What foods in Jamey's diet fall into these categories?

12. Use the ChooseMyPlate online tool (available from www.choosemyplate.gov; click on "Daily Food Plans" under "SuperTracker and Other Tools") to generate a customized daily food plan. Using this eating pattern, plan a 1-day menu for Jamey.

13. Now enter and assess the 1-day menu you planned for Jamey using the MyPlate SuperTracker online tool (http://www.choosemyplate.gov/supertracker-tools/supertracker.html). Does your menu meet macro- and micronutrient recommendations for Jamey?

14. Why did Dr. Lambert order a lipid profile and blood glucose tests? What lipid and glucose levels are considered altered (i.e., outside of normal limits) for the pediatric population? Evaluate Jamey's lab results.

IV. Nutrition Diagnosis

15. Select two nutrition problems and complete PES statements for each.

V. Nutrition Intervention

16. What behaviors associated with increased risk of overweight would you look for when assessing Jamey's and her family's diets? What aspects of Jamey's lifestyle place her at increased risk for overweight?

17. You talk with Jamey and her parents, who are friendly and cooperative. Jamey's mother asks if it would help for them to not let Jamey snack between meals and to reward her with dessert when she exercises. What would you tell the family regarding snacks between meals and rewards with dessert after exercise?

18. Identify one specific physical activity recommendation for Jamey.

19. For each PES statement written, establish an ideal goal (based on signs and symptoms) and an appropriate intervention (based on etiology).

20. Mr. and Mrs. Whitmer ask about gastric bypass surgery for Jamey. Based on the Evidence Analysis Library from the Academy of Nutrition and Dietetics or other evidenced-based guideline, what are the recommendations regarding gastric bypass surgery for the pediatric population?

VI.   Nutrition Monitoring and Evaluation

21. What is the optimal length of weight management therapy for Jamey?

22. Should her parents be included? Why or why not?

23. What would you assess during a follow-up counseling session? When should this occur?

Bibliography

Academy of Nutrition and Dietetics Evidence Based Library. Balanced Macronutrient Diet and Treating Childhood Obesity in Children Ages 6–12. AND Evidence Analysis Library. http://www.andeal.org/topic.cfm?cat =2914&conclusion_statement_id=250444. Accessed 02/10/15.

Academy of Nutrition and Dietetics Evidence Based Library. Effectiveness of using balanced macronutrient, reduced calorie (900–1200 kcal per day) dietary interventions for treating childhood obesity in children ages 6–12. AND Evidence Analysis Library. http://www.andeal.org/topic .cfm?cat=2914&conclusion_statement_id=250444. Accessed 02/10/15.

Academy of Nutrition and Dietetics Evidence Based Library. Effectiveness of using a program to increase physical activity as a part of an intervention program to treat childhood obesity. AND Evidence Analysis Library. http://www.andeal.org/topic .cfm?cat=2940&conclusion_statement_id=105. Accessed 02/10/15.

Academy of Nutrition and Dietetics. Pediatric Nutrition Care Manual, Overweight/Obesity. https://www.nutritioncaremanual.org/topic.cfm?ncm _category_id=13&lv1=144636&lv2=144783&ncm _toc_id=144783&ncm_heading=Nutrition%20Care. Accessed 02/10/15.

Academy of Nutrition and Dietetics Evidence Based Library. Pediatric Weight Management (PWM) Comprehensive, Multicomponent Weight Program for Treating Childhood Obesity. AND Evidence Analysis Library. http://www.andeal.org/template.cfm?template=guide _summary&key=1284. Accessed 02/10/15.

Academy of Nutrition and Dietetics Evidence Based Library. Pediatric Weight Management: Major Recommendations. AND Evidence Analysis Library. http://www.andeal.org/topic .cfm?menu=5296&cat=2724. Accessed 02/10/15.

Academy of Nutrition and Dietetics Evidence Based Library. Pediatric Weight Management (PWM) Physical Activity in the Treatment of Childhood and Adolescent Obesity. AND Evidence Analysis Library. http://www.andeal.org/template.cfm?template =guide_summary&key=1224. Accessed 02/10/15.

Academy of Nutrition and Dietetics Evidence Based Library. The Traffic Light Diet and Treating Childhood Obesity. AND Evidence Analysis Library. http://www.andeal.org/topic.cfm?menu=5296 &pcat=4162&cat=4184. Accessed 02/10/15.

Blüher S, Petroff D, Wagner A, et al. The one year exercise and lifestyle intervention program KLAKS: Effects on anthropometric parameters, cardiometabolic risk factors and glycemic control in childhood obesity. *Metabolism.* 2014;63:422–30.

Centers for Disease Control and Prevention, National Center for Health Statistics. CDC growth charts: United States. http://www.cdc.gov/growthcharts /. Accessed 02/10/15.

Dihingia A, Das A. Childhood obesity: Issues of the burden, its genesis and prevention. *SJAMS.* 2014;2:1700–1710.

Farajian P, Panagiotakos DB, Risvas G, Malisova O, Zampelas A. Hierarchical analysis of dietary, lifestyle and family environment risk factors for childhood obesity: The GRECO study. *Eur J Clin Nutr.* 2014;68:1107–12.

Let's Move! http://www.letsmove.gov/. Accessed 02/10/15.

National Academy of Sciences Food and Nutrition Board. *Dietary Reference Intakes for Energy, Carbohydrate, Fiber, Fat, Fatty Acids, Cholesterol, Protein, and Amino Acids.* Washington, DC: The National Academies Press; 2005.

Lacey K. Diseases and disorders of energy balance. In: Nelms M, Sucher K, Lacey K. *Nutrition Therapy and Pathophysiology.* 3rd ed. Belmont, CA: Wadsworth, Cengage Learning; 2016:250–291.

Noqueira I, Hrovat K. Adolescent bariatric surgery: Review on nutrition considerations. *Nutr Clin Pract.* 2014;29:740–746.

United States Department of Agriculture. Information for Health Care Professionals. MyPlate. http://www .choosemyplate.gov/information-healthcare-professionals.html. Accessed 02/10/15.

Internet Resources

American Academy of Pediatrics—Institute for Healthy Childhood Weight: https://ihcw.aap.org/Pages /default.aspx

American Sleep Apnea Association: http:// www.sleepapnea.org/

Baylor College of Medicine Children's Nutrition Research Center: https://www.bcm.edu /departments/pediatrics/sections-divisions-centers /childrens-nutrition-research-center/

Centers for Disease Control and Prevention, "Basics about Childhood Obesity": http://www.cdc.gov/obesity /childhood/basics.html

Centers for Disease Control and Prevention. Growth Charts: http://www.cdc.gov/growthcharts/

Case 2

Bariatric Surgery for Morbid Obesity

Objectives

After completing this case, the student will be able to:

1. Identify criteria that allow for an individual to qualify as a candidate for bariatric surgery.
2. Research and outline the health risks associated with morbid obesity.
3. Identify the current surgical procedures used for bariatric surgery.
4. Describe the potential physiological changes and nutrition problems that may occur after bariatric surgery.
5. Interpret nutrition assessment data to assist with the design of measurable goals, interventions, and strategies for monitoring and evaluation that address the nutrition diagnoses for the patient.

6. Understand current nutrition therapy guidelines for progression of oral intake after bariatric surgery.

Mr. McKinley is admitted for a Roux-en-Y gastric bypass surgery. He has suffered from type 2 diabetes mellitus, hyperlipidemia, hypertension, and osteoarthritis. Mr. McKinley has weighed over 250 lbs since age 15 with steady weight gain since that time. He has attempted to lose weight numerous times but the most weight he ever lost was 75 lbs, which he regained over a two-year period. He had recently reached his highest weight of 434 lbs, but since beginning the preoperative nutrition education program he has lost 24 lbs.

McKinley, Chris, Male, 37 y.o.
Allergies: NKA
Pt. Location: RM 703

Code: FULL
Physician: P Walker

Isolation: None
Admit Date: 2/23

Patient Summary: Patient is a morbidly obese 37-year-old white male who is admitted for Roux-en-Y gastric bypass surgery scheduled for 2/24. Patient has been obese his entire adult life with highest weight 6 months ago at 434 lbs. He has lost 24 lbs since that time as he has been attending the preoperative nutrition program at our clinic.

History:
Onset of disease: Lifelong obesity
Medical history: Type 2 diabetes mellitus, hypertension, hyperlipidemia, osteoarthritis
Surgical history: R total knee replacement 3 years previous
Medications at home: Metformin 1000 mg/twice daily; 35 u Lantus pm; Lasix 25 mg/day; Lovastatin 60 mg/day
Tobacco use: None
Alcohol use: Socially, 2–3 beers per week
Family history: Father: Type 2 DM, CAD, Htn, COPD; Mother: Type 2 DM, CAD, osteoporosis

Demographics:
Marital status: Single
Number of children: 0
Years education: Associate's degree
Language: English only
Occupation: Office manager for real estate office
Hours of work: 8–5 daily—sometimes on weekend
Household members: Lives with roommate
Ethnicity: Caucasian
Religious affiliation: None stated

Admitting History/Physical:
Chief complaint: "I am here for weight-loss surgery."
General appearance: Obese white male

Vital Signs: Temp: 98.9   Pulse: 85   Resp rate: 23
                   BP: 135/90   Height: 5'10"   Weight: 410 lbs
Heart: Normal rate, regular rhythm, normal heart; diminished distal pulses. Exam reveals no gallop and no friction rub.
HEENT: Head: WNL
          Eyes: PERRLA
          Ears: Clear
          Nose: WNL
          Throat: Moist mucous membranes without exudates or lesions
Genitalia: Normally developed 37-year-old male
Neurologic: Alert and oriented
Extremities: Ecchymosis, abrasions, petechiae on lower extremities, 2+ pitting edema

McKinley, Chris, Male, 37 y.o.
Allergies: NKA
Pt. Location: RM 703

Code: FULL
Physician: P Walker

Isolation: None
Admit Date: 2/23

Skin: Warm, dry to touch
Chest/lungs: Respirations WNL, clear to auscultation and percussion
Peripheral vascular: Diminished pulses bilaterally
Abdomen: Obese, rash present under skinfolds

Nursing Assessment	2/23
Abdominal appearance (concave, flat, rounded, obese, distended)	obese
Palpation of abdomen (soft, rigid, firm, masses, tense)	soft
Bowel function (continent, incontinent, flatulence, no stool)	continent
Bowel sounds (P=present, AB=absent, hypo, hyper)	
RUQ	P
LUQ	P
RLQ	P
LLQ	P
Stool color	lt brown
Stool consistency	formed
Tubes/ostomies	NA
Genitourinary	
Urinary continence	yes
Urine source	clean catch
Appearance (clear, cloudy, yellow, amber, fluorescent, hematuria, orange, blue, tea)	clear, yellow
Integumentary	
Skin color	pale
Skin temperature (DI=diaphoretic, W=warm, dry, CL=cool, CLM=clammy, CD+=cold, M=moist, H=hot)	W
Skin turgor (good, fair, poor, TENT=tenting)	good
Skin condition (intact, EC=ecchymosis, A=abrasions, P=petechiae, R=rash, W=weeping, S=sloughing, D=dryness, EX=excoriated, T=tears, SE=subcutaneous emphysema, B=blisters, V=vesicles, N=necrosis)	EC, A, R
Mucous membranes (intact, EC=ecchymosis, A=abrasions, P=petechiae, R=rash, W=weeping, S=sloughing, D=dryness, EX=excoriated, T=tears, SE=subcutaneous emphysema, B=blisters, V=vesicles, N=necrosis)	intact
Other components of Braden score: special bed, sensory pressure, moisture, activity, friction/shear (>18=no risk, 15–16=low risk, 13–14=moderate risk, ≤12=high risk)	15

McKinley, Chris, Male, 37 y.o.
Allergies: NKA
Pt. Location: RM 703

Code: FULL
Physician: P Walker

Isolation: None
Admit Date: 2/23

Orders:
Vital Signs, Routine, Every 4 hours
CBC with differential, comprehensive metabolic profile; PT/PTT; EKG; Urinalysis
NPO after midnight

Nutrition:
Meal type: NPO
Intake % of meals: NPO
Fluid requirement: 1800–2000 mL

MD Progress Note:
2/24
Subjective: Chris McKinley's previous 24 hours reviewed
Vitals: Temp: 98.9   Pulse: 78   Resp rate: 24   BP: 115/70
Urine output: 2230 mL   Point-of-Care Glu: 145

Physical Exam
HEENT: WNL
Neck: WNL
Heart: WNL
Lungs: Clear to auscultation
Abdomen: Obese, soft, some epigastric tenderness +BS × 4

Assessment/Plan:
POD#1 s/p Roux-en-Y gastric surgery—now with positive bowel sounds. Will progress to Stage 1 Bariatric Surgery Diet. If tolerated, discharge to home after nutrition consult. Schedule for postoperative visit in one week. P. Walker, MD

McKinley, Chris, Male, 37 y.o.
Allergies: NKA
Pt. Location: RM 703

Code: FULL
Physician: P Walker

Isolation: None
Admit Date: 2/23

Intake/Output 410 = 186.3636

Date			2/23 0701–2/24 0700			
Time			0701–1500	1501–2300	2301–0700	Daily total
IN		P.O.	0	60	100	160
		I.V.	680	680	680	2040
		(mL/kg/hr)	(0.45)	(0.45)	(0.45)	(0.45)
		I.V. piggyback	0	0	0	0
		TPN	0	0	0	0
		Total intake	680	740	780	2200
		(mL/kg)	(3.6)	(3.9)	(4.2)	(11.8)
OUT		Urine	700	710	820	2230
		(mL/kg/hr)	(0.47)	(0.47)	(0.55)	(0.50)
		Emesis output	0	0	0	0
		Other	0	0	0	0
		Stool	0	0	0	0
		Total output	700	710	820	2230
		(mL/kg)	(3.7)	(3.8)	(4.4)	(12.0)
Net I/O			−20	+30	−40	−30
Net since admission (2/23)			−20	+10	−30	−30

McKinley, Chris, Male, 37 y.o.
Allergies: NKA
Pt. Location: RM 703

Code: FULL
Physician: P Walker

Isolation: None
Admit Date: 2/23

Laboratory Results

	Ref. Range	2/23 1522
Chemistry		
Sodium (mEq/L)	136–145	138
Potassium (mEq/L)	3.5–5.1	5.8 !↑
Chloride (mEq/L)	98–107	99
Carbon dioxide (CO_2, mEq/L)	23–29	27
Bicarbonate (mEq/L)	23–28	25
BUN (mg/dL)	6–20	15
Creatinine serum (mg/dL)	0.6–1.1 F 0.9–1.3 M	0.9
BUN/Crea ratio	10.0–20.0	16.7:1
Uric acid (mg/dL)	2.8–8.8 F 4.0–9.0 M	5.2
Est GFR, non-Afr Amer (mL/min/1.73 m^2)	>60	95
Glucose (mg/dL)	70–99	145 ↑
Phosphate, inorganic (mg/dL)	2.2–4.6	3.9
Magnesium (mg/dL)	1.5–2.4	2.0
Calcium (mg/dL)	8.6–10.2	9.5
Osmolality (mmol/kg/H_2O)	275–295	289
Bilirubin total (mg/dL)	≤1.2	0.8
Bilirubin, direct (mg/dL)	<0.3	0.07
Protein, total (g/dL)	6–7.8	6.8
Albumin (g/dL)	3.5–5.5	4.2
Prealbumin (mg/dL)	18–35	22
Ammonia (NH_3, μmol/L)	6–47	11
Alkaline phosphatase (U/L)	30–120	118
ALT (U/L)	4–36	21
AST (U/L)	0–35	10
CPK (U/L)	30–135 F 55–170 M	220 !↑
Lactate dehydrogenase (U/L)	208–378	276
Cholesterol (mg/dL)	<200	320 !↑
HDL-C (mg/dL)	>59 F, >50 M	32 !↓

McKinley, Chris, Male, 37 y.o.
Allergies: NKA
Pt. Location: RM 703

Code: FULL
Physician: P Walker

Isolation: None
Admit Date: 2/23

Laboratory Results *(Continued)*

	Ref. Range	2/23 1522
VLDL (mg/dL)	7–32	45 !↑
LDL (mg/dL)	<130	232 !↑
LDL/HDL ratio	<3.22 F <3.55 M	7.5 !↑
Triglycerides (mg/dL)	35–135 F 40–160 M	245 !↑
T_4 (µg/dL)	5–12	6.1
T_3 (µg/dL)	75–98	82
HbA_{1C} (%)	<5.7	7.2 !↑
Coagulation (Coag)		
PT (sec)	11–13	12
INR	0.9–1.1	0.95
PTT (sec)	24–34	26
Hematology		
WBC ($\times$ 10^3/mm^3)	3.9–10.7	10.2
RBC ($\times$ 10^6/mm^3)	4.2–5.4 F 4.5–6.2 M	5.5
Hemoglobin (Hgb, g/dL)	12–16 F 14–17 M	14.5
Hematocrit (Hct, %)	37–47 F 41–51 M	42
Mean cell volume (µm^3)	80–96	82
Mean cell Hgb (pg)	28–32	29
Mean cell Hgb content (g/dL)	32–36	33
RBC distribution (%)	11.6–16.5	12.3
Platelet count ($\times$ 10^3/mm^3)	150–350	261
Transferrin (mg/dL)	250–380 F 215–365 M	279
Ferritin (mg/mL)	20–120 F 20–300 M	210
Iron (µg/dL)	65–165 F 75–175 M	110

(Continued)

McKinley, Chris, Male, 37 y.o.
Allergies: NKA
Pt. Location: RM 703

Code: FULL
Physician: P Walker

Isolation: None
Admit Date: 2/23

Laboratory Results *(Continued)*

	Ref. Range	2/23 1522
Total iron binding capacity (µg/dL)	240–460	269
Iron saturation (%)	15–50 F 10–50 M	15
Vitamin B$_{12}$ (ng/dL)	24.4–100	72
Folate (ng/dL)	5–25	15
Urinalysis		
Collection method	---	clean catch
Color	---	yellow
Appearance	---	clear
Specific gravity	1.001–1.035	1.004
pH	5–7	6.1
Protein (mg/dL)	Neg	Neg
Glucose (mg/dL)	Neg	Neg
Ketones	Neg	Neg
Blood	Neg	Neg
Bilirubin	Neg	Neg
Nitrites	Neg	Neg
Urobilinogen (EU/dL)	<1.0	0
Leukocyte esterase	Neg	Neg
Prot chk	Neg	Neg
WBCs (/HPF)	0–5	0
RBCs (/HPF)	0–2	0
Bact	0	0
Mucus	0	0
Crys	0	0
Casts (/LPF)	0	0
Yeast	0	0

Note*:* Values and units of measurement listed in these tables are derived from several resources. Substantial variation exists in the ranges quoted as "normal" and these may vary depending on the assay used by different laboratories.

Case Questions

I. Understanding the Diagnosis and Pathophysiology

1. Define the BMI and percent body fat criteria for the classification of obesity. What BMI is associated with morbid obesity?

2. List 10 health risks involved with untreated morbid obesity. What health risks does Mr. McKinley present with?

3. What are the standard adult criteria for consideration as a candidate for bariatric surgery? After reading Mr. McKinley's medical record, determine the criteria that allow him to qualify for surgery.

4. By performing an Internet search or literature review, find one example of a bariatric surgery program. Describe the information that is provided for the patient regarding qualification for surgery. Outline the personnel involved in the evaluation and care of the patient in this particular program.

5. Describe the following surgical procedures used for bariatric surgery, including advantages, disadvantages, and potential complications.

    a. Roux-en-Y gastric bypass

    b. Vertical sleeve gastrectomy

    c. Adjustable gastric banding (Lap-Band®)

    d. Vertical banded gastroplasty

    e. Duodenal switch

    f. Biliopancreatic diversion

6.   Mr. McKinley has had type 2 diabetes for several years. His physician shared with him that after surgery he will not be on any medications for his diabetes and that he may be able to stop his medications for diabetes altogether. Describe the proposed effect of bariatric surgery on the pathophysiology of type 2 diabetes. What, if any, other medical conditions might be affected by weight loss?

II.   Understanding the Nutrition Therapy

7.   How does the Roux-en-Y procedure affect digestion and absorption? Do other surgical procedures discussed in question #5 have similar effects?

8.   On post-op day one, Mr. McKinley was advanced to the Stage 1 Bariatric Surgery Diet. This consists of sugar-free clear liquids, broth, and sugar-free Jell-O. Why are sugar-free foods used?

9.   Over the next two months, Mr. McKinley will be progressed to a pureed-consistency diet with 6–8 small meals. Describe the major goals of this diet for the Roux-en-Y patient. How might the nutrition guidelines differ if Mr. McKinley had undergone a Lap-Band procedure?

10.   Mr. McKinley's RD has discussed the importance of hydration, protein intake, and intakes of vitamins and minerals, especially calcium, iron, and B_{12}. For each of these nutrients, describe why a deficiency may occur and explain the potential complications that could result from deficiency.

III.   Nutrition Assessment

11.   Assess Mr. McKinley's height and weight. Calculate his BMI and % usual body weight. What would be a reasonable weight goal for Mr. McKinley? Give your rationale for the method you used to determine this goal weight.

12.   After reading the physician's history and physical, identify any signs or symptoms that are most likely a consequence of Mr. McKinley's morbid obesity.

13.   Identify any abnormal biochemical indices and discuss the probable underlying etiology. How might they change after weight loss?

14. Determine Mr. McKinley's energy and protein requirements to promote weight loss. Explain the rationale for the method you used to calculate these requirements.

IV. Nutrition Diagnosis

15. Identify at least two pertinent nutrition problems and the corresponding nutrition diagnoses.

V. Nutrition Intervention

16. Determine the appropriate progression of Mr. McKinley's post–bariatric-surgery diet. Include recommendations for any supplementation that should be prescribed.

17. Describe any pertinent lifestyle changes that you would view as a priority for Mr. McKinley.

18. How would you assess Mr. McKinley's readiness for a physical activity plan? How does exercise assist in weight loss after bariatric surgery?

VI. Nutrition Monitoring and Evaluation

19. Identify the steps you would take to monitor Mr. McKinley's nutritional status postoperatively.

20. From the literature, what is the success rate of bariatric surgery? What patient characteristics may increase the likelihood for success?

21. Mr. McKinley asks you about the possibility of bariatric surgery for a young cousin who is 10 years old. What are the criteria for bariatric surgery in children and adolescents?

22. Write an ADIME note for your inpatient nutrition assessment with initial education for the Stage 1 and 2 (liquid) diet for Mr. McKinley.

Bibliography

Academy of Nutrition and Dietetics. Nutrition Care Manual. Bariatric surgery. https://www.nutritioncaremanual.org/topic.cfm?ncm_category_id=1&lv1=5545&lv2=16927&ncm_toc_id=16927. Accessed April 3, 2015.

Argyropoulos G. Bariatric surgery: Prevalence, predictors, and mechanisms of diabetes remission. *Curr Diab Rep.* 2015;15:15–24.

Bond DS, Thomas JG, King WC, et al. Exercise improves quality of life in bariatric surgery candidates: Results from the Bari-Active Trial. *Obesity.* 2015;23:536–542.

Bosnic G. Nutritional requirements after bariatric surgery. *Crit Care Nurs Clin N Am.* 2014;26:255–262.

Courcoulas AP, Yanovski SZ, Bonds D, et al. Long term outcomes of bariatric surgery: A National Institutes of Health symposium. *JAMA Surg.* 2014;149:1323–1329.

Egberts K, Brown WA, Brennan L, O'Brien PE. Does exercise improve weight loss after bariatric surgery? A systematic review. *Obes Surg.* 2012;22:335–341.

Handzlik-Orlik G, Holecki M, Orlik B, Wylezol M, Dulawa J. Nutrition management of the post-bariatric surgery patient. *Nutr Clin Pract.* 2014;29:18–739.

Ison KA, Andromalos L, Ariagno M, et al. Nutrition and metabolic support recommendations for the bariatric patient. *Nutr Clin Pract.* 2014;29:718–739.

Junior WS, Lopes do Amaral J, Nonino-Borges CB. Factors related to weight loss up to 4 years after bariatric surgery. *Obes Surg.* 2011;21:1724–1730.

Kalarchian M, Turk M, Elliott J, Gourash W. Lifestyle management for enhancing outcomes after bariatric surgery. *Curr Diab Rep.* 2014;14:530–539.

Lacey K. Diseases and disorders of weight balance. In: Nelms M, Sucher K, Lacey K, Long S. *Nutrition Therapy and Pathophysiology.* 3rd ed. Belmont, CA: Wadsworth, Cengage Learning; 2015:250–291.

Raftopoulos I, Bernstein B, O'Hara K, Ruby JA, Chhatrala R, Carty J. Protein intake compliance of morbidly obese patients undergoing bariatric surgery and its effect on weight loss and biochemical parameters. *Surgery for Obesity and Related Diseases.* 2011;7:733–742.

Shukla AP, Buniak WI, Aronne LJ. Treatment of obesity in 2015. *J CardioPulm Rehab Prev.* 2015;35:81–92.

Internet Resources

American Society for Metabolic and Bariatric Surgery: http://ASMBS.org

Bariatric Eating: www.bariatriceating.com

LapBand: www.lapband.com

Nutrition Care Manual: http://www.nutritioncaremanual.org

Obesity Help: www.obesityhelp.com

Realize: www.realize.com

Malnutrition Associated with Chronic Disease

Objectives

After completing this case, the student will be able to:

1. Identify the signs and symptoms associated with malnutrition.
2. Discern the physiological differences among starvation, chronic disease-related malnutrition, and malnutrition associated with acute disease.
3. Develop a nutrition care plan—with appropriate measurable goals, interventions, and strategies for monitoring and evaluation—that addresses the nutrition diagnoses for this case.

Harry Campbell is a 68-year-old male admitted to acute care for possible dehydration, weight loss, generalized weakness, and malnutrition.

Campbell, Harry, Male, 68 y.o.
Allergies: NKA
Pt. Location: RM 1119

Code: FULL
Physician: F. Connors

Isolation: None
Admit Date: 9/22

Patient Summary: Harry Campbell is a 68-year-old male admitted to acute care for possible dehydration, weight loss, generalized weakness, and malnutrition.

History:

Onset of disease: Patient diagnosed with squamous cell carcinoma of tongue five years ago. Patient previously treated with radiation therapy—no treatment × 3 years.
Medical history: Essential hypertension; hyperlipidemia; weight loss; primary tongue squamous cell carcinoma five years previous; peripheral vascular disease
Surgical history: s/p partial glossectomy five years ago
Medications at home: Lipitor 80 mg daily; Monopril 10 mg daily
Tobacco use: 1 ppd for 60 plus years
Alcohol use: 1–3 cans of beer per day
Family history: Mother died of pneumonia; father died of lung cancer.

Demographics:

Marital status: Married—lives with wife; *Spouse name*: Carol
Number of children: 2—alive, ages 42, 45
Years education: 9 years
Language: English only
Occupation: Electrician for 26 years; retired
Hours of work: N/A
Household members: Wife and patient
Ethnicity: Caucasian
Religious affiliation: Baptist

Admitting History/Physical:

Chief complaint: "I just feel weak all over and don't have the energy to do anything."
General appearance: Cachectic, appears older than 68 years of age

Vital Signs: Temp: 96.6   Pulse: 101   Resp rate: 20
                     BP: 122/77   Height: 6'3"   Weight: 156 lbs
Heart: Regular rate and rhythm
HEENT: Head: Noted temporal wasting
          Eyes: PERRLA
          Ears: Clear
          Nose: Dry mucous membranes with petechiae
          Throat: Dry mucous membranes without exudates or lesions
Genitalia: Deferred
Neurologic: Alert and oriented; strength reduced
Extremities: Decreased muscle tone with normal ROM; loss of lean mass noted quadriceps and gastrocnemius; 1+ pedal edema
Skin: Warm and dry with ecchymoses

Campbell, Harry, Male, 68 y.o.
Allergies: NKA
Pt. Location: RM 1119

Code: FULL
Physician: F. Connors

Isolation: None
Admit Date: 9/22

Chest/lungs: Respirations are shallow—clear to auscultation and percussion
Peripheral vascular: Diminished pulses bilaterally
Abdomen: Hypoactive bowel sounds × 4; nontender, nondistended

Nursing Assessment	9/22
Abdominal appearance (concave, flat, rounded, obese, distended)	flat
Palpation of abdomen (soft, rigid, firm, masses, tense)	soft
Bowel function (continent, incontinent, flatulence, no stool)	continent
Bowel sounds (P=present, AB=absent, hypo, hyper)	
RUQ	P, hypo
LUQ	P, hypo
RLQ	P, hypo
LLQ	P, hypo
Stool color	light brown
Stool consistency	soft
Tubes/ostomies	NA
Genitourinary	
Urinary continence	catheter
Urine source	catheter
Appearance (clear, cloudy, yellow, amber, fluorescent, hematuria, orange, blue, tea)	cloudy, amber
Integumentary	
Skin color	pale
Skin temperature (DI=diaphoretic, W=warm, dry, CL=cool, CLM=clammy, CD1=cold, M=moist, H=hot)	W, dry
Skin turgor (good, fair, poor, TENT=tenting)	TENT
Skin condition (intact, EC=ecchymosis, A=abrasions, P=petechiae, R=rash, W=weeping, S=sloughing, D=dryness, EX=excoriated, T=tears, SE=subcutaneous emphysema, B=blisters, V=vesicles, N=necrosis)	EC, D, T
Mucous membranes (intact, EC=ecchymosis, A=abrasions, P=petechiae, R=rash, W=weeping, S=sloughing, D=dryness, EX=excoriated, T=tears, SE=subcutaneous emphysema, B=blisters, V=vesicles, N=necrosis)	intact, D, P
Other components of Braden score: special bed, sensory pressure, moisture, activity, friction/shear (>18 = no risk, 15–16 = low risk, 13–14 = moderate risk, ≤12 = high risk)	friction/shear; 17

Orders:

0.9% sodium chloride with potassium chloride 20 mEq 125 mL/hr
Vancomycin 1 g in dextrose 200 mL IVPB

Campbell, Harry, Male, 68 y.o.
Allergies: NKA
Pt. Location: RM 1119

Code: FULL
Physician: F. Connors

Isolation: None
Admit Date: 9/22

Thiamin injection 100 mg daily
Multivitamin capsule 1 Cap daily
Metronidazole 500 mg in NaCl premix IVPB
Docusate capsule 100 mg twice daily
Lipitor 80 mg daily
Monopril 10 mg daily

Nutrition:

Meal type: Mechanical soft diet
Intake % of meals: <5%; sips of liquids
Fluid requirement: 2000–2500 mL
History: Patient states that he has lost over 60 lbs in past 1–2 years. He lost some weight when diagnosed with cancer 5 years ago but held steady at approximately 220 lbs even after completing radiation therapy until 1–2 years ago, when he began losing weight. He states that he gets full really easily and never feels hungry.
Usual intake (for past several months): AM—egg, coffee, few bites of toast; 10 am—½ can Ensure Complete; lunch—soup or ½ sandwich, milk; dinner – few bites of soft meat, potatoes or rice. Tries to drink the other ½ can of Ensure Complete.

Intake/Output

Date			9/22 0701–9/23 0700			
Time			0701–1500	1501–2300	2301–0700	Daily total
IN	P.O.		**sips**	**120**	**240**	**360**
	I.V. (mL/kg/hr)		**720** (1.3)	**720** (1.3)	**720** (1.3)	**2,160** (1.3)
	I.V. piggyback					
	TPN					
	Total intake (mL/kg)		**720** (10.2)	**840** (11.8)	**960** (13.5)	**2,520** (35.5)
OUT	Urine (mL/kg/hr)		**480** (0.8)	**320** (0.6)	**643** (1.1)	**1,443** (0.8)
	Emesis output					
	Other					
	Stool		1			1
	Total output (mL/kg)		**481** (6.8)	**320** (4.5)	**643** (9.1)	**1,444** (20.4)
Net I/O			**+239**	**+520**	**+317**	**+1,076**
Net since admission (9/22)			**+239**	**+759**	**+1,076**	**+1,076**

Campbell, Harry, Male, 68 y.o.
Allergies: NKA
Pt. Location: RM 1119

Code: FULL
Physician: F. Connors

Isolation: None
Admit Date: 9/22

Laboratory Results

	Ref. Range	9/22 1522
Chemistry		
Sodium (mEq/L)	136–145	150 !↑
Potassium (mEq/L)	3.5–5.1	3.5
Chloride (mEq/L)	98–107	106
Carbon dioxide (CO_2, mEq/L)	23–29	29
Bicarbonate (mEq/L)	23–28	24
BUN (mg/dL)	6–20	36 !↑
Creatinine serum (mg/dL)	0.6–1.1 F 0.9–1.3 M	1.4 !↑
Uric acid (mg/dL)	2.8–8.8 F 4.0–9.0 M	4.5
Glucose (mg/dL)	70–99	71
Phosphate, inorganic (mg/dL)	2.2–4.6	2.4
Magnesium (mg/dL)	1.5–2.4	1.9
Calcium (mg/dL)	8.6–10.2	8.4 !↓
Osmolality (mmol/kg/H_2O)	275–295	324 !↑
Protein, total (g/dL)	6–7.8	5.8 !↓
Albumin (g/dL)	3.5–5.5	1.8 !↓
Prealbumin (mg/dL)	18–35	9 !↓
Ammonia (NH_3, μg/L)	6–47	11
Alkaline phosphatase (U/L)	30–120	75
ALT (U/L)	4–36	31
AST (U/L)	0–35	24
CPK (U/L)	30–135 F 55–170 M	88
Cholesterol (mg/dL)	<200	112
HDL-C (mg/dL)	>59 F, >50 M	24 !↓
VLDL (mg/dL)	7–32	22
LDL (mg/dL)	<130	66
LDL/HDL ratio	<3.22 F <3.55 M	2.75

(Continued)

Campbell, Harry, Male, 68 y.o.
Allergies: NKA
Pt. Location: RM 1119

Code: FULL
Physician: F. Connors

Isolation: None
Admit Date: 9/22

Laboratory Results *(Continued)*

	Ref. Range	9/22 1522
Triglycerides (mg/dL)	35–135 F 40–160 M	112
T_4 (μg/dL)	5–12	5.8
T_3 (μg/dL)	75–98	81
HbA$_{1C}$ (%)	<5.7	5.3
Hematology		
WBC ($\times 10^3$/mm^3)	3.9–10.7	12.6 !↑
RBC ($\times 10^6$/mm^3)	4.2–5.4 F 4.5–6.2 M	2.4 !↓
Hemoglobin (Hgb, g/dL)	12–16 F 14–17 M	8.1 !↓
Hematocrit (Hct, %)	37–47 F 41–51 M	24.1 !↓
Mean cell volume (μm^3)	80–96	100.6 !↑
Mean cell Hgb (pg)	28–32	33.6 !↑
Mean cell Hgb content (g/dL)	32–36	33
RBC distribution (%)	11.6–16.5	18 !↑
Platelet count ($\times 10^3$/mm^3)	150–350	240
Transferrin (mg/dL)	250–380 F 215–365 M	382 !↑
Ferritin (mg/mL)	20–120 F 20–300 M	17 !↓
Hematology, Manual Diff		
Neutrophil (%)	40–70	55
Lymphocyte (%)	22–44	23
Monocyte (%)	0–7	4
Eosinophil (%)	0–5	0
Basophil (%)	0–2	0
Blasts (%)	3–10	4
Segs (%)	0–60	45
Bands (%)	0–10	10

Campbell, Harry, Male, 68 y.o.
Allergies: NKA
Pt. Location: RM 1119

Code: FULL
Physician: F. Connors

Isolation: None
Admit Date: 9/22

Laboratory Results *(Continued)*

	Ref. Range	9/22 1522
Urinalysis		
Collection method	—	clean catch
Color	—	dark amber
Appearance	—	cloudy
Specific gravity	1.001–1.035	1.036 !↑
pH	5–7	0.9
Protein (mg/dL)	Neg	+ !↑
Glucose (mg/dL)	Neg	Neg
Ketones	Neg	+ !↑
Blood	Neg	Neg
Bilirubin	Neg	Neg
Nitrites	Neg	Neg
Urobilinogen (EU/dL)	<1.0	Neg
Leukocyte esterase	Neg	Neg
Prot chk	Neg	+ !↑
WBCs (/HPF)	0–5	3–4
RBCs (/HPF)	0–2	1–2
Bact	0	+ !↑
Mucus	0	0
Crys	0	0
Casts (/LPF)	0	0
Yeast	0	0

Note: Values and units of measurement listed in these tables are derived from several resources. Substantial variation exists in the ranges quoted as "normal" and these may vary depending on the assay used by different laboratories.

Case Questions

I.   Understanding the Diagnosis and Pathophysiology

1. Outline the metabolic changes that occur during starvation/inadequate nutritional intake (not related to disease) that could result in weight loss.

2. Read the consensus statement of the Academy of Nutrition and Dietetics/American Society of Parenteral and Enteral Nutrition: Characteristics recommended for the identification and documentation of adult malnutrition. Explain the differences between malnutrition associated with chronic disease and malnutrition associated with acute illness and inflammation.

3. Find the current definitions of malnutrition in the United States using the ICD 10 codes. List all of them and describe the criteria for one of the diagnoses.

4. Current ICD definitions of malnutrition use biochemical markers as a component of the diagnostic criteria. Explain the effect of inflammation on visceral proteins and how that may impact the clinician's ability to diagnose malnutrition. What laboratory values may confirm the presence of inflammation?

II.   Understanding the Nutrition Therapy

5. Mr. Campbell was ordered a mechanical soft diet when he was admitted to the hospital. Describe how his meals will be modified with this diet order.

6. What is the Ensure Complete supplement that was ordered? Determine additional options for Mr. Campbell that would be appropriate for a high-calorie, high-protein beverage supplement.

III.   Nutrition Assessment

7. Assess Mr. Campbell's height and weight. Calculate his BMI and % usual body weight.

8. After reading the physician's history and physical, identify any signs or symptoms that support the diagnosis of malnutrition using the proposed definitions of malnutrition by AND/ASPEN malnutrition guidelines.

9.   Evaluate Mr. Campbell's initial nursing assessment. What important factors noted in his nutrition assessment may support the diagnosis of malnutrition?

10.   What is a Braden score? Assess Mr. Campbell's score. How does this relate to his nutritional status?

11.   Identify any signs (including laboratory values) or symptoms from the physician's history and physical and from the nursing assessment that are consistent with dehydration.

12.   Determine Mr. Campbell's energy and protein requirements. Explain the rationale for the method you used to calculate these requirements.

13.   Determine Mr. Campbell's fluid requirements. Compare this with the information on the intake/output report.

14.   From the nutrition history, assess Mr. Campbell's usual dietary intake. How does this compare to the requirements that you calculated for him? Can your evaluation of his dietary intake contribute to the evidence for diagnosing malnutrition?

IV.   Nutrition Diagnosis
15.   Identify the pertinent nutrition problems and the corresponding nutrition diagnoses and write at least two PES statements, with one focused on the clinical domain.

V.   Nutrition Intervention
16.   Determine the appropriate intervention for each nutrition diagnosis.

VI.   Nutrition Monitoring and Evaluation
17.   Identify the steps you would take to monitor Mr. Campbell's nutritional status while he is hospitalized. How would this differ if you were providing follow-up care through his physician's office?

18.   Write your ADIME note for this initial nutrition assessment for Mr. Campbell.

Bibliography

Corkins MR, Guenter P, DiMaria-Ghalilli RA, Jensen GL, et al. Malnutrition diagnoses in hospitalized patients: United States, 2010. *JPEN*. 2014;38:186–195.

Giannopoulous GA, Merriman LR, Ramsey A, Zweibel DS. Malnutrition coding 101: Financial impact and more. *Nutr Clin Pract*. 2013;28:698–709.

Jensen GL, Mirtallo J, Compher C, et al. Adult starvation and disease related malnutrition: A proposal for etiology-based diagnosis in the clinical practice setting from the International Consensus Guideline Committee. *Clinical Nutrition*. 2010;29:151–153.

Jensen GL, Wheeler D. A new approach to defining and diagnosing malnutrition in adult critical illness. *Curr Opin Crit Care*. 2012;18:206–211.

Malone A, Hamilton C. The Academy of Nutrition and Dietetics/The American Society for Parenteral and Enteral Nutrition Consensus Malnutrition Characteristics: Application in practice. *Nutr and Clin Pract*. 2013;28:639–650.

Nahikian-Nelms ML. Metabolic stress and the critically ill. In: Nelms M, Sucher K, Lacey K. *Nutrition Therapy and Pathophysiology*. 3rd ed. Belmont, CA: Cengage Learning; 2016:682–701.

Nahikian-Nelms ML, Habash D. Nutrition assessment: Foundation of the nutrition care process. In: Nelms M, Sucher K, Lacey K. *Nutrition Therapy and Pathophysiology*. 3rd ed. Belmont, CA: Cengage Learning; 2016:34–65.

Nicolo M, Compher C, Still C, Huseini M, Dayton S, Jensen GL. Feasibility of accessing data in hospitalized patients to support the diagnosis of malnutrition by the Academy-ASPEN malnutrition consensus recommended clinical characteristics. *Nutr Clin Pract*. 2013;28:639–650.

Tappendan KA, Quatrara B, Parkhurst ML, Malone AM, Fanjang G, Zeigler TR. Critical role of nutrition in improving quality of care: An interdisciplinary call to action to address adult hospital malnutrition. *JPEN*. 2013;17:482–497.

White JV, Guenter P, Jensen G, Malone A, Schofield M, Academy of Nutrition and Dietetics Malnutrition Work Group, A.S.P.E.N. Malnutrition Task Force, A.S.P.E.N. Board of Directors. Consensus statement of the Academy of Nutrition and Dietetics/American Society of Parenteral and Enteral Nutrition: Characteristics recommended for the identification and documentation of adult malnutrition. *J Acad Nutr Diet*. 2012;112:730–738.

Internet Resources

AND Evidence Analysis Library: http://www.adaevidencelibrary.com

Alliance to Advance Patient Nutrition: http://malnutrition.com

Prevention Plus Braden Scale: http://www.bradenscale.com

Centers for Medicare and Medicaid Services, ICD 10: http://cms.gov/Medicare/Coding/ICD10/index.html

Nutrition Care Manual: http://www.nutritioncaremanual.org

USDA SuperTracker: http://www.choosemyplate.gov/supertracker-tools/supertracker.html

Unit Two

NUTRITION THERAPY FOR CARDIOVASCULAR DISORDERS

Cardiovascular disease accounts for over 30% of all deaths in the United States. Risk factors for cardiovascular disease include dyslipidemia, smoking, diabetes mellitus, high blood pressure, obesity, and physical inactivity. Researchers estimate that more than 80 million Americans have one or more forms of cardiovascular disease; as a result, many patients that the health care team encounters will have conditions related to cardiovascular disease. Extensive health care costs for cardiovascular disease provide an important impetus to intervention and treatment with medical nutrition therapy.

This section includes three of the most common diagnoses: hypertension (HTN), myocardial infarction (MI), and heart failure (HF). All these diagnoses require a significant medical nutrition therapy component for their care.

Over 74 million people in the United States have hypertension. Stage One hypertension is defined as a systolic blood pressure of 140 mm Hg or higher and a diastolic pressure of 90 mm Hg or higher. Essential hypertension, which is the most common form of hypertension, is of unknown etiology. Case 4 focuses on lifestyle modifications as the first step in treatment of hypertension accompanied by dyslipidemia in a female patient. This case incorporates the pharmacological treatment of hypertension, and you will use the well-validated *Dietary Approaches to Stop Hypertension* (DASH) as the center of the medical nutrition therapy intervention. The 2015 *Dietary Guidelines* provide additional support for modification of sodium intake to assist with nutrition therapy.

Because cardiovascular disease is a complex, multifactorial condition, Case 4 provides the opportunity to evaluate these multiple risk factors through all facets of nutrition assessment. We specifically emphasize interpretation of laboratory indices for dyslipidemia. In this case, you will also determine the clinical classification and treatment of abnormal serum lipids, explore the use of drug therapy to treat dyslipidemias, and develop appropriate nutrition interventions using the most recent nutrition recommendations including the Mediterranean Diet.

Case 5 focuses on the acute care of an individual suffering a myocardial infarction (MI). Ischemia of the vessels within the heart results in death of the affected heart tissue. This case lets you evaluate pertinent assessment measures for the individual suffering an MI and then develop an appropriate nutrition care plan for lifestyle behavior change that complements the medical care for prevention of further cardiac deterioration.

Case 6 addresses the long-term consequences of cardiovascular disease in a patient suffering from heart failure (HF). In HF, the heart cannot pump effectively, and the lack of oxygen and nutrients affects the body's tissues. HF is a major public health problem in the United States, and its incidence is increasing. Without a heart transplant, long-term prognosis is poor. This advanced case requires you to integrate understanding of the physiology of several body systems as you address heart failure's metabolic effects including cardiac cachexia, with its significant effect on nutritional status.

Hypertension and Cardiovascular Disease

Objectives

After completing this case, the student will be able to:

1. Describe the physiology of blood pressure regulation.
2. Apply knowledge of the pathophysiology of hypertension and dyslipidemias to identify and explain common nutritional problems associated with these diseases.
3. Explain the role of nutrition therapy as an adjunct to pharmacotherapy, surgery, and other medical treatments of cardiovascular disease.
4. Interpret laboratory parameters for nutritional implications and significance.
5. Analyze nutrition assessment data to evaluate nutritional status and identify specific nutrition problems.
6. Determine nutrition diagnoses and write appropriate PES statements.
7. Develop a nutrition care plan—with appropriate measurable goals, interventions, and strategies for monitoring and evaluation—that addresses the nutrition diagnoses of this case.

Mrs. Margaret Moore is a 57-year-old retired nurse. For the past year, she has treated her newly diagnosed hypertension with lifestyle changes including diet, smoking cessation, and exercise. She is in to see her physician for further evaluation and treatment for essential hypertension. Blood drawn 2 weeks prior to this appointment shows an abnormal lipid profile.

Moore, Margaret Female, 57 y.o.

Allergies: No known allergies	**Code:** FULL	**Isolation:** None
Pt. Location: University Clinic	**Physician:** R. Evans	**Appointment Date:** 6/25

Patient Summary: 57-year-old female here for evaluation and treatment for essential hypertension and hyperlipidemia.

History:

Onset of disease: Mrs. Moore is a 57-year-old female who is a retired nurse. She was diagnosed 1 year ago with Stage 2 (essential) HTN. Treatment thus far has been focused on nonpharmacological measures. She began a walking program resulting in a 10-pound weight loss that she has been able to maintain during the past year. She walks 30 minutes 4–5 times per week, though she sometimes misses on weekends and on nights when she is volunteering for her church. She was given a nutrition information pamphlet in the MD office outlining a lower-Na diet. Mrs. Moore was a 2-pack-a-day smoker but quit ("cold turkey") when her HTN was diagnosed last year. No c/o of any symptoms related to HTN. Pt denies chest pain, SOB, syncope, palpitations, or myocardial infarction.

Medical history: Not significant before Dx of HTN

Surgical history: None

Medications at home: None

Tobacco use: No—quit 1 year ago

Alcohol use: 2–4 beers/wk

Family history: What? HTN. Who? Mother died of MI related to uncontrolled HTN.

Demographics:

Marital status: Married; *Spouse name:* Steve Moore, 60 yo

Number of children: Children are grown and do not live at home.

Years education: College degree

Language: English

Occupation: No employment outside of home—retired nurse

Hours of work: Varies—volunteers several times per month

Household members: 2

Ethnicity: African-American

Religious affiliation: Roman Catholic

MD Progress Note:

Review of Systems

Constitutional: Negative

Skin: Negative

Cardiovascular: No carotid bruits

Respiratory: Negative

Gastrointestinal: Negative

Neurological: Negative

Psychiatric: Negative

Physical Exam

General appearance: Healthy, middle-aged female who looks her age

Heart: Regular rate and rhythm, normal heart sounds—no clicks, murmurs, or gallops

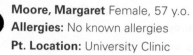

Moore, Margaret Female, 57 y.o.

Allergies: No known allergies   **Code:** FULL   **Isolation:** None

Pt. Location: University Clinic   **Physician:** R. Evans   **Appointment Date:** 6/25

HEENT: Eyes: No retinopathy, PERRLA

Genitalia: Normal female

Neurologic: Alert and oriented × 3

Extremities: Noncontributory

Skin: Smooth, warm, dry, excellent turgor, no edema

Chest/lungs: Lungs clear

Peripheral vascular: Pulse 4+ bilaterally, warm, no edema

Abdomen: Nontender, no guarding, normal bowel sounds

Vital Signs: Temp: 98.6   Pulse: 80   Resp rate: 15

 BP: 160/100   Height: 5'6"   Weight: 160 lbs   BMI: 25.8

Assessment and Plan:

Dx: Stage 2 HTN, heart disease, early COPD; here for initiation of pharmacologic therapy with thiazide diuretics and reinforcement of lifestyle modifications. R/O metabolic syndrome.

rule out

Medical Tx plan: Urinalysis; hematocrit; blood chemistry to include plasma glucose, potassium, BUN, creatinine, fasting lipid profile, triglycerides, calcium, uric acid; chest X-ray; nutrition consult; 25 mg hydrochlorothiazide daily; 2.5 mg Altace daily × 1 week; 5 mg Altace daily × 3 weeks and then 10 mg Altace daily thereafter; evaluate for initiation of HMG-CoA reductase inhibitor therapy; f/u 3 months

R. Evans, MD

Nutrition:

General: Mrs. Moore describes her appetite as "very good." She does the majority of grocery shopping and cooking, although Mr. Moore cooks breakfast on the weekends. She usually eats 3 meals each day, but on her volunteer nights, she may skip dinner. When she does this, she is really hungry when she gets home in the late evening, so she often eats a bowl of ice cream before going to bed. The Moores usually eat out on Friday and Saturday evenings at pizza restaurants or steakhouses (Mrs. Moore usually has 2 regular beers or 2 glasses of wine with these meals). She mentions that last year when her HTN was diagnosed, the MD's office gave her a sheet of paper with a list of foods to avoid for a lower-salt diet. She states that she certainly is familiar with a low-salt diet from when she practiced as an RN. She and her husband tried to comply with the diet guidelines, but they found foods bland and tasteless, and they soon abandoned the effort.

24-hour recall:

AM: 1 c coffee (black)

 Oatmeal (1 instant packet with 1 tsp margarine and 2 tsp sugar)

 1 c orange juice

Snack: 2 c coffee (black)

 1 glazed donut

Moore, Margaret Female, 57 y.o.

Allergies: No known allergies	**Code:** FULL	**Isolation:** None
Pt. Location: University Clinic	**Physician:** R. Evans	**Appointment Date:** 6/25

Lunch: 1 can Campbell's® tomato bisque soup prepared with milk
10 saltines
1 can diet cola

PM: 6 oz baked chicken (white meat, no skin; seasoned with salt, pepper, garlic)
1 large baked potato with 1 tbsp butter, salt, and pepper
1 c glazed carrots (1 tsp sugar, 1 tsp butter)
Dinner salad with ranch-style dressing (3 tbsp)—lettuce, spinach, croutons, sliced cucumber
2 regular beers

HS snack: 2 c buttered popcorn

Food allergies/intolerances/aversions: None
Previous nutrition therapy? Yes. If yes, when: 1 year ago. Where? MD's office.
Food purchase/preparation: Self and husband
Vit/min intake: Multivitamin/mineral daily

Laboratory Results

	Ref. Range	6/25	12/14 (6 mos. later)	3/15 (9 mos. later)
Chemistry				
Sodium (mEq/L)	136–145	137	138	137
Potassium (mEq/L)	3.5–5.1	4.5	3.6	3.9
Chloride (mEq/L)	98–107	102	100	101
Carbon dioxide (CO_2, mEq/L)	23–29	28	29	29
Bicarbonate (mEq/L)	23–28	25	25	26
BUN (mg/dL)	6–20	20	18	19
Creatinine serum (mg/dL)	0.6–1.1 F 0.9–1.3 M	0.9	1.1	1.1
Uric acid (mg/dL)	2.8–8.8 F 4.0–9.0 M	3.2	4.1	3.5
Est GFR, Afr-Amer (mL/min/1.73 m²)	>60	72	70	70
Glucose (mg/dL)	70–99	101 !↑	90	96
Phosphate, inorganic (mg/dL)	2.2–4.6	4.1	3.5	3.5
Magnesium (mg/dL)	1.5–2.4	2.1	2.3	2.4
Calcium (mg/dL)	8.6–10.2	9.2	9.1	9.5
Osmolality (mmol/kg/H_2O)	275–295	294	293	295
Bilirubin total (mg/dL)	≤1.2	1.1	0.8	0.9

Moore, Margaret Female, 57 y.o.
Allergies: No known allergies
Pt. Location: University Clinic

Code: FULL
Physician: R. Evans

Isolation: None
Appointment Date: 6/25

Laboratory Results *(Continued)*

	Ref. Range	6/25	12/14 (6 mos. later)	3/15 (9 mos. later)
Bilirubin, direct (mg/dL)	<0.3	0.1	0.12	0.11
Protein, total (g/dL)	6–7.8	7	6.2	6.9
Albumin (g/dL)	3.5–5.5	4.6	4.5	4.7
Prealbumin (mg/dL)	18–35	32	31	33
Ammonia (NH_3, μg/L)	6–47	19	18	21
Alkaline phosphatase (U/L)	30–120	120	100	101
ALT (U/L)	4–36	30	35	28
AST (U/L)	0–35	34	31	30
CPK (U/L)	30–135 F 55–170 M	100	125	130
Lactate dehydrogenase (U/L)	208–378	314	323	350
Cholesterol (mg/dL)	<200	270 !↑	230 !↑	210 !↑
HDL-C (mg/dL)	>59 F, >50 M	30 !↓	35 !↓	38 !↓
VLDL (mg/dL)	7–32	30	26	25
LDL (mg/dL)	<130	210 !↑	169 !↑	147 !↑
LDL/HDL ratio	<3.22 F <3.55 M	7.0 !↑	4.8 !↑	3.9 !↑
Apo A (mg/dL)	80–175 F 75–160 M	75 !↓	100	110
Apo B (mg/dL)	45–120 F 50–125 M	140 !↑	120	115
Triglycerides (mg/dL)	35–135 F 40–160 M	150 !↑	130	125
T_4 (μg/dL)	5–12	8.6	8.5	7.8
T_3 (μg/dL)	75-98	95	92	93
HbA_{1C} (%)	<5.7	4.9	5.0	5.1
Hematology				
WBC ($\times 10^3/mm^3$)	3.9–10.7	6.1	5.7	5.5
RBC ($\times 10^6/mm^3$)	4.2–5.4 F 4.5–6.2 M	5.3	5.0	5.25
Hemoglobin (Hgb, g/dL)	12–16 F 14–17 M	14.2	14.0	13.9

(Continued)

Moore, Margaret Female, 57 y.o.
Allergies: No known allergies
Pt. Location: University Clinic

Code: FULL
Physician: R. Evans

Isolation: None
Appointment Date: 6/25

Laboratory Results *(Continued)*

	Ref. Range	6/25	12/14 (6 mos. later)	3/15 (9 mos. later)
Hematocrit (Hct, %)	37–47 F 41–51 M	45	44	44
Urinalysis				
Collection method	—	rand. spec.	rand. spec.	rand. spec.
Color	—	pale yellow	pale yellow	pale yellow
Appearance	—	clear	clear	clear
Specific gravity	1.001–1.035	1.025	1.021	1.024
pH	5–7	7.0	5.0	6.0
Protein (mg/dL)	Neg	Neg	Neg	Neg
Glucose (mg/dL)	Neg	Neg	Neg	Neg
Ketones	Neg	Neg	Neg	Neg
Blood	Neg	Neg	Neg	Neg
Bilirubin	Neg	Neg	Neg	Neg
Nitrites	Neg	Neg	Neg	Neg
Urobilinogen (EU/dL)	<1.0	0.02	0.01	0.09
Leukocyte esterase	Neg	Neg	Neg	Neg
Prot chk	Neg	Neg	Neg	Neg
WBCs (/HPF)	0–5	0	0	0
RBCs (/HPF)	0–2	0	0	0
Bact	0	0	0	0
Mucus	0	0	0	0
Crys	0	0	0	0
Casts (/LPF)	0	0	0	0
Yeast	0	0	0	0

Note: Values and units of measurement listed in these tables are derived from several resources. Substantial variation exists in the ranges quoted as "normal" and these may vary depending on the assay used by different laboratories.

Case Questions

I. **Understanding the Disease and Pathophysiology**

1. Define arterial blood pressure (BP) and explain how it is measured.

2. Discuss briefly the mechanisms that regulate arterial blood pressure including the sympathetic nervous system, the renin–angiotensin–aldosterone system (RAAS), and renal function.

3. What is essential hypertension? What is the etiology?

4. What are the common symptoms of essential hypertension?

5. Using the JNC 8 guidelines, how is the diagnosis of hypertension made? What blood pressure readings are used to identify normal BP, stage 1 hypertension, and stage 2 hypertension?

6. List the risk factors for developing hypertension. What risk factors does Mrs. Moore currently have? Discuss the contribution of ethnicity to hypertension, especially for African Americans.

7. What are the four major modes of treatment for hypertension?

8. Dr. Evans indicated in his note that he will "rule out metabolic syndrome." What is metabolic syndrome?

9. What factors found in the medical and social history are pertinent for determining Mrs. Moore's coronary heart disease (CHD) risk category?

10. How is hypertension related to other cardiovascular disorders? What are the possible complications of uncontrolled or untreated hypertension?

II. Understanding the Nutrition Therapy

11. Briefly describe the DASH eating plan and discuss the major nutrients that are components of this nutrition therapy.

12. Using 2015 *Dietary Guidelines*, describe why decreased sodium intake is targeted as a focus to improve the health of Americans.

13. What do the current literature and the Evidence Analysis Library (EAL) indicate regarding the role of sodium intake in the control of hypertension? Is there a significant correlation between sodium intake and cardiovascular risk?

14. What is the Mediterranean diet? How might this dietary approach be appropriate for Mrs. Moore? Would this be culturally appropriate for her?

15. Lifestyle modifications reduce blood pressure, enhance the efficacy of antihypertensive medications, and decrease cardiovascular risk. List lifestyle modifications that have been shown to lower blood pressure.

III. Nutrition Assessment

16. What are the health implications of Mrs. Moore's body mass index (BMI)?

17. Calculate Mrs. Moore's energy and protein requirements.

18. Identify the major sources of sodium and saturated fat in Mrs. Moore's diet. Compare her typical diet to the components of the DASH diet.

19. What dietary assessment tools that target nutrients known to be associated with hypertension and CVD risk might be useful in assessing Mrs. Moore's diet?

20. From the information gathered within the intake domain, list possible nutrition problems using the diagnostic terms.

21. Dr. Evans ordered the laboratory tests listed in the following table. Complete the table with Mrs. Moore's values from 6/25 and the potential cause of any abnormalities.

Parameter	Normal Value	Pt's Value	Reason for Abnormality
Glucose	70–99 mg/dL		
BUN	6–20 mg/dL		
Creatinine	0.6–1.1 mg/dL		
Total cholesterol	<200 mg/dL		
HDL-cholesterol	>59 mg/dL		
LDL-cholesterol	<130 mg/dL		
Apo A	80–175 mg/dL		
Apo B	45–120 mg/dL		
Triglycerides	35–135 mg/dL		

22. Go to http://cvdrisk.nhlbi.nih.gov/. Using this online calculator, determine Mrs. Moore's risk of CVD based on her lipid profile. Are there other factors that contribute to her CVD risk?

23. How do Mrs. Moore's labs change between 6/25 and 3/15? What factors in her history may have made an impact on these?

24. Indicate the pharmacological differences among the antihypertensive agents listed below.

Medications	Mechanism of Action	Nutritional Side Effects and Contraindications
Diuretics		
Beta-blockers		
Calcium-channel blockers		
ACE inhibitors		
Angiotensin II receptor blockers		
Alpha-adrenergic blockers		

25. What are the most common nutritional implications of taking hydrochlorothiazide?

26. Mrs. Moore's physician has decided to prescribe an ACE inhibitor and an HMG-CoA reductase inhibitor (Zocor). What changes to Mrs. Moore's labs between 6/25 and 3/15, if any, would you attribute to Zocor use?

27. From the information gathered within the clinical domain, list possible nutrition problems using the diagnostic terms.

IV. Nutrition Diagnosis

28. Select two nutrition problems and complete the PES statement for each.

V. Nutrition Intervention

29. When you talk with Mrs. Moore on 3/15, you ask how much weight she would like to lose. She tells you she would like to weigh 125, which is what she weighed most of her adult life. Is this reasonable? What would you suggest as a goal for weight loss for Mrs. Moore? How quickly should Mrs. Moore lose this weight?

30. For each of the PES statements that you have written, establish an ideal goal (based on the signs and symptoms) and an appropriate intervention (based on the etiology).

31. List your major recommendations for dietary substitutions and/or other changes that would help Mrs. Moore reach her medical nutrition therapy goals, to be consistent with the DASH diet and sodium intake guidelines.

32. Your appointment with Mrs. Moore on 3/15 is concluded. What would you want to reevaluate at her next follow-up appointment?

Bibliography

Academy of Nutrition and Dietetics Evidence Analysis Library. Hypertension (HTN): Classification of Blood Pressure.

Academy of Nutrition and Dietetics Evidence Analysis Library. Hypertension Evidence-Based Nutrition Practice Guideline.

Academy of Nutrition and Dietetics Nutrition Care Manual. BMI and Weight Range Calculator.

Academy of Nutrition and Dietetics Nutrition Care Manual. Hypertension. http://nutritioncaremanual.

Brunner EJ, Thorogood M, Rees K, Hewitt G. Dietary advice for reducing cardiovascular risk. *Cochrane Database Syst Rev.* 2005;(4):CD002128.

Cook NR, Appel LJ, Whelton PK. Lower levels of sodium intake and reduced cardiovascular risk. *Circulation.* 2014;129:981–989.

Eckel RH, Jakicic JM, Ard, JD, et al. 2013 AHA/ACC guideline on lifestyle management to reduce cardiovascular risk: A report of the American College of Cardiology American/Heart Association Task Force on Practice Guidelines. *J Am Coll Cardiol.* 2014;63:2960–2984.

Go AS, Bauman M, King SM, et al. An effective approach to high blood pressure control: A science advisory from the American Heart Association, the American College of Cardiology, and the Centers for Disease Control and Prevention. *Hypertension.* 2014;63:878–885.

Graudal NA, Hubeck-Graudal T, Jurgens G. McCarron D. The significance of duration and amount of sodium reduction intervention in normotensivce and hypertensive individuals: A meta analysis. *Adv Nutr.* 2015;6:169–177.

Graudal NA, Hubeck-Graudal T, Jurgens G. Effects of low-sodium diet vs. high-sodium diet on blood pressure, renin, aldosterone, catacholamines, cholesterol, and triglyderide. *Am J Hypertens.* 2012;25:1–15.

Grosso G, Mistretta A, Frigiola A, et al. Mediterranean diet and cardiovascular risk factors: A systematic review. *Crit Rev Food Sci Nutr.* 2014;54:593–610.

Grundy SM, Brewer B, Cleeman JI, Smith SC, Lenfant C. Definition of metabolic syndrome: Report of the National Heart, Lung, and Blood Institute/American Heart Association Conference on scientific issues related to definition. *Circulation.* 2004;109:433–438.

Lacey K. The nutrition care process. In: Nelms M, Sucher K, Lacey K, Roth SL. *Nutrition Therapy and Pathophysiology.* 3rd ed. Belmont, CA: Cengage Learning; 2016:14–33.

National Institutes of Health, National Heart, Lung, and Blood Institutes. *DASH Eating Plan: Lower Your Blood Pressure.* U.S. Dept. of Health and Human Services, NIH Publication No. 06-4082. Originally printed 1998, revised October 2014. http://www.nhlbi.nih.gov/health/health-topics/topics/dash. Accessed 3/19/15.

National Institutes of Health, National Heart, Lung, and Blood Institutes. *What is metabolic syndrome?* U.S. Dept. of Health and Human Services, revised October 2011. http://www.nhlbi.nih.gov/health/health-topics/topics/ms. Accessed 3/19/15.

Nelms MN, Habash D. Nutrition assessment: Foundation of the nutrition care process. In: Nelms M, Sucher K, Lacey K. *Nutrition Therapy and Pathophysiology.* 3rd ed. Belmont, CA: Cengage Learning; 2016:34–65.

Pronsky ZM, Crowe JP. *Food and Medication Interaction,* 17th ed. Birchrunville, PA: Food-Medication Interactions; 2012.

Pujol TJ, Barnes J, Sucher K. Diseases of the cardiovascular system. In: Nelms M, Sucher K, Lacey K. *Nutrition Therapy and Pathophysiology.* 3rd ed. Belmont, CA: Cengage Learning; 2016:283–328.

Sacks FM, Svetkey LP, Vollmer WM, et al. Effects on blood pressure of reduced dietary sodium and the Dietary Approaches to Stop Hypertension (DASH) diet. DASH-Sodium Collaborative Research Group. *N Engl J Med.* 2001;344:3–10.

Strazzulo P, Leclercq C. Sodium. *Adv Nutr.* 2014;5:188–190.

Weber MA, Schiffrin EL, White WB, et al. Clinical practice guidelines for the management of hypertension in the community. A statement by the American Society of Hypertension and the International Society of Hypertension. *J Hypertens.* 2014;32:3–15.

Internet Resources

American Heart Association: www.heart.org

AHA/ACC Cardiovascular Risk Calculator: http://my.americanheart.org/professional/StatementsGuidelines/PreventionGuidelines/Prevention-Guidelines_UCM_457698_SubHomePage.jsp

NHLBI: Third Report of the Expert Panel on Detection, Evaluation, and Treatment of High Blood Cholesterol in Adults (Adult Treatment Panel III): www.nhlbi.nih.gov/health-pro/guidelines/current/cholesterol-guidelines

NHLBI: Your Guide to Lowering Your Blood Pressure with DASH: www.nhlbi.nih.gov/health/public/heart/hbp/dash/index.htm

National Cholesterol Education Program Provides clinical guidelines for treatment of dyslipidemia from the NHLBI: www.nhlbi.nih.gov/about/ncep

Medline Plus: Heart Diseases: www.nlm.nih.gov
    /medlineplus/heartdiseases.html
Calculate Your Body Mass Index: http://www.nhlbi.nih
    .gov/health/educational/lose_wt/BMI/bmicalc.htm
National Heart Lung Blood Institute: What is the DASH
    eating plan?: http://www.nhlbi.nih.gov/health
    /health-topics/topics/dash/

USDA Nutrient Data Laboratory: http://www.ars.usda
    .gov/main/site_main.htm?modecode=80-40-05-25
Office of Disease Prevention and Health Promotion:
    http://odphp.hhs.gov/
Scientific Report of the 2015 Dietary Guidelines
    Advisory Committee: http://www.health.gov
    /dietaryguidelines/2015-scientific-report/

Myocardial Infarction

Objectives

After completing this case, the student will be able to:

1. Understand the pathophysiology and initial medical and nutritional care of myocardial infarction.
2. Describe the progression of atherosclerosis and its role in the etiology of myocardial infarction.
3. Interpret laboratory parameters for nutritional implications and significance.
4. Analyze nutrition assessment data to evaluate nutritional status and identify specific nutrition problems.
5. Determine nutrition diagnoses and write appropriate PES statements.

6. Develop a nutrition care plan—with appropriate measurable goals, interventions, and strategies for monitoring and evaluation—that addresses the nutrition diagnoses of this case.

Mr. Garcia, a 61-year-old man, is admitted through the emergency department of University Hospital after experiencing a sudden onset of severe precordial pain on the way home from work. Mr. Garcia is found to have suffered a myocardial infarction and is treated with an emergency angioplasty of the infarct-related artery.

Garcia Jose, Male, 61 y.o.
Allergies: NKA
Pt. Location: RM 704

Code: FULL
Physician: RJ Warren

Isolation: None
Admit Date: 12/1

Patient Summary: Jose Garcia is a 61-year-old male admitted through the emergency department with diagnosis of unstable angina; s/p emergency coronary angiography with angioplasty of the infarct-related artery.

History:
Onset of disease: 61-yo male who noted the sudden onset of severe precordial pain on the way home from work. The pain is described as pressure-like pain radiating to the jaw and left arm. The patient has noted an episode of emesis and nausea. He denies palpitations or syncope. He denies prior history of pain. He admits to smoking cigarettes (1 pack/day for 40 years). He denies hypertension, diabetes, or high cholesterol. He denies SOB.
Medical history: Not significant before this admission
Surgical history: Surgery; cholecystectomy 10 years ago, appendectomy 30 years ago
Medications at home: None
Allergies: Sulfa drugs
Tobacco use: 40-year history, 1 pack /day
Alcohol use: 1 glass of wine per day
Family history: What? CAD. Who? Father—MI age 59.

Demographics:
Marital status: Married, *Spouse name*: Alice Garcia, 59 yo
Number of children: Daughter and two grandchildren live in the home.
Years education: AA degree
Language: English, Spanish
Occupation: IT network specialist
Hours of work: 40/wk
Household members: 5
Ethnicity: Mexican American
Religious affiliation: Catholic

MD Progress Note:
<u>Review of Systems</u>
Constitutional: Negative
Skin: Negative
Cardiovascular: No carotid bruits
Respiratory: Negative
Gastrointestinal: Negative
Neurological: Negative
Psychiatric: Negative

Garcia Jose, Male, 61 y.o.
Allergies: NKA   **Code:** FULL   **Isolation:** None
Pt. Location: RM 704   **Physician:** RJ Warren   **Admit Date:** 12/1

Physical Exam

General appearance: Mildly overweight male in acute distress from chest pain
Heart: PMI 5 ICS MCL focal. S1 normal intensity. S2 normal intensity and split. S4 gallop at the apex. No murmurs, clicks, or rubs.
HEENT: Head: Normocephalic
          Eyes: EOMI, fundoscopic exam WNL. No evidence of atherosclerosis, diabetic retinopathy, or early hypertensive changes.
          Ears: TM normal bilaterally
          Nose: WNL
          Throat: Tonsils not infected, uvula midline, gag normal
Genitalia: Grossly physiologic
Neurologic: No focal localizing abnormalities; DTR symmetric bilaterally
Extremities: No C, C, E
Skin: Diaphoretic and pale
Chest/lungs: Clear to auscultation and percussion
Peripheral vascular: PPP
Abdomen: RLQ scar and midline suprapubic scar. BS WNL. No hepatomegaly, splenomegaly, masses, inguinal lymph nodes, or abdominal bruits.

Vital Signs: Temp: 98.6   Pulse: 94   Resp rate: 23
                   BP: 140/99   Height: 5'10"   Weight: 215 lbs

Orders:
Early risk stratification: High risk
Activity: bed rest
Cardiac monitor
Vital signs q4h × 24 hours then q8h
Diet: house/no added salt/low saturated fat; low cholesterol
Call house officer for T >101, SBP >190 mm Hg or SBP <90 mm Hg, HR >120 bpm or HR <50 bpm, RR >30 or RR <10
Guaiac ALL stools while on heparin, LMWH, IIb/IIIa inhibitor
O$_2$: Nasal prongs (cannula) 2 L/min
Please call house officer for O$_2$ SAT <90%
Order for respiratory care O$_2$ SAT check q8h
ECG and repeat for recurrent chest pain
Troponin T/Troponin I: Now and every 6 hrs × 8 times
CK-MB: Now and every 6 hrs × 8 times
CBC, lipid profile, PTT, Chemistry (7) panel in AM – fasting
Aspirin 325 mg PO chewed, then 325 mg mg PO/d
Atenolol 75 mg/d
Nitroglycerin 1/150 (0.4 mg) 1 TAB SL q 5min × 3 prn chest pain; hold if: SBP <100 mm Hg

Garcia Jose, Male, 61 y.o.
Allergies: NKA
Pt. Location: RM 704

Code: FULL
Physician: RJ Warren

Isolation: None
Admit Date: 12/1

Eptifibatide 180 µg/kg IV bolus × 2, 10 min apart, followed by IV infusion of 2.0 µg/kg/min, reduce to 1.0 µg/kg/min if CrCl <50 mL/min

Enoxaparin 1 mg/kg SC q12h (if CrCl <30 mL/min, give 1 mg/kg every 24h)

PRN: Colace 100 mg po bid; Maalox plus ex str 15 mL q 6 h for indigestion; oxazepam 15-30 mg po qhs prn Insomnia; acetaminophen 650 mg po q 4h for headache; magnesium hydroxide 30 mL po qd for constipation; magnesium sulfate Sliding Scale IV qd; call house officer if serum Mg <1.2

Hold order for creatinine >1.9
If serum Mg <1.4 give 5 g MgSO$_4$ IV; if serum Mg <1.6 give 4 g MgSO$_4$ IV; if serum Mg <1.8 give 3 g MgSO$_4$ IV; if serum Mg <2.0 give 2 g MgSO$_4$ IV

Nutrition Consult: Patient admitted to cardiology ischemia pathway with known or suspected CAD. Please facilitate initial and outpatient education.

Social Service: Patient admitted to cardiology ischemia pathway with known or suspected CAD. Please assess and assist in need for outpatient support.

Nursing Assessment	12/1
Abdominal appearance (concave, flat, rounded, obese, distended)	rounded, obese
Palpation of abdomen (soft, rigid, firm, masses, tense)	soft
Bowel function (continent, incontinent, flatulence, no stool)	continent
Bowel sounds (P=present, AB=absent, hypo, hyper)	
RUQ	P
LUQ	P
RLQ	P
LLQ	P
Stool color	light brown
Stool consistency	soft
Tubes/ostomies	NA
Genitourinary	
Urinary continence	catheter
Urine source	catheter
Appearance (clear, cloudy, yellow, amber, fluorescent, hematuria, orange, blue, tea)	clear, yellow

Garcia Jose, Male, 61 y.o.
Allergies: NKA   **Code:** FULL   **Isolation:** None
Pt. Location: RM 704   **Physician:** RJ Warren   **Admit Date:** 12/1

Nursing Assessment *(Continued)*

Nursing Assessment	12/1
Integumentary	
Skin color	pale
Skin temperature (DI=diaphoretic, W=warm, dry, CL=cool, CLM=clammy, CD$_+$=cold, M=moist, H=hot)	DI, M
Skin turgor (good, fair, poor, TENT=tenting)	TENT
Skin condition (intact, EC=ecchymosis, A=abrasions, P−petechiae, R=rash, W=weeping, S=sloughing, D=dryness, EX−excoriated, T=tears, SE=subcutaneous emphysema, B=blisters, V=vesicles, N=necrosis)	intact
Mucous membranes (intact, EC=ecchymosis, A=abrasions, P=petechiae, R=rash, W=weeping, S=sloughing, D=dryness, EX=excoriated, T=tears, SE=subcutaneous emphysema, B=blisters, V=vesicles, N=necrosis)	intact
Other components of Braden score: special bed, sensory pressure, moisture, activity, friction/shear (>18=no risk, 15–16=low risk, 13–14=moderate risk, ≤12=high risk)	activity; 22

Nutrition:

Diet order: house/no added salt/low saturated fat; low cholesterol
History: Appetite good. Has been trying to change some things in his diet. Wife indicates that she has been using "corn oil" instead of butter and has tried not to fry foods as often.

24-hour recall:
Breakfast: Coffee with milk and sugar
Midmorning snack: Egg and cheese on English muffin from work cafeteria; 8 oz. orange juice, 2–3 c coffee with milk and sugar
Lunch: Leftovers from home; if eats in cafeteria: soup, salad, or sandwich. Had tomato soup and grilled cheese yesterday.
Dinner: Rice—1 c; black beans—1 c; roast pork with tomato and peppers— approx. 6 oz; cornbread—2 squares, each 2" wide
Snack: None yesterday but typically has cookies or ice cream

Food allergies/intolerances/aversions: None
Previous nutrition therapy? No
Food purchase/preparation: Spouse
Vit/min intake: None

Garcia Jose, Male, 61 y.o.
Allergies: NKA
Pt. Location: RM 704

Code: FULL
Physician: RJ Warren

Isolation: None
Admit Date: 12/1

Laboratory Results

	Ref. Range	12/1 1957	12/2 0630	12/3 0645
Chemistry				
Sodium (mEq/L)	136–145	141	142	138
Potassium (mEq/L)	3.5–5.1	4.2	4.1	3.9
Chloride (mEq/L)	98–107	103	102	100
Carbon dioxide (CO_2, mEq/L)	23–29	20 !↓	24	26
Bicarbonate (mEq/L)	23–28	24	23	24
BUN (mg/dL)	6–20	14	15	16
Creatinine serum (mg/dL)	0.6–1.1 F 0.9–1.3 M	1.1	1.1	1.1
BUN/Crea ratio	10.0–20.0	12.7	13.6	13.3
Uric acid (mg/dL)	2.8–8.8 F 4.0–9.0 M	5.1	5.7	6.1
Est GFR, non-Afr Amer (mL/min/1.73 m^2)	>60	68	68	68
Glucose (mg/dL)	70–99	136 !↑	106 !↑	104 !↑
Phosphate, inorganic (mg/dL)	2.2–4.6	3.1	3.2	3.0
Magnesium (mg/dL)	1.5–2.4	2.0	2.3	2.0
Calcium (mg/dL)	8.6–10.2	9.4	9.4	9.4
Osmolality (mmol/kg/H_2O)	275–295	292	290	291
Bilirubin total (mg/dL)	≤1.2	0.8	0.76	0.81
Bilirubin, direct (mg/dL)	< 0.3	0.10	0.11	0.14
Protein, total (g/dL)	6–7.8	6.0	5.9 !↓	6.1
Albumin (g/dL)	3.5–5.5	4.2	4.3	4.2
Prealbumin (mg/dL)	18–35	30	32	31
Ammonia (NH_3, µg/L)	6–47	26	22	25
Alkaline phosphatase (U/L)	30–120	75	70	68
ALT (U/L)	4–36	30	215 !↑	185 !↑
AST (U/L)	0–35	25	245 !↑	175 !↑
CPK (U/L)	30–135 F 55–170 M	75	500 !↑	335 !↑
CPK-MB (U/L)	0	0	75 !↑	55 !↑
Lactate dehydrogenase (U/L)	208–378	325	685 !↑	365
Troponin I (ng/dL)	<0.2	2.4 !↑	2.8 !↑	3.1 !↑

Garcia Jose, Male, 61 y.o.
Allergies: NKA
Pt. Location: RM 704

Code: FULL
Physician: RJ Warren

Isolation: None
Admit Date: 12/1

Laboratory Results *(Continued)*

	Ref. Range	12/1 1957	12/2 0630	12/3 0645
Troponin T (ng/dL)	<0.03	2.1 !↑	2.7 !↑	3.2 !↑
Cholesterol (mg/dL)	<200	235 !↑	226 !↑	214 !↑
HDL–C (mg/dL)	>59 F, >50 M	30 !↓	32 !↓	33 !↓
VLDL (mg/dL)	7–32	44 !↑	49 !↑	51 !↑
LDL (mg/dL)	<130	160 !↑	150 !↑	141 !↑
LDL/HDL ratio	<3.22 F <3.55 M	5.3 !↑	4.7 !↑	4.3 !↑
Apo A (mg/dL)	80–175 F 75–160 M	72 !↓	80	98
Apo B (mg/dL)	45–120 F 50–125 M	115	110	105
Triglycerides (mg/dL)	35–135 F 40–160 M	220 !↑	245 !↑	257 !↑
HbA$_{1c}$ (%)	<5.7	5.9 !↑		
Hematology				
WBC ($\times$ 10^3/mm^3)	3.9–10.7	11.0 !↑	9.32	8.8
RBC ($\times$ 10^6/mm^3)	4.2–5.4 F 4.5–6.2 M	4.7	4.75	4.68
Hemoglobin (Hgb, g/dL)	12–16 F 14–17 M	15	14.8	14.4
Hematocrit (Hct, %)	37–47 F 41–51 M	45	45	44
Mean cell volume (µm^3)	80–96	91	92	90
Mean cell Hgb (pg)	28–32	30	31	30
Mean cell Hgb content (g/dL)	32–36	33	32	33
RBC distribution (%)	11.6–16.5	13.2	12.8	13.0
Platelet count ($\times$ 10^3/mm^3)	150–350	320	295	280
Hematology, Manual Diff				
Neutrophil (%)	40–70	55	58	62
Lymphocyte (%)	22–44	22	23	35
Monocyte (%)	0–7	4	4	7
Eosinophil (%)	0–5	0	0	0
Basophil (%)	0–2	0	0	0

(Continued)

Garcia Jose, Male, 61 y.o.
Allergies: NKA
Pt. Location: RM 704

Code: FULL
Physician: RJ Warren

Isolation: None
Admit Date: 12/1

Laboratory Results *(Continued)*

	Ref. Range	12/1 1957	12/2 0630	12/3 0645
Blasts (%)	3–10	3	3	4
Segs (%)	0–60	45	47	52
Bands (%)	0–10	15 !↑	17 !↑	8
Urinalysis				
Collection method	---	catheter	catheter	catheter
Color	---	pale yellow	pale yellow	pale yellow
Appearance	---	clear	clear	clear
Specific gravity	1.001–1.035	1.020	1.015	1.018
pH	5–7	5.8	5.0	6
Protein (mg/dL)	Neg	+ !↑	Neg	Neg
Glucose (mg/dL)	Neg	+ !↑	Neg	Neg
Ketones	Neg	Trace !↑	Neg	Neg
Blood	Neg	Neg	Neg	Neg
Bilirubin	Neg	Neg	Neg	Neg
Nitrites	Neg	Neg	Neg	Neg
Urobilinogen (EU/dL)	<1.0	0	0	0
Leukocyte esterase	Neg	Neg	Neg	Neg
Prot chk	Neg	Neg	Neg	Neg
WBCs (/HPF)	0–5	0	0	0
RBCs (/HPF)	0–2	1	0	0
Bact	0	0	0	0
Mucus	0	0	0	0
Crys	0	0	0	0
Casts (/LPF)	0	0	0	0
Yeast	0	0	0	0

Note: Values and units of measurement listed in these tables are derived from several resources. Substantial variation exists in the ranges quoted as "normal" and these may vary depending on the assay used by different laboratories.

Case Questions

I.   Understanding the Disease and Pathophysiology

1.   Mr. Garcia had a myocardial infarction. Explain what happened to his heart muscle and vascular system.

2.   Mr. Garcia's chest pain resolved after two sublingual NTG at 3-minute intervals and 2 mg of IV morphine. In the cardiac catherization lab he was *"found to have a totally occluded distal right coronary artery and a 70% occlusion in the left circumflex coronary artery. The left anterior descending was patent. Angioplasty of the distal right coronary artery resulted in a patent infarct-related artery with near-normal flow. A stent was left in place to stabilize the patient and limit infarct size. Left ventricular ejection fraction was normal at 42%, and a posterobasilar scar was present with hypokinesis."* Explain angioplasty and stent placement. What is the purpose of this medical procedure?

3.   Mr. Garcia and his wife are concerned about the future of his heart health. What role does cardiac rehabilitation play in his return to normal activities and in determining his future heart health?

II.   Understanding the Nutrition Therapy

4.   What are the current recommendations for nutritional intake during a hospitalization following a myocardial infarction?

5.   List the risk factors indicated in his medical record that can be addressed through nutrition therapy.

6.   The RDN plans to talk about the Mediterranean diet with Mr. Garcia and his wife. What are the basic principles of the Mediterranean diet? What does the literature say in regards to the relationship between Mediterranean dietary principles and future heart health?

III.   Nutrition Assessment

7.   What is the healthy weight range for an individual of Mr. Garcia's height?

8.   Mr. Garcia works in a sedentary job, but he does get some exercise daily. He walks his dog outside for about 15 minutes at a leisurely pace each day and plays with his grandchildren. Calculate his energy and protein requirements.

9. Using Mr. Garcia's 24-hour recall, estimate the total number of kilocalories he consumed as well as the energy distribution of kilocalories for protein, carbohydrate, and fat using the food lists for diabetes.

10. Examine the laboratory results for Mr. Garcia. Which labs are consistent with the MI diagnosis? Explain. Why were the levels higher on 12/2?

11. Mr. Garcia may be at risk for metabolic syndrome. What is this? Does he have any laboratory values that would support this diagnosis?

12. List the abnormal values that are found in his lipid profile. What are the long-term implications? What are the possible treatment options for these abnormalities?

13. Mr. Garcia was prescribed the following medications on discharge. What are the rationale and the food-medication interactions for each of these medications?

    Lopressor 50 mg daily:

    Lisinopril 10 mg daily:

    Nitro-Bid 9.0 mg twice daily:

    NTG 0.4 mg sl prn chest pain:

    ASA 81 mg daily:

14. You talk with Mr. Garcia and his wife. They are friendly and appear interested in your information. They are both anxious to learn what they can do to prevent another heart attack. What are examples of questions that you can ask them to assess how to best help them?

15. Are there other issues besides diet that should be addressed to support successful lifestyle changes for Mr. Garcia? If yes, please list them.

16. From the information gathered within the assessment, list possible nutrition problems using the correct diagnostic terms.

IV. Nutrition Diagnosis

17. Select two of the identified nutrition problems and complete the PES statement for each.

V. Nutrition Intervention

18. For each of the PES statements you have written, establish an ideal goal (based on the signs and symptoms) and an appropriate intervention (based on the etiology).

19. Mr. Garcia and his wife ask about supplements. "My roommate here in the hospital told me I should be taking fish oil pills." What does the research say about omega-3-fatty acid supplementation for this patient?

VI. Nutrition Monitoring and Evaluation

20. What would you want to assess in three to four weeks when he and his wife return for additional counseling? (Hint: Your follow-up assessment should be based on signs and symptoms in your PES statements.)

Bibliography

Academy of Nutrition and Dietetics Evidence Analysis Library. Disorders of lipid metabolism (DLM) and nutrition monitoring and evaluation. http://www.andeal.org/template.cfm?template=guide_summary&key=2999. Accessed 02/12/15.

Academy of Nutrition and Dietetics Evidence Analysis Library. Disorders of lipid metabolism (DLM) and referral to a registered dietitian for medical nutrition therapy. http://www.andeal.org/template.cfm?template=guide_summary&key=2875. Accessed 02/12/15.

Academy of Nutrition and Dietetics Evidence Analysis Library. Is waist-to-hip ratio an independent predictor of CHD? http://www.andeal.org/topic.cfm?cat=1395&conclusion_statement_id=298&highlight=waist%20to%20hip%20ratio%20and%20chd&home=1. Accessed 02/12/15.

Academy of Nutrition and Dietetics Evidence Analysis Library. Recommendation summary: Disorders of lipid metabolism (DLM) and nutrition assessment. http://www.andeal.org/template.cfm?template=guide_summary&key=2990. Accessed 02/12/15.

Academy of Nutrition and Dietetics Evidence Analysis Library. Recommendation summary: Disorders of lipid metabolism (DLM) and omega-3 fatty acids. http://www.andeal.org/template.cfm?template=guide_summary&key=2876. Accessed 02/12/15.

Academy of Nutrition and Dietetics Nutrition Care Manual. BMI and Weight Range Calculator. https://www.nutritioncaremanual.org/calculators.cfm?calculator_type=CalcBMI. Accessed 2/12/15.

Artinian NT, Fletcher GJ, Mozaffarian D, et al.; on behalf of the American Heart Association Prevention Committee of the Council on Cardiovascular Nursing. Interventions to promote physical activity and dietary lifestyle changes for cardiovascular risk factor reduction in adults: A scientific statement from the American Heart Association. *Circulation.* 2010;122:406–441.

Booth JN, Levita EB, Brown TM, et al. Effect of sustaining lifestyle modifications (nonsmoking, weight reduction, physical activity, and Mediterranean diet) after healing of myocardial infarction, percutaneous intervention, or coronary bypass (from the Reasons for geographic and racial differences in stroke study). *Am J Cardiol.* 2014;113:1933–1940.

Bruckert E, Masana L, Chapman MJ, Descamps O, Bosi E, Allaert FA. Dietary supplementation contributes to lifestyle improvement in hypercholesterolemic patients in real-life contexts. *Curr Med Res Opin.* 2014;30:1309–1316.

Dalen JE, Devries S. Diets to prevent coronary heart disease 1957–2013: What have we learned? *Am J Med.* 2014;127:364–369.

DiNicolantonio JJ, Niazi AK, McCarty MF, O'Keefe JH, Meier P, Lavie CJ. Omega-3s and cardiovascular health. *The Ochsner Journal.* 2014;14:399–412.

Franklin BA, Durstine JL, Roberts CK, Barnard RJ. Impact of diet and exercise on lipid management in the modern era. *Best Practice and Res Clin Endocrinol Metab.* 2014;28:405–421.

Gardener H, Wright CB, Gu Y, et al. Mediterranean-style diet and risk of ischemic stroke, myocardial infarction, and vascular death: The Northern Manhattan Study. *Am J Clin Nutr.* 2011;94:1458–1464.

Hemilä H, Miller ER. Evidenced-based medicine and vitamin E supplementation. *Am J Clin Nutr.* 2007;86:261–262.

Lopez-Garcia E, Rodriguez-Artalejo F, Li TY, et al. The Mediterranean-style dietary pattern and mortality among men and women with cardiovascular disease. *Am J Clin Nutr.* 2014;99:172–180.

Nelms MN. Nutrition assessment: Foundation of the nutrition care process. In: Nelms M, Sucher K, Lacey K. *Nutrition Therapy and Pathophysiology.* 3rd ed. Belmont, CA: Cengage Learning; 2016:36–71.

Pronsky ZM, Crowe JP. *Food and Medication Interaction.* 17th ed. Birchrunville, PA: Food-Medication Interactions; 2012.

Pujol TJ, Barnes JT, Sucher K. Diseases of the cardiovascular system. In: Nelms M, Sucher K, Lacey K. *Nutrition Therapy and Pathophysiology.* 3rd ed. Belmont, CA: Cengage Learning; 2016:292–341.

Roger VL, Go AS, Lloyd-Jones DM, et al.; on behalf of the American Heart Association Statistics Committee and Stroke Statistics Subcommittee. Heart disease and stroke statistics—2012 update: A report from the American Heart Association. *Circulation.* 2012;125:e2–e220. http://circ.ahajournals.org/content/125/1/e2. Accessed 02/12/15.

Salisbury AC, Amin AP, Harris WS, et al. Predictors of omega-3-index in patients with acute myocardial infarction. *Mayo Clin Proc.* 2011;86:626–632.

U.S. National Library of Medicine. MedlinePlus. Fish oil. http://www.nlm.nih.gov/medlineplus/druginfo/natural/993.html. Accessed 02/12/15.

🌐 Internet Resources

AND Evidence Analysis Library: https://www.andeal.org/
The Cleveland Clinic: Acute Myocardial Infarction: http://www.clevelandclinicmeded.com/medicalpubs/diseasemanagement/cardiology/acute-myocardial-infarction/

Drug Bank: http://www.drugbank.ca/
Nutrition Care Manual: http://www.nutritioncaremanual.org
USDA Nutrient Data Laboratory: http://www.ars.usda.gov/ba/bhnrc/ndl

Heart Failure with Resulting Cardiac Cachexia

Objectives

After completing this case, the student will be able to:

1. Explain the basic pathophysiology of heart failure and the subsequent effects on pulmonary, renal, and liver function.
2. Correlate a patient's signs and symptoms with the pathophysiology of heart failure.
3. Demonstrate understanding of heart failure's potential effects on an individual's nutritional status.
4. Identify the roles of pharmacologic intervention in the treatment of heart failure and drug–nutrient interactions.
5. Use nutrition assessment information to determine baseline nutritional status and identify factors that may suggest malnutrition.
6. Determine appropriate nutritional interventions for the patient with heart failure.

Katherine Maney, a 65-year-old female, is admitted with acute symptoms related to her heart failure. Mrs. Maney has a long history of cardiac disease, including a previous myocardial infarction and mitral valve disease.

Maney, Katherine, Female, 65 y.o.
Allergies: Shellfish
Pt. Location: RM 1952

Code: DNR
Physician: DL Levine

Isolation: None
Admit Date: 2/14

Patient Summary: Katherine Maney has a past medical history of being treated for CAD, mitral valve replacement, HTN, and HF.

History:

Onset of disease: HF × 2 yrs
Medical history: Long-standing history of CAD, HTN, mitral valve insufficiency, previous anterior MI
Surgical history: s/p mitral valve replacement
Medications at home: Lanoxin 0.125 mg once daily, Lasix 80 mg twice daily, Aldactone 25 mg once daily, lisinopril 30 mg po once daily, Lopressor 25 mg once daily, Zocor 20 mg once daily, Metamucil 1 tbsp twice daily, calcium carbonate 500 mg twice daily, Centrum 2 tablets once daily
Tobacco use: No
Alcohol use: No
Family history: What? HTN, CAD. Who? Parents.

Demographics:

Marital status: Married—lives with husband; *Spouse name:* Robert
Number of children: 4
Years education: High school
Language: English only
Occupation: Retired caterer
Hours of work: N/A
Ethnicity: Caucasian
Religious affiliation: Lutheran

Admitting History/Physical:

Chief complaint: Patient collapsed at home and was brought to the emergency room by ambulance.
General appearance: Older female in acute distress

Vital Signs: Temp: 98   Pulse: 110   Resp rate: 24
                BP: 90/70   Height: 5'2"   Weight: 105 lbs

Heart: Diffuse PMI in AAL in LLD; Grade II holosystolic murmur at the apex radiating to the left sternal border; first heart sound diminished and second heart sound preserved; third heart sound present
HEENT: Head: Temporal wasting
         Eyes: Ophthalmoscopic exam reveals AV crossing changes and arteriolar spasm
         Ears: WNL
         Nose: WNL
         Throat: Jugular venous distension in sitting position with a positive hepatojugular reflux
Genitalia: WNL
Neurologic: WNL

Maney, Katherine, Female, 65 y.o.
Allergies: Shellfish
Pt. Location: RM 1952

Code: DNR
Physician: DL Levine

Isolation: None
Admit Date: 2/14

Extremities: 2 + pedal edema; weak hand grip
Skin: Gray, moist
Chest/lungs: Rales in both bases posteriorly
Peripheral vascular: WNL
Abdomen: Ascites, no masses, liver tender to A&P

Nursing Assessment	2/14
Abdominal appearance (concave, flat, rounded, obese, distended)	distended
Palpation of abdomen (soft, rigid, firm, masses, tense)	firm
Bowel function (continent, incontinent, flatulence, no stool)	continent
Bowel sounds (P=present, AB=absent, hypo, hyper)	
RUQ	P
LUQ	P
RLQ	P
LLQ	P
Stool color	light brown
Stool consistency	formed
Tubes/ostomies	NA
Genitourinary	
Urinary continence	catheter
Urine source	catheter
Appearance (clear, cloudy, yellow, amber, fluorescent, hematuria, orange, blue, tea)	clear, yellow
Integumentary	
Skin color	gray
Skin temperature (DI=diaphoretic, W=warm, dry, CL=cool, CLM=clammy, CD1=cold, M=moist, H=hot)	M
Skin turgor (good, fair, poor, TENT=tenting)	fair
Skin condition (intact, EC=ecchymosis, A=abrasions, P=petechiae, R=rash, W=weeping, S=sloughing, D=dryness, EX=excoriated, T=tears, SE=subcutaneous emphysema, B=blisters, V=vesicles, N=necrosis)	intact
Mucous membranes (intact, EC=ecchymosis, A=abrasions, P=petechiae, R=rash, W=weeping, S=sloughing, D=dryness, EX=excoriated, T=tears, SE=subcutaneous emphysema, B=blisters, V=vesicles, N=necrosis)	intact
Other components of Braden score: special bed, sensory pressure, moisture, activity, friction/shear (>18 = no risk, 15–16 = low risk, 13–14 = moderate risk, ≤12 = high risk)	activity, 15

Maney, Katherine, Female, 65 y.o.
Allergies: Shellfish   **Code:** DNR   **Isolation:** None
Pt. Location: RM 1952   **Physician:** DL Levine   **Admit Date:** 2/14

Orders:
Admit to CCU
Parenteral dopamine and IV diuretics
100 mg thiamin IV
Telemetry
Vitals every 1 hr × 8, every 2 hrs × 8 for first 24 hours
Daily ECG and chest X-rays
Echocardiogram
Chem 24
Urinalysis
Strict I&Os

Nutrition:
Meal type: 2 g Na$^+$ 1500 mL fluid restriction
Intake % of meals: <5%, sips of liquids for past 24 hrs
Fluid requirement: 1,500 mL
History: Husband reports that Mrs. Maney's appetite has been poor for the last 6 months, but with no real weight loss that he can determine. "It's very hard to know the difference between her real weight and any fluid she is retaining." Husband also states that he thinks her arms, shoulders, and face are "skinnier" than normal. She describes difficulty eating due to SOB and nausea.
Usual dietary intake: Generally likes all foods but has recently been eating only soft foods, esp. ice cream. Tries to drink 2 cans Boost each day.
Food allergies/intolerances/aversions: Shellfish
Previous nutrition therapy? Not specifically, but has monitored salt intake for the past 2 years as well as followed a low-fat, low-cholesterol diet for at least the previous 10 years
Food purchase/preparation: Self and spouse
Vit/min intake: Centrum Silver 2×/day, calcium supplement 1000 mg/day

Laboratory Results

	Ref. Range	2/14 1952	2/16 0645	2/20 0630
Chemistry				
Sodium (mEq/L)	136–145	132 !↓	133 !↓	135 !↓
Potassium (mEq/L)	3.5–5.1	3.7	3.6	3.8
Chloride (mEq/L)	98–107	98	100	99
Carbon dioxide (CO_2, mEq/L)	23–29	26	24	25
Bicarbonate (mEq/L)	23–28	25	24	27
BUN (mg/dL)	6–20	32 !↑	34 !↑	30 !↑
Creatinine serum (mg/dL)	0.6–1.1 F 0.9–1.3 M	1.6 !↑	1.7 !↑	1.5 !↑
BUN/Crea ratio	10.0–20.0	20	20	20

Maney, Katherine, Female, 65 y.o.
Allergies: Shellfish
Pt. Location: RM 1952

Code: DNR
Physician: DL Levine

Isolation: None
Admit Date: 2/14

Laboratory Results *(Continued)*

	Ref. Range	2/14 1952	2/16 0645	2/20 0630
Uric acid (mg/dL)	2.8–8.8 F 4.0–9.0 M	5.1	5.0	5.5
Est GFR, non-Afr Amer (mL/min/1.73 m²)	>60	34 !↓		
Glucose (mg/dL)	70–99	110 !↑	106 !↑	102 !↑
Phosphate, inorganic (mg/dL)	2.2–4.6	2.4	2.5	2.5
Magnesium (mg/dL)	1.5–2.4	2.0	1.9	1.8
Calcium (mg/dL)	8.6–10.2	9.0	8.8	8.9
Osmolality (mmol/kg/H₂O)	275–295	281	284	286
Bilirubin total (mg/dL)	≤1.2	1.4 !↑	1.7 !↑	1.8 !↑
Bilirubin, direct (mg/dL)	<0.3	1.0 !↑	1.1 !↑	0.9 !↑
Protein, total (g/dL)	6–7.8	5.8 !↓	5.6 !↓	5.5 !↓
Albumin (g/dL)	3.5–5.5	2.8 !↓	2.7 !↓	2.6 !↓
Prealbumin (mg/dL)	18–35	15 !↓	11 !↓	10 !↓
Ammonia (NH₃, µg/L)	6–47	32	30	33
Alkaline phosphatase (U/L)	30–120	112	115	118
ALT (U/L)	4–36	100 !↑	120 !↑	115 !↑
AST (U/L)	0–35	70 !↑	80 !↑	85 !↑
CPK (U/L)	30–135 F 55–170 M	180 !↑	200 !↑	205 !↑
Lactate dehydrogenase (U/L)	208–378	350	450 !↑	556 !↑
Troponin I (ng/L)	<0.2	0.026 !↑	0.028 !↑	0.027 !↑
Troponin T (ng/L)	<0.03	0.035 !↑	0.037 !↑	0.036 !↑
BNP (pg/mL)	<100	975 !↑	983 !↑	1025 !↑
CRP (mg/L)	<1.0	225 !↑	240 !↑	338 !↑
Cholesterol (mg/dL)	<200	150	162	149
HDL-C (mg/dL)	>59 F, >50 M	30 !↓	31 !↓	30 !↓
VLDL (mg/dL)	7–32	15	16	15
LDL (mg/dL)	<130	180 !↑	160 !↑	152 !↑
LDL/HDL ratio	<3.22 F <3.55 M	5.00 !↑	5.23 !↑	4.97 !↑
Triglycerides (mg/dL)	35–135 F 40–160 M	78	82	78
HbA₁c (%)	<5.7	4.9		

(Continued)

Maney, Katherine, Female, 65 y.o.
Allergies: Shellfish
Pt. Location: RM 1952

Code: DNR
Physician: DL Levine

Isolation: None
Admit Date: 2/14

Laboratory Results *(Continued)*

	Ref. Range	2/14 1952	2/16 0645	2/20 0630
Coagulation (Coag)				
INR	0.9–1.1	0.98		
Hematology				
WBC ($\times 10^3$/mm^3)	3.9–10.7	12.7 !↑	13.4 !↑	10.5
RBC ($\times 10^6$/mm^3)	4.2–5.4 F 4.5–6.2 M	3.8 !↓	3.7 !↓	3.72 !↓
Hemoglobin (Hgb, g/dL)	12–16 F 14–17 M	10.5 !↓	10.7 !↓	10.1 !↓
Hematocrit (Hct, %)	37–47 F 41–51 M	31 !↓	30 !↓	29 !↓
Platelet count ($\times 10^3$/mm^3)	150–350	286	245	278
Transferrin (mg/dL)	250–380 F 215–365 M	406 !↑	414 !↑	412 !↑
Ferritin (mg/mL)	20–120 F 20–300 M	11 !↓		
Iron (µg/dL)	65–165 F 75–175 M	42 !↓		
Vitamin B$_{12}$ (ng/dL)	24.4–100	55		
Folate (ng/dL)	5–25	17		
Hematology, Manual Diff				
Neutrophil (%)	40–70	74 !↑		
Lymphocyte (%)	22–44	22		
Monocyte (%)	0–7	2		
Eosinophil (%)	0–5	0		
Basophil (%)	0–2	0		
Blasts (%)	3–10	3		
Segs (%)	0–60	1		
Bands (%)	0–10	3		
Urinalysis				
Collection method	—	catheter		
Color	—	amber		
Appearance	—	cloudy		

Maney, Katherine, Female, 65 y.o.
Allergies: Shellfish
Pt. Location: RM 1952

Code: DNR
Physician: DL Levine

Isolation: None
Admit Date: 2/14

Laboratory Results *(Continued)*

	Ref. Range	2/14 1952	2/16 0645	2/20 0630
Specific gravity	1.001–1.035	1.036 !↑		
pH	5–7	5.5		
Protein (mg/dL)	Neg	+ !↑		
Glucose (mg/dL)	Neg	Neg		
Ketones	Neg	Neg		
Blood	Neg	Neg		
Bilirubin	Neg	Neg		
Nitrites	Neg	Neg		
Urobilinogen (EU/dL)	<1.0	0.002		
Leukocyte esterase	Neg	Neg		
Prot chk	Neg	+		
WBCs (/HPF)	0–5	0		
RBCs (/HPF)	0–2	0		
Bact	0	0		
Mucus	0	0		
Crys	0	0		
Casts (/LPF)	0	0		
Yeast	0	0		
Arterial Blood Gases (ABGs)				
pH	7.35–7.45	7.41	7.44	7.43
pCO$_2$ (mm Hg)	35–45	46 !↑	47 !↑	47 !↑
SO$_2$ (%)	≥95	84 !↓	96	96
CO$_2$ content (mmol/L)	25–30	35 !↑	31 !↑	30
O$_2$ content (%)	15–22	14 !↓	17	18
pO$_2$ (mm Hg)	≥80	84	82	85
HCO$_3^-$ (mEq/L)	21–28	29 !↑	28	27

Note: Values and units of measurement listed in these tables are derived from several resources. Substantial variation exists in the ranges quoted as "normal" and these may vary depending on the assay used by different laboratories.

Maney, Katherine, Female, 65 y.o.
Allergies: Shellfish
Pt. Location: RM 1952

Code: DNR
Physician: DL Levine

Isolation: None
Admit Date: 2/14

Intake/Output

Date		2/14 0701–2/15 0700			
Time		0701–1500	1501–2300	2301–0700	Daily total
IN	P.O.	10	15	0	25
	I.V. (mL/kg/hr)	336 (0.88)	336 (0.88)	336 (0.88)	1008 (0.88)
	I.V. piggyback				
	TPN				
	Total intake (mL/kg)	346 (7.3)	351 (7.4)	336 (7.0)	1033 (21.7)
OUT	Urine (mL/kg/hr)	200 (0.52)	175 (0.46)	250 (0.66)	625 (0.55)
	Emesis output				
	Other				
	Stool				
	Total output (mL/kg)	200 (4.2)	175 (3.7)	250 (5.2)	625 (13.1)
Net I/O		+146	+176	+86	+408
Net since admission (2/14)		+146	+322	+408	+408

Case Questions

I.   Understanding the Disease and Pathophysiology

1.   Outline the typical pathophysiology of heart failure. Onset of heart failure usually can be traced to damage from an MI and atherosclerosis. Is this consistent with Mrs. Maney's history?

2.   Identify specific signs and symptoms in the patient's physical examination that are consistent with heart failure. For any three of these signs and symptoms, write a brief discussion that connects them to physiological changes that you described in question #1.

3.   Heart failure is often described as R-sided failure or L-sided failure. What is the difference? How are the clinical manifestations different?

II.   Understanding the Nutrition Therapy

4.   Mrs. Maney's husband states that they have monitored their salt intake for several years. What is the role of sodium restriction in the treatment of heart failure? What level of sodium restriction is recommended for the outpatient with heart failure? What difficulties may a patient have in following a sodium restriction?

5.   Why is Mrs. Maney placed on a fluid restriction? How will this assist with the treatment of her heart failure? What specific foods are typically "counted" as a fluid?

6.   Identify any common nutrient deficiencies found in patients with heart failure.

III.   Nutrition Assessment

7.   Identify factors that would affect interpretation of Mrs. Maney's weight and body composition. Look at the I/O record. What will likely happen to Mrs. Maney's weight if this trend continues?

8.   Calculate Mrs. Maney's energy and protein requirements. Explain your rationale for the weight you have used in your calculation.

9. Do you have any evidence that Mrs. Maney may be malnourished? Identify factors that may support a diagnosis of malnutrition using the latest AND/ASPEN proposed guidelines for malnutrition diagnosis.

10. Malnutrition in heart failure is often referred to as cardiac cachexia. What is cardiac cachexia? What are the characteristic symptoms? Explain the role of the underlying heart disease in the development of malnutrition.

11. Do you feel that Mrs. Maney may benefit from enteral feeding? What guidelines would you use to make this decision? Outline a nutrition therapy regimen for her that includes formula choice, total volume, and goal rate.

12. Identify any abnormal biochemical values associated with Mrs. Maney's heart failure or CVD and assess them using the following table:

Name of Laboratory Value	Normal Value	Pt's Value & Date	Reason for Abnormality

13. The following drugs/supplements were prescribed for Mrs. Maney. Give the medical rationale for the use of each. In addition, describe any nutritional concerns for Mrs. Maney while she is taking these medications.

Lanoxin:

Lasix:

Dopamine:

Thiamin:

IV.   Nutrition Diagnosis

14. Select two nutrition problems and complete a PES statement for each.

V.   Nutrition Intervention

15. Mrs. Maney was not able to tolerate the enteral feeding because of nursing report for diarrhea. What recommendations could be made to improve tolerance to the tube feeding?

16. The tube feeding was discontinued because of continued intolerance. Parenteral nutrition was not initiated. What recommendations could you make to optimize Mrs. Maney's oral intake?

17. Outline steps you would take to assist Mrs. Maney as she prepares for discharge. Include the specific nutrition education that you would include.

Bibliography

Academy of Nutrition and Dietetics Evidence Analysis Library. Heart failure recommendations summary DM: Intervention options 2008. http://www.andeal.org/template.cfm?template=guide_summary&key=2114. Accessed 02/22/15.

Academy of Nutrition and Dietetics Nutrition Care Manual. Heart failure. https://www.nutrition caremanual.org/topic.cfm?ncm_category_id=1&lv1=5803&lv2=8585&ncm_toc_id=8585&ncm_heading=Nutrition%20Care. Accessed 02/22/15.

Arnett DK, Goodman RA, Halperin JL, Anderson JL, Parekh AK, Zoghbi WA. AHA/ACC/HHS strategies to enhance application of clinical practice guidelines in patients with cardiovascular disease and comorbid conditions: From the American Heart Association, American College of Cardiology, and U.S. Department of Health and Human Services. *Circulation.* 2014;130(18):1662–1667.

Basuray A, Dolansky M, Josephson R, et al. Dietary sodium adherence is poor in heart failure patients. *J Card Fail.* 2015; 21: 323–328.

Bonow RO, Ganiats TG, Beam CT, et al. ACCF/AHA/AMA-PCPI 2011 performance measures for adults with heart failure: A report of the American College of Cardiology Foundation/American Heart Association Task Force on Performance Measures and the American Medical Association–Physician Consortium for Performance Improvement. *J Am Coll Cardiol.* 2012;59:1812–1832.

Dumitru I. Heart failure. Medscape Web site. http://emedicine.medscape.com/article/163062-overview. Updated October 1, 2013. Accessed 03/01/15.

Haehling S, Stepney R, Anker S. Advances in understanding and treating cardiac cachexia: Highlights from the 5th Cachexia Conference. *International J Cardiol.* 2010;144:347–349.

Hummel Sl, Seymour M, Brook RD, et al. Low sodium DASH diet improves diastolic function and ventricular-arterial coupling in hypertensive heart failure with preserved ejection fraction. *Clin Heart Fail.* 2013;6:1165–1171.

Hunt SA, Abraham WT, Chin MH, et al. 2009 Focused update incorporated into the ACC/AHA 2005 guidelines for the diagnosis and management of heart failure in adults: A report of the American College of Cardiology Foundation/American Heart Association Task Force on Practice Guidelines. *Circulation.* 2009;119:e391–e479.

Kociol RD, Pang PS, Gheorghiade M, Fonarow GC, O'Connor CM, Felker GM. Troponin elevation in patients with heart failure. *J Am Coll Cardiol.* 2010;56:1071–1078.

Martins T, Vitorino R, Amado F, Duarte JA, Ferreira R. Biomarkers for cardiac cachexia: Reality or utopia. *Clinica Chimica Acta.* 2014;436:323–328.

Philipson H, Ekman I, Forslund HB, Swedberg K, Schaufelberger M. Salt and fluid restriction is effective in patients with chronic heart failure. *Eur J Heart Fail.* 2013;15:1304–1310.

Pujol TJ, Barnes JT, Sucher, K. Diseases of the cardiovascular system. In: Nelms M, Sucher K, Lacey K. *Nutrition Therapy and Pathophysiology.* 3rd ed. Belmont, CA: Cengage Learning; 2016:292–341.

Ray KK, Kastelein JJ, Boekholdt SM, et al. The ACC/AHA 2013 guideline on the treatment of blood cholesterol to reduce atherosclerotic cardiovascular disease risk in adults: The good the bad and the uncertain: A comparison with ESC/EAS guidelines for the management of dyslipidaemias 2011. *Eur Heart J.* 2014;35(15):960–968.

Ukleja A, Freeman KL, Gilbert K, et al. Standards for nutrition support. Adult hospitalized patients. *Nutr Clin Pract.* 2010;25:403–414.

Vader JM, Drazner MH. Clinical assessment of heart failure: Utility of symptoms, signs, and daily weights. *Heart Fail Clin.* 2009;5(2):149–160.

Weiss BD. Sodium restriction in heart failure: How low should we go? *Am Fam Phys.* 2014;89:509–510.

Wessler JD, Hummel SL, Maurer MS. Dietary interventions for heart failure in older adults: Re-emergence of the hedonic shift. *Prog in Cardio Dis.* 2014;57:160–167.

Internet Resources

Academy of Nutrition and Dietetics: Nutrition Care Manual (by subscription): www.nutritioncaremanual.org

American Heart Association: http://www.heart.org/HEARTORG/Conditions/HeartFailure/Heart-Failure_UCM_002019_SubHomePage.jsp

Heart Failure (animation): http://medmovie.com/library_id/3255/topic/ahaw_0079a/

Heart Failure Society of America: http://www.hfsa.org/

Heart Failure Online: www.heartfailure.org

MedlinePlus: Heart Failure Overview: www.nlm.nih.gov/medlineplus/ency/article/000158.htm

WebMD: Cardiac Cachexia: http://www.webmd.com/heart-disease/heart-failure/tc/cardiac-cachexia-topic-overview

Unit Three

NUTRITION THERAPY FOR UPPER GASTROINTESTINAL DISORDERS

The seven cases presented in Units Three and Four cover a wide array of diagnoses that ultimately affect normal digestion and absorption. These conditions use medical nutrition therapy as a cornerstone of their treatment.

In some disorders, such as celiac disease, medical nutrition therapy is the *only* treatment. With other GI problems, it is important to understand that, because of the symptoms the patient experiences, nutritional status is often in jeopardy. Nausea, vomiting, diarrhea, constipation, and malabsorption are common with these disorders. Interventions in these cases are focused on treating such symptoms in order to restore nutritional health.

Case 7 targets gastroesophageal reflux disease (GERD). More than 20 million Americans suffer from symptoms of gastroesophageal reflux daily, and more than 100 million suffer occasional symptoms. Gastroesophageal reflux disease most frequently results from lower esophageal sphincter (LES) incompetence. Factors that influence LES competence include both physical and lifestyle factors. This case identifies the common symptoms of GERD and challenges you to develop and analyze both nutritional and medical care for this patient.

Case 8 addresses the disorder gastroparesis, which is defined as delayed gastric emptying. Individuals with gastroparesis are at high risk of malnutrition, due to the inability to consume adequate nutrients, and/or frequent vomiting, with subsequent dehydration and electrolyte imbalances.

Case 9 focuses on peptic ulcer disease (PUD) treated pharmacologically and surgically. Peptic ulcer disease involves ulcerations that penetrate the submucosa, usually in the antrum of the stomach or in the duodenum. Erosion may proceed to other levels of tissue and can eventually result in perforation. The breakdown in tissue allows continued insult by the highly acidic environment of the stomach. *Helicobacter pylori* is established as a major cause of chronic gastritis and peptic ulcer disease. This case describes the complications of PUD resulting in hemorrhage and perforation that require surgical intervention. Nutritional complications, such as dumping syndrome and malabsorption, often accompany gastric surgery. This case also introduces the transition from enteral nutrition support to the appropriate oral diet for discharge.

Case 7

Gastroesophageal Reflux Disease

Objectives

After completing this case, the student will be able to:

1. Apply knowledge of the pathophysiology of gastroesophageal reflux disease (GERD) in order to identify and explain common nutritional problems associated with this disease.

2. Describe basic principles of drug action required for medical treatment of GERD.

3. Understand the potential complications of untreated GERD.

4. Discuss the rationale for nutrition recommendations to minimize adverse symptoms of GERD.

5. Interpret pertinent laboratory parameters for nutritional implications and significance.

6. Analyze nutrition assessment data to evaluate nutritional status and identify specific nutrition problems.

7. Determine nutrition diagnoses and write appropriate PES statements.

8. Develop a nutrition care plan—with appropriate measurable goals, interventions, and strategies for monitoring and evaluation—that addresses the nutrition diagnoses of this case.

Krishna Gupta, a 48-year-old Indian male, visited his physician for evaluation of increasing complaints of severe indigestion. He was scheduled for a variety of tests, including intraesophageal pH monitoring and a barium esophagram, that support a diagnosis of gastroesophageal reflux disease.

75

Gupta, Krishna, Male, 48 y.o.
Allergies: NKA
Pt. Location: University Gastroenterology Clinic   **Physician:** Jen Li   **Date:** 11/1

Patient Summary: 48-yo male here for evaluation and treatment for increased indigestion

History:
Onset of disease: Patient has been experiencing increased indigestion over last year. Previously it was only at night but now he experiences indigestion almost constantly. He has been taking Tums several times daily and also tried the herb fenugreek and turmeric for relief of symptoms. Mr. Gupta has gained almost 30 lbs since he had knee surgery 3 years ago, which he attributes to a decrease in his ability to run and not being able to find a consistent replacement for this form of exercise. Patient states he plays with his children on the weekends, but that is the extent of his physical activity. He states he probably has been eating and drinking more over the last year, which he attributes to stress. He is worried about his family history of heart disease, which is why he takes an aspirin each day. He has not changed his diet in any way except for the addition of fenugreek and turmeric.
Medical history: Essential HTN—Dx 1 year ago
Surgical history: s/p R knee arthroplasty 5 years ago
Medications at home: Atenolol 50 mg daily; 325 mg aspirin daily; multivitamin daily; 500 mg ibuprofen twice daily for last month
Tobacco use: No
Alcohol use: Yes; 1–2 beers 1–2 times/week
Family history: What? CAD. Who? Father.

Demographics:
Marital status: Married—lives with wife and 2 sons
Spouse name: Saanvi
Number of children: 2 (ages 8 and 12)
Years education: BA
Language: English and Hindi
Occupation: Retail manager of local department store
Hours of work: M–F, works consistently in evenings and on weekends as well
Ethnicity: Indian
Religious affiliation: Hinduism

MD Progress Note:
Review of Systems
Constitutional: Negative
Skin: Negative
Cardiovascular: No carotid bruits
Respiratory: Negative
Gastrointestinal: Heme + stool
Neurological: Negative
Psychiatric: Negative

Gupta, Krishna, Male, 48 y.o.
Allergies: NKA
Pt. Location: University Gastroenterology Clinic   **Physician:** Jen Li   **Date:** 11/1

Physical Exam

General appearance: Mildly obese 48-year-old Indian male in mild distress
Heart: Noncontributory
HEENT: Noncontributory
Genitalia: WNL
Neurologic: Oriented × 4
Extremities: No edema; normal strength, sensations, and DTR
Skin: Warm, dry
Chest/lungs: Lungs clear to auscultation and percussion
Peripheral vascular: Pulses full—no bruits
Abdomen: No distention. BS present in all regions. Liver percusses approx 8 cm at the midclavicular line, one fingerbreadth below the right costal margin. Epigastric tenderness without rebound or guarding.

Vital Signs: Temp: 98.6   Pulse: 90   Resp rate: 16
                    BP: 119/75   Height: 5'9"   Weight: 215 lbs

142

Assessment and Plan:

Dx: Gastroesophageal reflux disease, HTN

Medical Tx plan: Hematology, Chem 24, Ambulatory 48-hour pH monitoring with Bravo™ pH Monitoring System, Barium esophagram—request radiologist to attempt to demonstrate reflux using abdominal pressure and positional changes; Endoscopy with biopsy to r/o *H. pylori* infection; Begin omeprazole 30 mg every am; Decrease aspirin to 75 mg daily; D/C self-medication of ibuprofen daily; Nutrition consult
.J.Li,.M.D...

Nutrition:

History: Patient relates he has gained almost 30 lbs since his knee surgery. He attributes this to a decrease in his ability to run, and he has not found a consistent replacement for this form of exercise. He plays with his children on weekends, but that is the extent of his physical activity. He states he probably has been eating and drinking more over the last year, which he attributes to stress with his busy lifestyle and long work hours. He is worried about his family history of heart disease, which is why he takes an aspirin each day. He has not really followed any diet restrictions for health concerns. He eats a combination of traditional Indian foods along with more American-style food choices. He has lived in the United States since his high school years so he does not follow any strict dietary practices related to his religious background of Hinduism.

Gupta, Krishna, Male, 48 y.o.
Allergies: NKA
Pt. Location: University Gastroenterology Clinic   **Physician:** Jen Li   **Date:** 11/1

Usual dietary intake:

AM: 1½–2 c hot cereal; ½–¾ c skim milk on cereal; sometimes egg
                                        and naan
                                        16–32 oz orange juice
                                        Hot tea with milk and sugar

Lunch: Fast food burger with fries, Diet Coke (or leftovers from previous
                                        evening)

Snack when he comes home: Handful of crackers, cookies, or chips, 1 12-oz beer

PM: Typically eats traditional Indian foods at home for evening meal:
                                        3–4 oz of meat (chicken primarily) or tofu (grilled or cooked on top
                                        of stove) cooked with rice and vegetables; chapattis; hot chai or
                                        black tea;
                                        Relates that his family's schedule has been increasingly busy, so
                                        they sometimes (1–2 times per week) order pizza or stop for fast
                                        food instead of cooking.

Late PM: Ice cream, popcorn, or crackers. Drinks 3–4 12-oz diet sodas daily
                                        as well as hot tea.

24-hr recall:

(at home PTA):   2 scrambled eggs, naan; hot black tea

At work: 3 12-oz Diet Pepsis

Lunch: Leftover curry with spinach, chickpeas, rice—2 c
                                        Hot black tea

Late afternoon: 2 c chips, 1 beer

Dinner: Lentil dal—2 c over approx. 2 c rice
                                        2 slices naan
                                        2 c hot chai tea

Bedtime: 2 c ice cream mixed with 1 c skim milk for milkshake

Food allergies/intolerances/aversions: Fried foods seem to make the indigestion worse
Previous nutrition therapy? No
Food purchase/preparation: Wife or eats out
Vit/min intake: One-A-Day for Men multivitamin daily

Gupta, Krishna, Male, 48 y.o.
Allergies: NKA
Pt. Location: University Gastroenterology Clinic   **Physician:** Jen Li   **Date:** 11/1

Laboratory Results

	Ref. Range	11/1 0700
Chemistry		
Sodium (mEq/L)	136–145	144
Potassium (mEq/L)	3.5–5.1	4.5
Chloride (mEq/L)	98–107	102
Carbon dioxide (CO_2, mEq/L)	23–29	25
Bicarbonate (mEq/L)	23–28	24
BUN (mg/dL)	0–20	8
Creatinine serum (mg/dL)	0.6–1.1 F 0.9–1.3 M	0.9
Uric acid (mg/dL)	2.8–8.8 F 4.0–9.0 M	5.1
Est GFR, non-Afr Amer (mL/min/1.73 m²)	>60	117
Glucose (mg/dL)	70–99	91
Phosphate, inorganic (mg/dL)	2.2–4.6	3.8
Magnesium (mg/dL)	1.5–2.4	1.9
Calcium (mg/dL)	8.6–10.2	8.9
Bilirubin total (mg/dL)	≤1.2	0.9
Bilirubin, direct (mg/dL)	<0.3	0.05
Protein, total (g/dL)	6–7.8	6.3
Albumin (g/dL)	3.5–5.5	4.5
Prealbumin (mg/dL)	18–35	31
Alkaline phosphatase (U/L)	30–120	83
ALT (U/L)	4–36	11
AST (U/L)	0–35	9
CPK (U/L)	30–135 F 55–170 M	71
Lactate dehydrogenase (U/L)	208–378	210
Cholesterol (mg/dL)	<200	245 !↑
HDL-C (mg/dL)	>59 F, >50 M	52
VLDL (mg/dL)	7–32	35 !↑
LDL (mg/dL)	<130	157 !↑
LDL/HDL ratio	<3.22 F <3.55 M	3.02

(Continued)

Gupta, Krishna, Male, 48 y.o.
Allergies: NKA
Pt. Location: University Gastroenterology Clinic   **Physician:** Jen Li   **Date:** 11/1

Laboratory Results *(Continued)*

	Ref. Range	11/1 0700
Triglycerides (mg/dL)	35–135 F 40–160 M	178 !↑
HbA$_{1C}$ (%)	<5.7	5.1
Hematology		
WBC (× 10^3/mm^3)	3.9–10.7	5.6
RBC (× 10^6/mm^3)	4.2–5.4 F 4.5–6.2 M	5.2
Hemoglobin (Hgb, g/dL)	12–16 F 14–17 M	14.0
Hematocrit (Hct, %)	37–47 F 41–51 M	43
Mean cell volume (μm^3)	80–96	85
Mean cell Hgb (pg)	28–32	28
Mean cell Hgb content (g/dL)	32–36	32
RBC distribution (%)	11.6–16.5	15.5
Platelet count (× 10^3/mm^3)	150–350	345
Hematology, Manual Diff		
Neutrophil (%)	40–70	55
Lymphocyte (%)	22–44	28
Monocyte (%)	0–7	6
Eosinophil (%)	0–5	0
Basophil (%)	0–2	0
Blasts (%)	3–10	3
Urinalysis		
Collection method	—	Clean catch
Color	—	Pale yellow
Appearance	—	Clear
Specific gravity	1.001–1.035	1.006
pH	5–7	6.1
Protein (mg/dL)	Neg	Neg
Glucose (mg/dL)	Neg	Neg
Ketones	Neg	Neg
Blood	Neg	Neg
Bilirubin	Neg	Neg

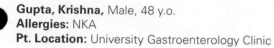

Gupta, Krishna, Male, 48 y.o.
Allergies: NKA
Pt. Location: University Gastroenterology Clinic   **Physician:** Jen Li   **Date:** 11/1

Laboratory Results *(Continued)*

	Ref. Range	11/1 0700
Nitrites	Neg	Neg
Urobilinogen (EU/dL)	<1.0	0.009
Leukocyte esterase	Neg	Neg
Prot chk	Neg	Neg
WBCs (/HPF)	0–5	1
RBCs (/HPF)	0–2	0.5
Bact	0	0
Mucus	0	0
Crys	0	0
Casts (/LPF)	0	0
Yeast	0	0

Note: Values and units of measurement listed in these tables are derived from several resources. Substantial variation exists in the ranges quoted as "normal" and these may vary depending on the assay used by different laboratories.

Case Questions

I. **Understanding the Disease and Pathophysiology**

1. How and where is acid produced and controlled within the gastrointestinal tract?

2. What role does the lower esophageal sphincter (LES) pressure play in the etiology of gastroesophageal reflux disease? What factors affect LES pressure?

3. What are the complications of gastroesophageal reflux disease?

4. The physician biopsied for *H. pylori*. What is this?

5. Identify the patient's signs and symptoms that could suggest the diagnosis of gastroesophageal reflux disease.

6. Describe the diagnostic tests performed for this patient.

7. What risk factors does the patient present with that might contribute to his diagnosis? (Be sure to consider lifestyle, medical, and nutritional factors.)

8. The MD has decreased the patient's dose of daily aspirin and recommended discontinuing his ibuprofen. Why? How might aspirin and other NSAIDs affect gastroesophageal disease?

9. The MD has prescribed omeprazole. What class of medication is this? What is the basic mechanism of the drug? What other drugs are available in this class? What other groups of medications are used to treat GERD?

II. **Understanding the Nutrition Therapy**

10. Summarize the current recommendations for nutrition therapy for GERD.

III. **Nutrition Assessment**

11. Calculate the patient's %UBW and BMI. What does this assessment of weight tell you? In what ways may this contribute to his diagnosis?

12. Calculate energy and protein requirements for Mr. Gupta. How would this recommendation be modified to support a gradual weight loss?

13. Mr. Gupta and his wife are originally from India. Are there components of their traditional diet that may aggravate his symptoms of GERD?

14. What considerations related to Hinduism should you keep in mind when assessing Mr. Gupta's diet?

15. Estimate his caloric intake from his 24-hour recall. How does this compare to your calculated energy requirements?

16. Are there any abnormal labs that should be addressed to improve Mr. Gupta's overall health? Explain.

17. Mr. Gupta's history includes the use of fenugreek and turmeric as alternative treatments for his symptoms of GERD. Examine the evidence regarding these supplements. What could you tell Mr. Gupta? Are there any concerns with the ingestion of these supplements?

18. What other components of lifestyle modification would you address in order to help in treating his disorder?

IV. Nutrition Diagnosis

19. Identify pertinent nutrition problems and corresponding nutrition diagnoses and write at least two PES statements for them.

V. Nutrition Intervention

20. Determine the appropriate intervention for each nutrition diagnosis.

21. Does the long-term use of proton pump inhibitors have nutritional effects? Are there specific interventions that you might implement to address these effects?

Bibliography

Academy of Nutrition and Dietetics Nutrition Care Manual. https://www.nutritioncaremanual.org/client_ed.cfm?ncm_client_ed_id=165. Accessed 03/25/15.

Bredenoord AJ. Mechanisms of reflux perception in gastroesophageal reflux disease: A review. *Am J Gastroenterol.* 2012;107:8–15.

Esmaillzadeh A, Keshteli AH, Feizi A. Zaribaf F, Feinle-Bisset C, Adibi P. Patterns of diet-related practices and prevalence of gastro-esophageal reflux disease. *Neurogastro Motil.* 2013;25:831–e638.

Katz PO, Gerson LB, Vila MF. Diagnosis and management of gastroesophageal disease. *Am J Gastroenterol.* 2013;108:308–328.

Khan N, Bukhari S, Lakha A, et al. Gastroesophageal reflux disease: The case for improving patient education in primary care. *J Fam Prac.* 2013;63:719–723.

Kittler P, Sucher K, Nelms M. Food and religion. In: Kittler P, Sucher K, Nelms M. *Food and Culture* 6th ed. Belmont, CA: Cengage Learning; 2011:94–97.

National Digestive Diseases Information Clearinghouse. Bethesda, MD: National Digestive Diseases Information Clearinghouse; May 2007; last updated April 30, 2012. Heartburn, gastroesophageal reflux (GER), and gastroesophageal reflux disease (GERD); NIH Publication No. 07-0882: http://www.niddk.nih.gov/health-information/health-topics/digestive-diseases/ger-and-gerd-in-children-and-adolescents/Pages/facts.aspx. Accessed 03/25/15.

Nelms MN, Habash D. Nutrition assessment: Foundation of the nutrition care process. In: Nelms M, Sucher K, Lacey K. *Nutrition Therapy and Pathophysiology.* 3rd ed. Belmont, CA: Cengage Learning; 2016:36–71.

Nelms MN. Diseases of the upper gastrointestinal tract. In: Nelms M, Sucher K, Lacey K. *Nutrition Therapy and Pathophysiology.* 3rd ed. Belmont, CA: Cengage Learning; 2016: 342–378.

Patrick L. Gastroesophageal reflux disease (GERD): A review of conventional and alternative treatments. *Altern Med Rev.* 2011;16(2):116–133.

Pronsky ZM. *Food-Medication Interactions.* 17th ed. Birchrunville, PA: Food-Medication Interactions; 2012.

Queensland Government. Health care provider' handbook on Hindu patients. *Queensland Health.* 2011. Available from: http://www.health.qld.gov.au/multicultural/support_tools/hbook-hindu.pdf. Accessed: 03/25/15.

Singh M, Lee J, Gupta N, et al. Weight loss can lead to resolution of gastroesophageal reflux disease of symptoms: A prospective intervention trial. *Obesity.* 2013;21:284–290.

Internet Resources

American College of Gastroenterology: Acid Reflux: http://patients.gi.org/topics/acid-reflux/

National Center for Complementary and Integrative Health: https://nccih.nih.gov/

National Institute of Diabetes and Digestive and Kidney Diseases: Digestive Diseases A–Z: http://digestive.niddk.nih.gov

Medline Plus: GERD: http://www.nlm.nih.gov/medlineplus/gerd.html

Gastroparesis

Objectives

After completing this case, the student will be able to:

1. Apply knowledge of the pathophysiology of gastroparesis in order to identify and explain common nutritional problems associated with this condition.
2. Identify the common signs and symptoms associated with gastroparesis.
3. Understand the potential nutritional complications of gastroparesis.
4. Discuss the rationale for nutrition recommendations to minimize adverse symptoms of gastroparesis and to improve nutritional outcomes.
5. Interpret pertinent laboratory parameters for nutritional implications and significance.

6. Analyze nutrition assessment data to evaluate nutritional status and identify specific nutrition problems.
7. Determine nutrition diagnoses and write appropriate PES statements.
8. Develop a nutrition care plan—with appropriate measurable goals, interventions, and strategies for monitoring and evaluation—that addresses the nutrition diagnoses of this case.

Mrs. Williams is here for a follow-up appointment with her gastroenterologist and the clinic's registered dietitian. She has recently been diagnosed with gastroparesis and needs assistance with nutrition therapy for this condition.

Williams, Dorothy, Female, 49 y.o.
Allergies: NKA
Pt. Location: University Gastroenterology Clinic   **Physician:** R Levin   **Date:** 6/5

Patient Summary: 49-year-old female here for evaluation and treatment for recently diagnosed gastroparesis.

History:
Onset of disease: Patient has been experiencing increased nausea over the past 6 months. She has had some indigestion in the past and has been diagnosed with a hiatal hernia. Mrs. Williams recently underwent a scintigraphy gastric emptying test. Test results determined that 85% of the test meal was retained after 2 hours. She has now been referred to the outpatient gastroenterology clinic.
Medical history: Indigestion; hiatal hernia
Surgical history: s/p hysterectomy 2 years previous secondary to endometriosis
Medications at home: Ranitidine 80 mg Tab; omeprazole 20 mg Cap DR
Tobacco use: None
Alcohol use: None
Family history: What? CAD, diabetes, cancer. Who? Parents, sister, and brother.

Demographics:
Marital status: Married—lives with husband and 4 children
Spouse name: Sam
Number of children: 4—ages 9, 11, 14, 16
Years education: High school
Language: English
Occupation: Administrative assistant for local elementary school
Hours of work: M–F, works consistently in evenings and on weekends as well
Ethnicity: African American
Religious affiliation: African Methodist Episcopal

MD Progress Note:

Review of Systems
Constitutional: Negative
Skin: Negative
Cardiovascular: No carotid bruits
Respiratory: Negative
Gastrointestinal: Nausea, bloating, abdominal pain
Neurological: Negative
Psychiatric: Negative

Physical Exam
General appearance: No acute distress. Well nourished.
Heart: S1S2, normal rate, no m/r/g

Williams, Dorothy, Female, 49 y.o.
Allergies: NKA
Pt. Location: University Gastroenterology Clinic   **Physician:** R Levin   **Date:** 6/5

HEENT: Head is normocephalic and atraumatic. Pupils are equal and reactive to light. Extraocular muscles are intact. Sclerae are anicteric. Conjunctivae are pink. There is no obvious hearing loss. The oropharynx exam reveals the mucous membranes to be moist. The tongue is midline. The uvula elevates with phonation. The teeth are in good state of repair.
Neck: Supple without lymphadenopathy, thyromegaly, or JVD.
Genitalia: WNL
Neurologic: Oriented × 4. The patient is alert and fully oriented with an appropriate affect.
Extremities: No edema; normal strength, sensations, and DTR
Skin: Warm, dry, no rash or jaundice
Chest/lungs: Lungs clear to auscultation and percussion. The AP diameter is normal.
Peripheral vascular: Pulses full—no bruits
Abdomen: The abdomen is soft and nontender to palpation. There is no guarding, rebound tenderness, or rigidity. Normal, active bowel sounds are heard in all quadrants. No masses or organomegaly are noted.

Vital Signs: Temp: 98.6   Pulse: 72   Resp rate: 122
                     BP: 128/82   Height: 5'6"   Weight: 126 lbs

Assessment and Plan:

Dx: Gastroesophageal reflux disease, gastroparesis, hiatal hernia

Medical Tx plan: Increase ranitidine 150 mg Tab; omeprazole 60 mg Cap DR daily; metoclopramide 10 mg four times daily. Nutrition consult.
.... E Levin, MD

Nuclear Medicine Result
Exam: Gastric Emptying NSSCAN=W
Comparison: No prior gastric emptying scintigraphy studies are available for comparison.
Clinical history: 49-year-old woman who presents with nausea and vomiting. The study is requested for evaluation of gastric emptying.
Relevant medications taken by patient within 2 days prior to this study (as reported by the patient): None
Technique: 0.534 mCi of Tc-99m sulfur colloid was mixed with 120 g of EggBeaters (commercial egg white preparation; equivalent to two eggs) and subsequently scrambled. The patient consumed this radiolabeled meal orally along with 2 slices of dry toast, 30 g of jam, and 120 mL of water. Images of the abdomen in anterior and posterior projections were acquired immediately after meal consumption and at 1 and 2 hours after meal consumption. Region of interest analysis (via geometric mean) was used to calculate percent retained gastric activity at 1 and 2 hours after meal consumption.

Williams, Dorothy, Female, 49 y.o.
Allergies: NKA
Pt. Location: University Gastroenterology Clinic   **Physician:** R Levin   **Date:** 6/5

Findings: At 60 minutes after meal consumption, 95% of initial gastric contents were retained within the stomach (normal range, 30–90%). At 120 minutes after meal consumption, 85% of initial gastric contents were retained within the stomach (normal range, <60%).
Reference: Abell TL et al. Consensus Recommendations for Gastric Emptying Scintigraphy: A Joint Report of the American Neurogastroenterology and Motility Society and the Society of Nuclear Medicine. *Am J Gastroenterology* 2007;102:1–11.
Electronically signed by: Smith L. (Physician) 5/26
Impression: Scintigraphic findings are abnormal at both 1 hour and at 2 hours. Dx: gastroparesis.

Nutrition:

History: Patient relates she has lost more than 40 lbs over the previous year. She describes constant nausea and occasional vomiting over the previous 6 months. She states that she is never hungry but has to make herself eat. She cooks regularly for her family and she tries to eat a little bit whenever she prepares these meals. She takes soup or leftovers for lunch at her job. She has stopped eating meats as they cause a lot of abdominal pain. Mrs. Williams states that she tolerates drinking beverages better than she does eating solid foods.

Usual dietary intake:

AM:	Approx. ½ scrambled egg, few bites of toast; coffee with milk and sugar
Lunch:	Soup—chicken noodle—½ c; Sprite
Snack when she comes home:	Yogurt or 4 oz chocolate milk
PM:	½ c pasta with cheese; mashed potatoes or vegetables
Late PM:	½ can Ensure or 4 oz milk

Food allergies/intolerances/aversions: Meats, spicy foods, fried foods make symptoms worse
Previous nutrition therapy? No
Food purchase/preparation: Self
Vit/min intake: None

Williams, Dorothy, Female, 49 y.o.
Allergies: NKA
Pt. Location: University Gastroenterology Clinic   **Physician:** R Levin   **Date:** 6/5

Laboratory Results

	Ref. Range	6/5
Chemistry		
Sodium (mEq/L)	136–145	138
Potassium (mEq/L)	3.5–5.1	4.1
Chloride (mEq/L)	98–107	101
Carbon dioxide (CO_2, mEq/L)	23–29	23
Bicarbonate (mEq/L)	23–28	25
BUN (mg/dL)	6–20	6
Creatinine serum (mg/dL)	0.6–1.1 F 0.9–1.3 M	0.6
Uric acid (mg/dL)	2.8–8.8 F 4.0–9.0 M	2.9
Est GFR, non-Afr Amer (mL/min/1.73 m²)	>60	89
Glucose (mg/dL)	70–99	78
Phosphate, inorganic (mg/dL)	2.2–4.6	2.4
Magnesium (mg/dL)	1.5–2.4	1.5
Calcium (mg/dL)	8.6–10.2	8.98
Bilirubin total (mg/dL)	≤1.2	0.4
Bilirubin, direct (mg/dL)	<0.3	0.01
Protein, total (g/dL)	6–7.8	6.0
Albumin (g/dL)	3.5–5.5	3.5
Prealbumin (mg/dL)	18–35	21
Alkaline phosphatase (U/L)	30–120	81
ALT (U/L)	4–36	5
AST (U/L)	0–35	11
CPK (U/L)	30–135 F 55–170 M	62
Lactate dehydrogenase (U/L)	208–378	217
Cholesterol (mg/dL)	<200	150
HDL-C (mg/dL)	>59 F, >50 M	62
VLDL (mg/dL)	7–32	15
LDL (mg/dL)	<130	82
LDL/HDL ratio	<3.22 F <3.55 M	1.58

(Continued)

Williams, Dorothy, Female, 49 y.o.
Allergies: NKA
Pt. Location: University Gastroenterology Clinic   **Physician:** R Levin   **Date:** 6/5

Laboratory Results (Continued)

	Ref. Range	6/5
Triglycerides (mg/dL)	35–135 F 40–160 M	78
HbA$_{1c}$ (%)	<5.7	5.3
Hematology		
WBC ($\times 10^3$/mm^3)	3.9–10.7	6.2
RBC ($\times 10^6$/mm^3)	4.2–5.4 F 4.5–6.2 M	4.8
Hemoglobin (Hgb, g/dL)	12–16 F 14–17 M	10.5 !↓
Hematocrit (Hct, %)	37–47 F 41–51 M	34 !↓
Mean cell volume (μm^3)	80–96	71 !↓
Mean cell Hgb (pg)	28–32	22 !↓
Mean cell Hgb content (g/dL)	32–36	24 !↓
RBC distribution (%)	11.6–16.5	17.5 !↑
Hematology, Manual Diff		
Neutrophil (%)	40–70	42
Lymphocyte (%)	22–44	22
Monocyte (%)	0–7	3
Eosinophil (%)	0–5	0
Basophil (%)	0–2	0
Blasts (%)	3–10	3
Urinalysis		
Collection method	—	Clean catch
Color	—	Amber
Appearance	—	Clear
Specific gravity	1.001–1.035	1.034
pH	5–7	6.3
Protein (mg/dL)	Neg	Neg
Glucose (mg/dL)	Neg	Neg
Ketones	Neg	+ !↑
Blood	Neg	Neg
Bilirubin	Neg	Neg

Williams, Dorothy, Female, 49 y.o.
Allergies: NKA
Pt. Location: University Gastroenterology Clinic   **Physician:** R Levin   **Date:** 6/5

Laboratory Results (*Continued*)

	Ref. Range	6/5
Nitrites	Neg	Neg
Urobilinogen (EU/dL)	<1.0	0.009
Leukocyte esterase	Neg	Neg
Prot chk	Neg	+ !↑
WBCs (/HPF)	0–5	0
RBCs (/HPF)	0–2	0
Bact	0	0
Mucus	0	0
Crys	0	0
Casts (/LPF)	0	0
Yeast	0	0

Note: Values and units of measurement listed in these tables are derived from several resources. Substantial variation exists in the ranges quoted as "normal" and these may vary depending on the assay used by different laboratories.

Case Questions

I.   Understanding the Disease and Pathophysiology

1. Identify the major physiological controls for gastric emptying.

2. List and discuss physiological factors that may lead to the diagnosis of gastroparesis.

3. According to the American College of Gastroenterology, scintigraphy is the gold standard for diagnosis of gastroparesis. This test was performed on Mrs. Williams. Explain this test and discuss how her results confirm her diagnosis. Are there other diagnostic tests that could be used?

4. What are the common signs and symptoms of gastroparesis? Explain how they may lead to nutritional deficits.

II.   Understanding the Nutrition Therapy

5. Summarize the current recommendations for nutrition therapy for gastroparesis. Choose at least 3 of the recommended dietary modifications and explain why each may assist with control of symptoms or improve nutritional status.

6. If a patient with gastroparesis is not able to meet his or her nutritional needs orally, what type of enteral feeding recommendations are appropriate?

III.   Nutrition Assessment

7. Calculate the patient's %UBW and BMI. What does this assessment of weight tell you?

8. Calculate energy and protein requirements for Mrs. Williams. Explain how you determined these recommendations.

9. Estimate her caloric intake from her usual dietary intake. How does this compare to your calculated energy requirements?

10. Are there any abnormal labs that should be addressed to improve Mrs. Williams's overall health? Explain the possible cause(s) for each abnormal lab result.

IV.   Nutrition Diagnosis

11. Identify the most pertinent nutrition problems and corresponding nutrition diagnoses and write at least two PES statements for them.

V.   Nutrition Intervention

12. Determine the appropriate intervention for each nutrition diagnosis.

VI.   Evaluation and Monitoring

13. Identify measurable outcomes for each of your interventions. What are possible nutrition concerns that you may want to address in a follow-up visit with Mrs. Williams?

Bibliography

Academy of Nutrition and Dietetics Nutrition Care Manual. https://www.nutritioncaremanual.org/client_ed.cfm?ncm_client_ed_id=165. Accessed 03/25/15.

Acosta A, Camilleri C. Prokinetics in gastroparesis. *Gastroenterology Clinics of North America*. 2015;44:97–111.

Bouras EP, Vazquez Roque MI, Aranda-Michel J. Gastroparesis: From concepts to management. *Nutr Clin Prac*. 2013;28:437–447.

Camilleri M, Parkman H, Shafi M, Abell T, Gerson L. Clinical guideline: Management of gastroparesis. *Am J Gastroenterol*. 2013;108:18–37.

Hasler WL. Symptomatic management for gastroparesis. *Gastroenterology Clinics of North America*. 2015;44:113–126.

Homko CJ, Duffy F, Friedenberg FK, Boden G, Parkman HP. Effect of dietary fat and food consistency on gastroparesis symptoms in patients with gastroparesis. *Neurogastroenterol Motil*. 2015;27:501-508.

Lee LA, Chen J, Yin J. Complementary and alternative medicine for gastroparesis. *Gastroenterology Clinics of North America*. 2015;44:137–150.

Nelms MN, Habash D. Nutrition assessment: Foundation of the nutrition care process. In: Nelms M, Sucher K, Lacey K. *Nutrition Therapy and Pathophysiology*. 3rd ed. Belmont, CA: Cengage Learning; 2016:36–71.

Nelms MN. Diseases of the upper gastrointestinal tract. In: Nelms M, Sucher K, Lacey K. *Nutrition Therapy and Pathophysiology*. 3rd ed. Belmont, CA: Cengage Learning; 2016:342–378.

Nguyen LA, Snape WJ. Clinical presentation and pathophysiology of gastroparesis. *Gastroenterology Clinics of North America*. 2015;44:21–30.

Pronsky Z. M. *Food-Medication Interactions*. 17th ed . Birchrunville, PA: Food-Medication Interactions; 2012.

Rees-Parrish C. Nutritional considerations in the patient with gastroparesis. *Gastroenterology Clinics of North America*. 2015;44:83–95.

Internet Resources

American College of Gastroenterology: Gastroparesis: http://patients.gi.org/topics/gastroparesis/

Mayo Clinic: Gastroparesis: http://www.mayoclinic.org/diseases-conditions/gastroparesis/basics/definition/con-20023971

National Institute of Diabetes and Digestive and Kidney Diseases: Gastroparesis: http://www.niddk.nih.gov/health-information/health-topics/digestive-diseases/gastroparesis/Pages/facts.aspx

University of Virginia Digestive Health Center: Diet Intervention for Gastroparesis: https://uvahealth.com/services/digestive-health/images-and-docs/gastroparesis-diet.pdf

Ulcer Disease: Medical and Surgical Treatment

Objectives

After completing this case, the student will be able to:

1. Discuss the etiology and risk factors for development of ulcer disease.
2. Identify classes of medications used to treat ulcer disease and determine possible drug–nutrient interactions.
3. Describe surgical procedures used to treat refractory ulcer disease and explain common nutritional problems associated with this treatment.
4. Apply knowledge of nutrition therapy guidelines for ulcer disease and gastric surgery.
5. Analyze nutrition assessment data to evaluate nutritional status and identify specific nutrition problems.
6. Determine nutrition diagnoses and write appropriate PES statements.
7. Calculate enteral nutrition prescriptions.
8. Evaluate a standard enteral nutritional regimen.
9. Develop a nutrition care plan—with appropriate measurable goals, interventions, and strategies for monitoring and evaluation—that addresses the nutrition diagnoses of this case.

Maria Rodriguez is a 38-year-old female who has been treated as an outpatient for her gastro-esophageal reflux disease. Her increasing symptoms of hematemesis, vomiting, and diarrhea lead her to be admitted for further gastrointestinal workup. She undergoes a gastrojejunostomy to treat her perforated duodenal ulcer.

Rodriguez, Maria, Female, 38 y.o.
Allergies: Codeine causes N/V
Pt. Location: RM 1145

Code: FULL
Physician: S. Sharma

Isolation: None
Admit Date: 8/30

Patient Summary: Maria Rodriguez is a 38-year-old female admitted through ED for a surgical consult for possible perforated duodenal ulcer.

History:

Onset of disease: Diagnosed with GERD approx. 11 months ago; diagnosed with duodenal ulcer 2 weeks ago

Medical history: Gravida 2 para 2. No other significant history except history of GERD.

Surgical history: She is s/p endoscopy (2 weeks ago as an outpatient) that revealed 2-cm duodenal ulcer with generalized gastritis and a positive biopsy for *Helicobacter pylori*.

Medications at home: She has completed 10 days of a 14-day course of bismuth subsalicylate 525 mg 4 × daily, metronidazole 250 mg 4 × daily, tetracycline 500 mg 4 × daily, and omeprazole 20 mg 2 × daily, prescribed for total of 28 days

Tobacco use: Yes

Alcohol use: No

Family history: What? DM, PUD. Who? DM: maternal grandmother; PUD: father and grandfather.

Demographics:

Marital status: Widowed—lives with 2 daughters ages 12 and 14

Number of children: 2

Years education: Associate's degree

Language: English and Spanish

Occupation: Computer programmer

Hours of work: M–F 9–5

Ethnicity: Hispanic

Religious affiliation: Catholic

MD Note 9/2 POD#2: s/p gastrojejunostomy secondary to perforated duodenal ulcer.

General appearance: 38-year-old Hispanic female—thin, pale, and in acute distress

Physical exam:

Heart: Regular rate and rhythm, heart sounds normal

HEENT: Noncontributory

Genitalia: WNL

Neurologic: Oriented × 4

Extremities: Noncontributory

Skin: Warm and dry to touch

Chest/lungs: Rapid breath sounds, lungs clear

Peripheral vascular: Pulses full—no bruits

Abdomen: Tender with guarding, absent bowel sounds

24 hr. Vital Signs:

Temp: 99
BP: 101/72

Pulse: 78
Height: 5'2"

Resp rate: 32
Weight: 110 lbs

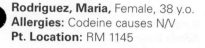

Rodriguez, Maria, Female, 38 y.o.
Allergies: Codeine causes N/V
Pt. Location: RM 1145

Code: FULL
Physician: S. Sharma

Isolation: None
Admit Date: 8/30

Assessment and Plan:
38-yo female 2 days post-op gastrojejunostomy secondary to perforated duodenal ulcer. Pain well controlled.

Plan:
NPO with ice chips
Enteral nutrition via jejunostomy feeding tube placed during surgery. Receiving Pivot 1.5@25 mL/hr via continuous drip.
Continue with PT for ambulation.
Wound care.

.... S. Sharma, MD

Nutrition:
History: Patient relates that she understands about the feeding she is receiving through her tube. She explains that she has eaten very little since her ulcer was diagnosed and wonders how long it will be before she can eat again. Her physicians have told her they might like her to try something by mouth in the next few days.

Usual dietary intake (prior to current illness)*:*
AM: Coffee, 1 slice dry toast. On weekends, cooked large breakfasts for family, which included omelets, rice, pozole, or pancakes, waffles, fruit.
Lunch: Sandwich from home (2 oz turkey on whole-wheat bread with mustard); 1 piece of raw fruit, cookies (2–3 Chips Ahoy)
Dinner: 2 c rice, some type of meat (2–3 oz chicken), fresh vegetables (steamed tomatoes, peppers, and onions—1 c), coffee
Usual intake includes 8–10 c coffee and 1–2 soft drinks (12-oz cans) daily

24-hr recall: Has been NPO since admission.
Food allergies/intolerances/aversions: See nutrition history.
Previous nutrition therapy? No
Food purchase/preparation: Self and daughters
Vit/min intake: None

Rodriguez, Maria, Female, 38 y.o.
Allergies: Codeine causes N/V
Pt. Location: RM 1145

Code: FULL
Physician: S. Sharma

Isolation: None
Admit Date: 8/30

Intake/Output

Date			9/2 0701 – 9/3 0700			
Time			0701–1500	1501–2300	2301–0700	Daily total
IN	Tube feeding: Formula		150	100	200	450
	Tube feeding: Flush		50	50	50	150
	(mL/kg/hr)		(0.5)	(0.38)	(0.63)	(0.5)
	I.V.		**400**	**400**	**380**	**1180**
	(mL/kg/hr)		(1)	(1)	(0.95)	(0.98)
	I.V. piggyback					
	TPN					
	Total intake		**600**	**550**	**630**	**1780**
	(mL/kg)		(12)	(11)	(12.6)	(35.6)
OUT	Urine		**550**	**200**	**480**	**1230**
	(mL/kg/hr)		(1.38)	(0.5)	(1.2)	(1.03)
	Emesis output					
	Other: Drains		**275**	**320**	**220**	**815**
	Stool		**200**		**128**	**328**
	Total output		**1025**	**520**	**828**	**2373**
	(mL/kg)		(20.5)	(10.4)	(16.56)	(47.46)
Net I/O			**−425**	**+30**	**−198**	**−593**
Net since admission (8/30)			**−425**	**−395**	**−593**	**−593**

Laboratory Results

	Ref. Range	8/30 0800	9/2 0600
Chemistry			
Sodium (mEq/L)	136–145	141	140
Potassium (mEq/L)	3.5–5.1	4.5	4.2
Chloride (mEq/L)	98–107	103	101
Carbon dioxide (CO_2, mEq/L)	23–29	26	24
Bicarbonate (mEq/L)	23–28	24	23
BUN (mg/dL)	6–20	18	15
Creatinine serum (mg/dL)	0.6–1.1 F 0.9–1.3 M	1.1	0.9
BUN/Crea ratio	10.0–20.0	16.3	16.6
Uric acid (mg/dL)	2.8–8.8 F 4.0–9.0 M	3.2	4.4

Rodriguez, Maria, Female, 38 y.o.
Allergies: Codeine causes N/V
Pt. Location: RM 1145

Code: FULL
Physician: S. Sharma

Isolation: None
Admit Date: 8/30

Laboratory Results *(Continued)*

	Ref. Range	8/30 0800	9/2 0600
Est GFR, non-Afr Amer (mL/min/1.73 m²)	>60	56 !↓	70
Glucose (mg/dL)	70–99	80	128 !↑
Phosphate, inorganic (mg/dL)	2.2–4.6	3.7	3.5
Magnesium (mg/dL)	1.5–2.4	1.9	1.7
Calcium (mg/dL)	8.6–10.2	9.0	8.7
Osmolality (mmol/kg/H₂O)	275–295	293	292
Bilirubin total (mg/dL)	≤1.2	1.7 !↑	1.0
Bilirubin, direct (mg/dL)	<0.3	1.3 !↑	0.6 !↑
Protein, total (g/dL)	6–7.8	5.7 !↓	5.8 !↑
Albumin (g/dL)	3.5–5.5	3.0 !↓	3.3 !↓
Prealbumin (mg/dL)	18–35	15 !↓	14 !↓
Ammonia (NH₃, μg/L)	6–47	11	10
Alkaline phosphatase (U/L)	30–120	98	90
ALT (U/L)	4–36	30	24
AST (U/L)	0–35	30	17
CPK (U/L)	30–135 F 55–170 M	155 !↑	135
Lactate dehydrogenase (U/L)	208–378	351	321
Coagulation (Coag)			
PT (sec)	11–13	11.5	12.1
PTT (sec)	24–34	25.5	24
Hematology			
WBC (× 10³/mm³)	3.9–10.7	16.3 !↑	12.5 !↑
RBC (× 10⁶/mm³)	4.2 5.4 F 4.5–6.2 M	4.9	5.0
Hemoglobin (Hgb, g/dL)	12–16 F 14–17 M	11.2 !↓	10.2 !↓
Hematocrit (Hct, %)	37–47 F 41–51 M	33 !↓	31 !↓
Mean cell volume (μm³)	80–96	91	86
Mean cell Hgb (pg)	28–32	25.9 !↓	25.5 !↓
Mean cell Hgb content (g/dL)	32–36	31 !↓	28.5 !↓
RBC distribution (%)	11.6–16.5	17.2 !↑	

(Continued)

Rodriguez, Maria, Female, 38 y.o.
Allergies: Codeine causes N/V
Pt. Location: RM 1145

Code: FULL
Physician: S. Sharma

Isolation: None
Admit Date: 8/30

Laboratory Results *(Continued)*

	Ref. Range	8/30 0800	9/2 0600
Platelet count ($\times 10^3/mm^3$)	150–350	267	
Transferrin (mg/dL)	250–380 F 215–365 M	401 !↑	
Ferritin (mg/mL)	20–120 F 20–300 M	15 !↓	
Iron (μg/dL)	65–165 F 75–175 M	63 !↓	
Vitamin B_{12} (ng/dL)	24.4–100	45	
Folate (ng/dL)	5–25	15	
Hematology, Manual Diff			
Neutrophil (%)	40–70	45	55
Lymphocyte (%)	22–44	22	30
Monocyte (%)	0–7	5	4
Eosinophil (%)	0–5	2	3
Basophil (%)	0–2	0	1
Blasts (%)	3–10	4	5
Segs (%)	0–60	87 !↑	78 !↑

Note: Values and units of measurement listed in these tables are derived from several resources. Substantial variation exists in the ranges quoted as "normal" and these may vary depending on the assay used by different laboratories.

Case Questions

I.   Understanding the Disease and Pathophysiology

1.   Identify the patient's risk factors for ulcer disease.

2.   How is smoking related to ulcer disease?

3.   What role does *H. pylori* play in ulcer disease?

4.   Four different medications were prescribed for treatment of this patient's *H. pylori* infection: metronidazole, tetracycline, bismuth subsalicylate, and omeprazole. Identify the drug functions/mechanisms of each.

5.   What are the possible drug–nutrient side effects from Mrs. Rodriguez's prescribed regimen? (See question #4.) Which drug–nutrient side effects are most pertinent to her current nutritional status?

6.   Explain the surgical procedure the patient received.

7.   How may the normal digestive process change with this procedure?

II.   Understanding the Nutrition Therapy

8.   The most common physical side effects from this surgery are development of early or late dumping syndrome. Describe each of these syndromes, including symptoms the patient might experience, etiology of the symptoms, and standard interventions for preventing/treating the symptoms.

9.   What potential nutritional deficiencies may occur after this surgical procedure? Why might Mrs. Rodriguez be at risk for iron-deficiency anemia, pernicious anemia, and/or megaloblastic anemia?

10.   Should Mrs. Rodriguez be on any type of vitamin/mineral supplementation at home when she is discharged? Would you make any recommendations for specific types? Explain.

III.   Nutrition Assessment

11. Prior to being diagnosed with GERD, Mrs. Rodriguez weighed 145 lbs. Calculate %UBW and BMI. Which of these is the most pertinent in identifying the patient's nutrition risk? Why?

12. What other anthropometric measures could be used to further confirm her nutritional status?

13. Calculate energy and protein requirements for Mrs. Rodriguez.

14. This patient was started on an enteral feeding postoperatively. What type of enteral formula is Pivot 1.5? Using the current ASPEN guidelines for initiation of nutrition support, state whether you agree with this choice and provide a rationale for your response.

15. Why was the enteral formula started at 25 mL/hr?

16. Is the current enteral prescription meeting this patient's nutritional needs? Compare her energy and protein requirements to what is provided by the formula. If her needs are not being met, what should be the goal for her enteral support?

17. What would the RD assess to monitor tolerance to the enteral feeding?

18. Using the intake/output record for 9/2, how much enteral nutrition did the patient receive? How does this comparc to what was prescribed?

19. As the patient is advanced to solid food, what modifications in diet would the RD address? Why? What would be a typical first meal for this patient?

20. What other advice would you give to Mrs. Rodriguez to maximize her tolerance of solid food?

21. Using her admission chemistry and hematology values, which biochemical measures are abnormal?

    a. Which values can be used to further assess her nutritional status? Explain.

    b. Which laboratory measures are related to her diagnosis of a duodenal ulcer? Why would they be abnormal?

22. Do you think this patient is malnourished? If so, what criteria can be used to support a diagnosis of malnutrition? Using the guidelines proposed by ASPEN and AND, what type of malnutrition can be suggested as the diagnosis for this patient?

IV. Nutrition Diagnosis

23. Select two nutrition problems and complete the PES statement for each.

V. Nutrition Intervention

24. For each of the PES statements that you have written, establish an ideal goal (based on the signs and symptoms) and an appropriate intervention (based on the etiology).

25. Mrs. Rodriguez asks to speak with you because she is concerned about having to follow a special diet forever. What might you tell her? What nutrition education should this patient receive prior to discharge?

26. Do any lifestyle issues need to be addressed with this patient? Explain.

Bibliography

Academy of Nutrition and Dietetics Nutrition Care Manual. Diseases and conditions of the upper GI tact—peptic ulcers. http://nutritioncaremanual.org /topic.cfm?ncm_toc_id=20009. Accessed 02/2015.

McClave SA, Martindale RG, Vanek VW, et al. Guidelines for the provision and assessment of nutrition support therapy in the adult critically ill patient: Society of Critical Care Medicine (SCCM) and American Society for Parenteral and Enteral Nutrition (A.S.P.E.N.). *JPEN J Parenter Enteral Nutr.* 2009;33:277–316.

Nelms MN. Diseases of the upper gastrointestinal tract. In: Nelms M, Sucher K, Lacey K. *Nutrition Therapy and Pathophysiology.* 3rd ed. Belmont, CA: Cengage Learning; 2016:342–378.

Nelms MN. Enteral and parenteral nutrition support. In Nelms M, Sucher K, Lacey K. *Nutrition Therapy and Pathophysiology.* 3rd ed. Belmont, CA: Cengage Learning; 2016:88–113.

Nelms MN. Nutrition assessment: Foundation of the nutrition care process. In: Nelms M, Sucher K, Lacey K. *Nutrition Therapy and Pathophysiology.* 3rd ed. Belmont, CA: Cengage Learning; 2016:36–71.

Pronsky ZM. Food-Medication Interactions, 18th ed. Birchrunville, PA: Food-Medication Interactions; 2012.

Tack J, Deloose E. Complications of bariatric surgery: Dumping syndrome, reflux and vitamin deficiencies. *Obesity and the Gastrointestinal Tract.* 2014;28:741–749.

White JV, Guenter P, Jensen G, Malone A, Schofield M, Academy of Nutrition and Dietetics Malnutrition Work Group, A.S.P.E.N. Malnutrition Task Force, A.S.P.E.N. Board of Directors. Consensus statement of the Academy of Nutrition and Dietetics/American Society of Parenteral and Enteral Nutrition: Characteristics recommended for the identification and documentation of adult malnutrition (undernutrition). *J Acad Nutr Diet.* 2012;112:730–738.

Internet Resources

American Association for Clinical Chemistry Lab Tests Online: Complete Blood Count: http://labtestsonline. org/understanding/analytes/cbc/

Mayo Clinic: Peptic Ulcer: http://www.mayoclinic.org /diseases-conditions/peptic-ulcer/basics/definition /con-20028643

Medline Plus: Peptic Ulcer: http://www.nlm.nih.gov /medlineplus/pepticulcer.html

Medscape: Peptic Ulcer Disease: http://emedicine .medscape.com/article/181753-overview

National Institute of Diabetes and Digestive and Kidney Diseases: Peptic Ulcer Disease: http://digestive.niddk .nih.gov/ddiseases/pubs/pepticulcers_ez/

NUTRITION THERAPY FOR LOWER GASTROINTESTINAL DISORDERS

The next four cases explore conditions affecting the small and large intestines. These conditions, whose etiologies are all different, involve the symptoms of diarrhea, constipation, and sometimes malabsorption. In all four cases, nutrition therapy is a crucial component of the patient's care.

Celiac disease, explored in Case 10, is an autoimmune disease triggered by exposure to gliadin, a protein found in the gluten portion of wheat, rye, and barley. This case explores an atypical presentation of celiac disease, diagnostic procedures for celiac disease, secondary malabsorption syndromes, and the use of the gluten-free diet as medical nutrition therapy.

Case 11 examines irritable bowel syndrome (IBS), which is the most common gastrointestinal complaint in the United States and Canada. The improved recognition and understanding of IBS in recent years has allowed for development of additional treatments. This case addresses the FODMAP diet as a component of care for IBS.

Case 12 targets inflammatory bowel disease. Crohn's disease and ulcerative colitis are two conditions that fall under the diagnosis of inflammatory bowel disease. Both of these conditions dramatically affect nutritional status and often require nutritional support during periods of exacerbation. This case involves the effects of Crohn's disease on digestion and absorption, the diagnosis of malnutrition, and parenteral nutrition support.

Case 13 allows the student to explore the consequences of gastrointestinal surgery and the nutritional care for the individual with an ostomy. The case provides reinforcement for understanding the normal physiology of the lower gastrointestinal tract and the consequences when it is surgically resected.

Celiac Disease

Objectives

After completing this case, the student will be able to:

1. Apply knowledge of the pathophysiology of celiac disease to identify and explain common nutritional problems associated with the disease.

2. Apply knowledge of nutrition therapy for celiac disease.

3. Analyze nutrition assessment data to evaluate nutritional status and identify specific nutrition problems.

4. Determine nutrition diagnoses and write appropriate PES statements.

5. Develop a nutrition care plan—with appropriate measurable goals, interventions, and strategies for monitoring and evaluation—that addresses the nutrition diagnoses of this case.

After she experiences abdominal pain, diarrhea, and then joint pain, Mrs. Kelly Talbot's family physician refers her to the outpatient gastroenterology clinic, where she is evaluated for a possible diagnosis of celiac disease.

Talbot, Kelly, Female, 26 y.o.
Allergies: NKA
Pt. Location: University Gastroenterology Clinic   **Physician:** R. Smith   **Date:** 1/5

Patient Summary: 26-year-old female here for evaluation of symptoms of abdominal pain, diarrhea, and joint pain

History:

Onset of disease: Patient relates having diarrhea off and on since high school but it is worse now. She has occasional abdominal pain and now has joint pain. These symptoms have made it hard for her to work, and she generally feels uncomfortable. She visited her family physician, who, after conducting screening tests, referred Mrs. Talbot to the gastroenterologist for follow-up care.
Medical history: 2 pregnancies—1 live birth, 1 miscarriage at 22 weeks. No other significant medical history.
Surgical history: N/A
Medications at home: Vitamins
Tobacco use: Yes
Alcohol use: No
Family history: What? CAD. Who? Father.

Demographics:

Marital status: Married—lives with husband and 1 son; *Spouse name*: Michael
Number of children: 1
Years education: Bachelor's degree
Language: English only
Occupation: Kindergarten teacher
Hours of work: 7:30–3:30
Ethnicity: Caucasian
Religious affiliation: None

Physical Exam
General appearance: Pale woman who complains of fatigue, diarrhea, abdominal pain, and recent onset of joint pain.
HEENT: Eyes: PERRLA sclera pale; fundi benign
             Throat: Pharynx clear without postnasal drainage
Genitalia: Deferred
Neurologic: Intact; alert and oriented
Extremities: No edema, strength 4/5
Skin: Pale
Chest/lungs: Lungs clear to percussion and auscultation
Peripheral vascular: Pulses full—no bruits
Abdomen: Not distended; bowel sounds present

Vital Signs: Temp: 98.2   Pulse: 78   Resp rate: 17
                    BP: 108/72   Height: 5'3"   Weight: 125 lbs

Talbot, Kelly, Female, 26 y.o.
Allergies: NKA
Pt. Location: University Gastroenterology Clinic   **Physician:** R. Smith   **Date:** 1/5

Assessment and Plan:
26-year-old female with fatigue, diarrhea, and abdominal pain with new joint pain.

Dx: R/O Celiac disease and anemia

Medical Tx plan: IgA-tTG, total serum IgA, IgG-tTG, Chem 24, hematology with differential
Gluten-free diet
Nutrition consult

.... R. Smith, MD

Nutrition:
History: Pt denies any specific problems with appetite or individual foods. States her greatest nonpregnant weight was prior to her last pregnancy, when she weighed 150 lbs. She gained 25 lbs with her pregnancy, and her full-term son weighed 6 lbs 6 oz.

Usual dietary intake: Likes a variety of foods.

24-hr recall (prior to admission):
AM: Toast—ww 2 slices, 1 tsp butter, hot tea with 2 tsp sugar
Lunch: 1 c chicken noodle soup, peanut butter & jelly sandwich (2 slices ww bread, 2 tbsp peanut butter, 2 tsp grape jelly), 1 c applesauce, 12 oz Sprite
Dinner: 1 c ww pasta, ½ c marinara sauce (no meat), 1 c sautéed green beans, 1 slice garlic bread, ½ c rainbow sherbet

Food allergies/intolerances/aversions: Maybe NutraSweet?
Previous nutrition therapy? No
Food purchase/preparation: Self
Vit/min intake: Multivitamin/mineral

Talbot, Kelly, Female, 26 y.o.
Allergies: NKA
Pt. Location: University Gastroenterology Clinic   **Physician:** R. Smith   **Date:** 1/5

Laboratory Results

	Ref. Range	1/5
Chemistry		
Sodium (mEq/L)	136–145	141
Potassium (mEq/L)	3.5–5.1	3.7
Chloride (mEq/L)	98–107	101
Carbon dioxide (CO_2, mEq/L)	23–29	27
Bicarbonate (mEq/L)	23–28	27
BUN (mg/dL)	6–20	9
Creatinine serum (mg/dL)	0.6–1.1 F 0.9–1.3 M	0.7
BUN/Crea ratio	10.0–20.0	12.85
Uric acid (mg/dL)	2.8–8.8 F 4.0–9.0 M	4.3
Est GFR, non-Afr Amer (mL/min/1.73 m²)	>60	120
Glucose (mg/dL)	70–99	72
Phosphate, inorganic (mg/dL)	2.2–4.6	2.7
Magnesium (mg/dL)	1.5–2.4	1.6
Calcium (mg/dL)	8.6–10.2	9.1
Osmolality (mmol/kg/H_2O)	275–295	294
Bilirubin total (mg/dL)	≤1.2	1.0
Bilirubin, direct (mg/dL)	<0.3	0.2
Protein, total (g/dL)	6–7.8	6.0
Albumin (g/dL)	3.5–5.5	3.5
Prealbumin (mg/dL)	18–35	16 !↓
Ammonia (NH_3, µg/L)	6–47	10
Alkaline phosphatase (U/L)	30–120	125 !↑
ALT (U/L)	4–36	12
AST (U/L)	0–35	8
CPK (U/L)	30–135 F 55–170 M	128
Lactate dehydrogenase (U/L)	208–378	354
Cholesterol (mg/dL)	<200	117
tTg IgA antibody (U/mL)	<4	11 !↑
tTg IgG antibody (U/mL)	<6	8 !↑

Talbot, Kelly, Female, 26 y.o.
Allergies: NKA
Pt. Location: University Gastroenterology Clinic   **Physician:** R. Smith   **Date:** 1/5

Laboratory Results *(Continued)*

	Ref. Range	1/5
T_4 (µg/dL)	5–12	9.1
T_3 (µg/dL)	75–98	81
HbA_{1c} (%)	<5.7	5.1
Hematology		
WBC ($\times 10^3$/mm³)	3.9–10.7	8.5
RBC ($\times 10^6$/mm³)	4.2–5.4 F 4.5–6.2 M	3.9 !↓
Hemoglobin (Hgb, g/dL)	12–16 F 14–17 M	10.5 !↓
Hematocrit (Hct, %)	37–47 F 41–51 M	34 !↓
Mean cell volume (µm³)	80–96	71 !↓
Mean cell Hgb (pg)	28–32	22 !↓
Mean cell Hgb content (g/dL)	32–36	24 !↓
RBC distribution (%)	11.6–16.5	17.1 !↑
Platelet count ($\times 10^3$/mm³)	150–350	289
Transferrin (mg/dL)	250–380 F 215–365 M	395 !↑
Ferritin (ng/mL)	20–120 F 20–300 M	17 !↓
Iron (mg/dL)	65–165 F 75–175 M	54 !↓
Vitamin B_{12} (ng/dL)	24.4–100	65
Folate (ng/dL)	5–25	18

Note: Values and units of measurement listed in these tables are derived from several resources. Substantial variation exists in the ranges quoted as "normal" and these may vary depending on the assay used by different laboratories.

Case Questions

I.   Understanding the Disease and Pathophysiology

1. What is the etiology of celiac disease? Is anything in Mrs. Talbot's history typical of patients with celiac disease? Explain. The prevalence of celiac disease appears to be increasing. What does the current literature suggest as contributors to this change in celiac disease prevalence?

2. tTG antibodes are used in serological testing to diagnose celiac disease. Each test is sensitive and specific for the antibody it measures. The tTG test has a sensitivity of more than 90%. What does this mean? It also has a specificity of more than 95%. What does this mean?

3. Mrs. Talbot presents with some nondescript symptoms of celiac disease. List the nongastrointestinal as well as the gastrointestinal clinical manifestations of celiac disease.

4. Biopsy of the small intestine continues to be the "gold standard" for diagnosis of celiac disease. Briefly describe the procedure.

5. How does celiac disease damage the small intestine?

II.   Understanding the Nutrition Therapy

6. Gluten restriction is the major component of the medical nutrition therapy for celiac disease. What is gluten? Where is it found?

7. Can patients on a gluten-free diet tolerate oats?

8. Are there any known health benefits of following a gluten-free diet if a person does not have celiac disease?

9. Can patients with celiac disease also be lactose intolerant?

10. There is a high prevalence of anemia among individuals with celiac disease. How can this be explained? What tests are used for anemia?

III. Nutrition Assessment

11. Calculate this patient's total energy and protein needs.

12. Evaluate Mrs. Talbot's laboratory measures for nutritional significance. Identify all laboratory values that are indicative of a potential nutrition problem.

13. Are the abnormalities identified in question #12 related to the consequences of celiac disease? Explain.

14. Are any symptoms from Mrs. Talbot's physical examination consistent with her laboratory values? Explain.

IV. Nutrition Diagnosis

15. Select two nutrition problems and complete the PES statement for each.

V. Nutrition Intervention

16. For each of the PES statements that you have written, establish an ideal goal (based on the signs and symptoms) and an appropriate intervention (based on the etiology).

17. What type of diet would you initially prescribe, considering the possibility that Mrs. Talbot has suffered intestinal damage?

VI. Nutrition Monitoring and Evaluation

18. Evaluate the following excerpt from Mrs. Talbot's food diary. Identify the foods that might not be tolerated on a gluten-/gliadin-free diet. For each food identified, provide an appropriate substitute.

AM—cornflakes, milk, banana, coffee with half and half

LUNCH—hot dog on bun, French fries, chocolate milk

DINNER—stir-fry chicken nuggets with soy sauce, mixed vegetables on rice; pudding, iced tea

SNACK—gluten-free graham crackers with peanut butter; cookie dough ice cream

19. Mrs. Talbot asks what steps she should take to keep herself from being exposed to gluten in her kitchen since her family does not have celiac disease. What advice would you give her? Are there other potential environmental sources of gluten that you would alert Mrs. Talbot to?

Bibliography

Academy of Nutrition and Dietetics Nutrition Care Manual. https://www.nutritioncaremanual.org/topic.cfm?ncm_toc_id=22684. Accessed 02/21/15.

Guandalini S, Newland C. Differentiating food allergies from food intolerances. *Curr Gastroenterol Rep.* 2011;13:426–434.

Latorre M, Lagana SM, Freedberg DE, et al. Endoscopic biopsy technique in the diagnosis of celiac disease: One bite or two? *Gastrointestinal Endoscopy.* 2015;81:1–6.

Lebwohl B, Ludvigsson J, Green P. Editorial: The unfolding story of Celiac disease risk factors. *Clinical Gastroenterology and Hepatology.* 2014;12:632–634.

Medeiros D, Wildman R. *Advanced Human Nutrition.* 3rd ed. Burlington, MA: Jones & Bartlett Learning; 2015.

Nelms MN, Habash D. Nutrition assessment: Foundation of the nutrition care process. In: Nelms M, Sucher K, Lacey K. *Nutrition Therapy and Pathophysiology.* 3rd ed. Belmont, CA: Cengage Learning; 2016:36–71.

Nelms MN. Diseases of the lower gastrointestinal tract. In: Nelms M, Sucher K, Lacey K. *Nutrition Therapy and Pathophysiology.* 3rd ed. Belmont, CA: Cengage Learning; 2016:379–435.

Pronsky ZM. *Food-Medication Interactions*, 18th ed. Birchrunville, PA: Food-Medication Interactions; 2012.

Riddle MS, Murray JA, Porter CK. The incidence and risk of celiac disease in a healthy US adult population. *Am J Gastroenterol.* 2012;107:1248–1255.

Rubio-Tapia A, Ludvigsson JF, Brantner TL, Murray JA, Everhart JE. The prevalence of celiac disease in the United States. *Am J Gastroenterol.* 2012;107:1538–1544.

Stordal K, Haugen M, Brantsaeter A, Lundin K, Stene L. Association Between Maternal Iron Supplementation During Pregnancy and Risk of Celiac Disease in Children. *Clinical Gastroenterology and Hepatology.* 2014;12(4):624–631.

Tonutti E, Bizzaro N. Diagnosis and classification of celiac disease and gluten sensitivity. *Autoimmunity Reviews.* 2014;13:472–476.

Internet Resources

Celiac Disease Center at Columbia University: http://celiacdiseasecenter.columbia.edu/

Celiac Disease Foundation: http://www.celiac.org/

Celiac Support Association: http://www.csaceliacs.info/celiac_disease.jsp

National Digestive Diseases Information Clearinghouse (NDDIC): http://www.niddk.nih.gov/health-information/health-topics/digestive-diseases/celiac-disease/Pages/ez.aspx

National Library of Medicine/National Institutes of Health Medline Plus: http://www.nlm.nih.gov/medlineplus/celiacdisease.html

University of Chicago Celiac Disease Center: http://www.cureceliacdisease.org/

USDA Nutrient Data Laboratory: http://www.ars.usda.gov/nutrientdata

Case 11

Irritable Bowel Syndrome (IBS)

Objectives

After completing this case, the student will be able to:

1. Describe the proposed etiologies of IBS.
2. Use the current medical diagnostic criteria to identify IBS signs and symptoms found within the patient's history and physical exam.
3. Assess the nutritional status for an individual with IBS.
4. Understand the proposed mechanisms of avoidance of fermentable carbohydrates as a component of FODMAP nutrition therapy.

5. Develop a nutrition care plan—with appropriate measurable goals, interventions, and strategies for monitoring and evaluation—that addresses the nutrition diagnoses for this case.

Alicia Clarke is a 42-year-old female who presents to the gastroenterology clinic with generalized stomach and intestinal complaints.

Clarke, Alicia, Female, 42 y.o.
Allergies: NKA
Pt. Location: Gastroenterology Clinic

Code: FULL
Physician: A. Mohammed MD

Isolation: None
Date: 3/30

Patient Summary: Alicia Clarke is a 42-year-old female who presents to outpatient gastroenterology clinic with stomach and intestinal complaints.

History:

Onset of disease: Patient presents upon referral from her family practice physician after experiencing both diarrhea and constipation for many years. Family physician found negative stool cultures. Colonoscopy negative for active disease.

Medical history: Hypothyroidism, gastroesophageal reflux disease, obesity

Surgical history: Caesarean × 2

Medications at home: Omeprazole 50 mg twice daily; levothyroxine 25 mcg; vitamin D 600 IU; 800 mg calcium; Lomotil prn

Tobacco use: 1 ppd × 10 years—quit at age 30

Alcohol use: 3–4 × per week

Family history: Father—HTN, atherosclerosis; mother, sister—hypothyroidism, type 2 DM

Demographics:

Marital status: Divorced; 2 children—ages 12 and 14

Years education: 16 years

Language: English only

Occupation: Kindergarten teacher

Hours of work: 8–4 weekdays

Household members: Self, two children, and mother. Ex-husband lives in same city and shares custody of children.

Ethnicity: Caucasian

Religious affiliation: Methodist

History/Physical:

Chief complaint: "I am here for a workup of my stomach and intestinal problems. My family doctor did some tests but did not find anything. I have always had a 'funny' stomach, I think. As far back as I can remember, I have had times when I had diarrhea and others when I would go for days without going to the bathroom. The diarrhea is much worse now and I have had several accidents when I didn't make it to the bathroom. This is really interfering with my daily life." Patient describes ongoing abdominal pain almost every day with alternating constipation and diarrhea. She also describes having significant bloating and gas on some days. Diarrhea has been more predominant lately with several episodes per day.

General appearance: Obese, anxious-appearing female

Vital Signs: Temp: 98.6   Pulse: 100   Resp rate: 16
                   BP: 128/72   Height: 5'5"   Weight: 191 lbs

Heart: Regular rate and rhythm

Clarke, Alicia, Female, 42 y.o.
Allergies: NKA   **Code:** FULL   **Isolation:** None
Pt. Location: Gastroenterology Clinic   **Physician:** A. Mohammed MD   **Date:** 3/30

HEENT: Head: WNL
               Eyes: PERRLA
               Ears: Clear
               Nose: Clear
               Throat: Dry mucous membranes without exudates or lesions
Genitalia: Deferred
Neurologic: Alert and oriented × 3
Extremities: WNL
Skin: Warm and dry
Chest/lungs: WNL—clear to auscultation and percussion
Peripheral vascular: Pulse 4 + bilaterally, warm, no edema
Abdomen: Hyperactive bowel sounds × 4; no organomegaly or masses—lower abdominal tenderness

Assessment/Plan:

Patient meets Rome III criteria for IBS. Will begin Elavil 25 mg daily. Initiate Metamucil 1 tbsp in 8 oz of liquid twice daily; Lomotil PRN as needed. Schedule laboratory for hydrogen breath test, anti-tTG. Nutrition consult. Patient return to clinic in four weeks.

.... A. Mohammed, MD

Nutrition:

History: Patient states that her appetite is good even with her abdominal pain and diarrhea. She has steadily gained weight since her pregnancies and in the last 5 years has gained over 20 lbs. She feels that there is not any one food that causes diarrhea more than others. She does notice more gas after eating foods like broccoli or cauliflower. She likes most foods—likes to cook and prepares most meals at home. Patient states that she has been trying to follow a high-fiber diet so that it might help with her gastrointestinal symptoms. Patient also asks if her yogurt intake will provide enough probiotics as she has heard she needs to balance the bacteria in her intestines. She does admit that she isn't quite sure what that means.

AM:	Homemade yogurt smoothie with 1 c fresh fruit (peaches and cherries), 1 8-oz yogurt, or dry cereal with dried fruit, nuts mixed with yogurt; 2–3 c coffee with half and half and artificial sweetener
Mid-morning:	Diet Pepsi, ½ c dried fruit and nuts
Lunch:	Salad with kidney beans or lentils, cheese, tomatoes, carrots, asparagus; wheat crackers—approx. 12–15, Diet Pepsi
PM:	Some type of meat—varies, but mostly chicken; pasta or potatoes, variety of vegetables, some type of bread or roll with butter
Snacks:	Ice cream, cake, or cookies, usually each night but lately has been trying to eat sugar-free candies to help with weight loss. Wine or beer—2–3 times per week.

Clarke, Alicia, Female, 42 y.o.
Allergies: NKA
Pt. Location: Gastroenterology Clinic

Code: FULL
Physician: A. Mohammed MD

Isolation: None
Date: 3/30

FODMAP Assessment

Food	In an average week, how often do you:	Daily or several × per week	Some-times (1×/week)	Rarely (1×/ month)	Never
Meals	1. Eat meals from sit-down or take-out restaurants?		X		
Grains	2. Eat wheat or white breads?	X			
	3. Eat wheat pasta and/or noodles?	X			
	4. Eat wheat-based breakfast cereals?	X			
	5. Eat wheat-based cookies, cakes, and/or crackers?	X			
Fruit	6. Eat apples, pears, guava, honeydew melon, mango, papaya, quince, star fruit, and/or watermelon?		X		
	7. Eat stone fruits such as apricots, peaches, cherries, plums, and/or nectarines?		X		
	8. Eat grapes, persimmons, and/or lychee?		X		
	9. Eat dried fruits?	X			
	10. Drink fruit juice?	X			
Vegetables	11. Eat onion, leeks, asparagus, artichokes, cabbage, Brussels sprouts, and/or green beans?	X			
Dairy	12. Drink milk (whole, 1%, 2%, or skim)?	X			
	13. Drink coconut milk?				X
	14. Eat ice cream, yogurt, and/or cream-based products?		X		
Protein	15. Eat legumes such as baked beans, kidney beans, lentils, black-eyed peas, chickpeas, and/or butter beans?	X			

Clarke, Alicia, Female, 42 y.o.
Allergies: NKA
Pt. Location: Gastroenterology Clinic

Code: FULL
Physician: A. Mohammed MD

Isolation: None
Date: 3/30

FODMAP Assessment *(Continued)*

Food	In an average week, how often do you:	Daily or several × per week	Some-times (1×/week)	Rarely (1×/ month)	Never
Sweets	16. Eat products with high-fructose corn syrup such as fruit drinks, carbonated sugar drinks, pancake syrup, jams, and/or jellies?	X			
	17. Add fructose to your food?				X
	18. Add honey to your food or beverages?	X			
	19. Use foods or medicines with artificial sweeteners such as sorbitol, mannitol, isomalt, and/or xylitol?	X			
Beverages	20. Drink carbonated beverages?	X			
	21. Drink fortified wines such as port wines and/or sherry?				X
	22. Drink chicory-based coffee substitute?				X
Condiments	23. Eat catsup, tomato paste, chutney, pickle relish, plum sauce, sweet and sour sauce, and/or barbecue sauce?		X		

Laboratory Results

	Ref. Range	3/30 0800
Chemistry		
Sodium (mEq/L)	136–145	141
Potassium (mEq/L)	3.5–5.1	3.7
Chloride (mEq/L)	98–107	101
Carbon dioxide (CO_2, mEq/L)	23–29	25
Bicarbonate (mEq/L)	23–28	24
BUN (mg/dL)	6–20	11
Creatinine serum (mg/dL)	0.6–1.1 F 0.9–1.3 M	0.7
BUN/Crea ratio	10.0–20.0	15.7

(Continued)

Clarke, Alicia, Female, 42 y.o.
Allergies: NKA
Pt. Location: Gastroenterology Clinic

Code: FULL
Physician: A. Mohammed MD

Isolation: None
Date: 3/30

Laboratory Results *(Continued)*

	Ref. Range	3/30 0800
Uric acid (mg/dL)	2.8–8.8 F 4.0–9.0 M	4.2
Est GFR, non-Afr Amer (mL/min/1.73 m^2)	>60	124
Glucose (mg/dL)	70–99	115 !↑
Phosphate, inorganic (mg/dL)	2.2–4.6	3.1
Magnesium (mg/dL)	1.5–2.4	1.8
Calcium (mg/dL)	8.6–10.2	10.1
Osmolality (mmol/kg/H$_2$O)	275–295	292
Bilirubin total (mg/dL)	≤1.2	0.2
Bilirubin, direct (mg/dL)	<0.3	0.1
Protein, total (g/dL)	6–7.8	6.2
Albumin (g/dL)	3.5–5.5	4.1
Prealbumin (mg/dL)	18–35	22
Ammonia (NH$_3$, µg/L)	6–47	11
Alkaline phosphatase (U/L)	30–120	35
ALT (U/L)	4–36	6
AST (U/L)	0–35	1
CPK (U/L)	30–135 F 55–170 M	114
Lactate dehydrogenase (U/L)	208–378	271
Cholesterol (mg/dL)	<200	201 !↑
HDL-C (mg/dL)	>59 F, >50 M	42 !↓
VLDL (mg/dL)	7–32	36
LDL (mg/dL)	<130	122
LDL/HDL ratio	<3.22 F <3.55 M	2.90
Triglycerides (mg/dL)	35–135 F 40–160 M	181 !↑
T$_4$ (µg/dL)	5–12	6
T$_3$ (µg/dL)	75–98	79
HbA$_{1C}$ (%)	<5.7	6.1 !↑
Hematology		
WBC (× 10^3/mm^3)	3.9–10.7	5.5

Clarke, Alicia, Female, 42 y.o.
Allergies: NKA
Pt. Location: Gastroenterology Clinic

Code: FULL
Physician: A. Mohammed MD

Isolation: None
Date: 3/30

Laboratory Results (Continued)

	Ref. Range	3/30 0800
RBC ($\times 10^6$/mm^3)	4.2–5.4 F 4.5–6.2 M	5.1
Hemoglobin (Hgb, g/dL)	12–16 F 14–17 M	12.1
Hematocrit (Hct, %)	37–47 F 41–51 M	37
Urinalysis		
Collection method	—	Clean catch
Color	—	Yellow
Appearance	—	Clear
Specific gravity	1.001–1.035	1.004
pH	5–7	5.1
Protein (mg/dL)	Neg	Neg
Glucose (mg/dL)	Neg	Neg
Ketones	Neg	Neg
Blood	Neg	Neg
Bilirubin	Neg	Neg
Nitrites	Neg	Neg
Urobilinogen (EU/dL)	<1.0	Neg
Leukocyte esterase	Neg	Neg
Prot chk	Neg	Neg
WBCs (/HPF)	0–5	0
RBCs (/HPF)	0–2	0
Bact	0	0
Mucus	0	0
Crys	0	0
Casts (/LPF)	0	0
Yeast	0	0

Note: Values and units of measurement listed in these tables are derived from several resources. Substantial variation exists in the ranges quoted as "normal" and these may vary depending on the assay used by different laboratories.

Case Questions

I.   Understanding the Diagnosis and Pathophysiology

1. IBS is considered to be a functional disorder. What does this mean? How does this relate to Mrs. Clarke's history of having a colonoscopy and her physician's order for a hydrogen breath test and measurements of anti-tTG?

2. What are the Rome III criteria that were used as part of Dr. Mohammed's diagnosis? Using the information from Mrs. Clarke's history and physical, determine how Dr. Mohammed made his diagnosis of IBS.

3. Discuss the primary factors that may be involved in IBS etiology. You must include in your discussion the possible roles of genetics, infection, and serotonin.

4. Mrs. Clarke's physician prescribed two medications for her IBS. What are they and what is the proposed mechanism of each? She discusses the potential use of Lotronex if these medications do not help. What is this medication and what is its mechanism? Identify any potential drug–nutrient interactions for these medications.

II.   Understanding the Nutrition Therapy

5. For each of the following foods, outline the possible effect on IBS symptoms.

   a. lactose

   b. fructose

   c. sugar alcohols

6. What is FODMAP? What does the current literature tell us about this intervention?

7. Define the terms *prebiotic* and *probiotic*. What does the current research indicate regarding their use for treatment of IBS? What guidance would you give Mrs. Clarke for choosing a probiotic?

III.   Nutrition Assessment

8.   Assess Mrs. Clarke's weight and BMI. What is her desirable weight?

9.   Identify any abnormal laboratory values measured at this clinic visit and explain their significance for the patient with IBS.

10.   List Mrs. Clarke's other medications and identify the rationale for each prescription.

11.   Determine Mrs. Clarke's energy and protein requirements. Be sure to explain what standards you used to make this estimation.

12.   Assess Mrs. Clarke's recent diet history. How does this compare to her estimated energy and protein needs? Identify foods that may potentially aggravate her IBS symptoms.

IV.   Nutrition Diagnosis

13.   Prioritize two nutrition problems and complete the PES statement for each.

V.   Nutrition Intervention

14.   The RD that counsels Mrs. Clarke discusses the use of an elimination diet. How may this be used to treat Mrs. Clarke's IBS?

15.   The RD discusses the use of the FODMAP assessment to identify potential trigger foods. Describe the use of this approach for Mrs. Clarke. How might a food diary help her determine which foods she should avoid?

16.   Mrs. Clarke is interested in trying other types of treatment for IBS including acupuncture, herbal supplements, and hypnotherapy. What would you tell her about the use of each of these in IBS? What is the role of the RD in discussing complementary and alternative therapies?

VI.   Nutrition Monitoring and Evaluation

17.   Write an ADIME note for your initial nutrition assessment with your plans for education and follow-up.

Bibliography

Academy of Nutrition and Dietetics Nutrition Care Manual. Irritable Bowel Syndrome. https://www .nutritioncaremanual.org/topic.cfm?ncm_cat egory_id=1&lv1=5522&lv2=145209&ncm_toc _id=19589&ncm_heading=Nutrition%20Care. Accessed 3/30/15.

Barrett JS, Gibson PR. Development and validation of a comprehensive semi-quantitative food frequency questionnaire that includes FODMAP and glycemic index. *J Am Diet Assoc.* 2010;110:1469–1470.

Barrett JS, Gibson PR. Fermentable oligosaccharides, disaccharides, monosaccharides and polyols (FOD-MAPs) and nonallergic food intolerance: FOD-MAPs or food chemicals? *Therap Adv Gastroenterol.* 2012;5:261–268.

Brenner DM, Moeller MJ, Chey WD, Schoenfield PS. The utility of probiotics in the treatment of irritable bowel syndrome: A systematic review. *Am J Gastroenterol.* 2009;104:1033–1049.

Camilleri M. Pharmacology of the new treatments for lower gastrointestinal motility disorders and irritable bowel syndrome. *Nature.* 2012;91:44–59.

Camilleri M, Lasch K, Zhou W. Irritable bowel syndrome; methods, mechanisms, and pathophysiology: the confluence of increased permeability, inflammation, and pain is irritable bowel syndrome. *Am J Physiol Gastrointest Liver Physiol.* 2012;303:G775–G785.

Chey WD, Eswaran S, Kurlander J. JAMA patient page. Irritable bowel syndrome. *JAMA.* 2015;313:982.

Clarke G, Cryan JF, Dinan TG, Quigley EM. Review article: Probiotics for the treatment of irritable bowel syndrome: Focus on lactic acid bacteria. *Aliment Pharmacol Ther.* 2012;35:403–413.

Crowell MD. Role of serotonin in the pathophysiology of the irritable bowel syndrome. *Br J Pharmacol.* 2004;141(8):1285–1293.

Douglas LC, Sanders ME. Probiotics and prebiotics in dietetics practice. *J Am Diet Assoc.* 2008;108:510–521.

El-Salhy M, Ostgaard H, Gundersen D, Hatlebakk JG, Hausen T. The role of diet in the pathogenesis and management of irritable bowel syndrome (Review). *Int J Mol Med.* 2012;29:723–731.

Ford AC, Moayyedi P, Lacy BE, et al. American College of Gastroenterology monograph on the management of irritable bowel syndrome and chronic idiopathic constipation. *Am J Gastroenterol.* 2014;109 Suppl 1:S2–S26.

Ford AC, Quigley EM, Lacy BE, et al. Efficacy of prebiotics, probiotics, and synbiotics in irritable bowel syndrome and chronic idiopathic constipation: Systematic review and meta-analysis. *Am J Gastroenterol.* 2014;109(10):1547–1561.

Gibson PR, Shepherd SJ. Food choice as a key management strategy for functional gastrointestinal symptoms. *Am J Gastroenterol.* 2012;107:657–666.

Gibson PR, Varney J, Malakar S, Muir JG. Food components and irritable bowel syndrome. *Gastroenterol.* 2015;Feb 10. Date of Electronic Publication: 2015 Feb 10.

Halmos EP, Christophersen CT, Bird AR, et al. Diets that differ in their FODMAP content alter the colonic luminal microenvironment. *Gut.* 2015;64:93–100.

Halmos EP, Power VA, Shepherd SG, et al. A diet low in FODMAPs reduces symptoms of irritable bowel syndrome. *Gastroenterology.* 2014;146:67–75.

Hungin AP, Molloy-Bland M, Claes R, et al. Systematic review: The perceptions, diagnosis and management of irritable bowel syndrome in primary care—a Rome Foundation working team report. *Aliment Pharmacol Ther.* 2014;40(10):1133–1145.

Khan M, Nawras A, Bielefeldt K. Low FODMAP diet for irritable bowel syndrome: Is it ready for prime time? *Dig Dis Sci.* 2014;Nov 20. Date of Electronic Publication: 2014 Nov 20.

Lacy BE. The science, evidence and practice of dietary interventions in irritable bowel syndrome. *Clin Gastroenter Hep.* 2015;Mar 10. pii: S1542-3565(15)00248-7. doi: 10.1016/j.cgh.2015.02.043. [Epub ahead of print]

Lim B, Manheimer E, Lao L, et al. Acupuncture for treatment of irritable bowel syndrome. *Cochrane Database Syst Rev.* 2006;(4):CD005111.

Liu JP, Yang M, Liu YX, Wei ML, Grimsgaard S. Herbal medicines for treatment of irritable bowel syndrome. *Cochrane Database Syst Rev.* 2006;(4):CD005111.

Lorenzo-Zúñiga V, Llop E, Suárez C, et al. I.31, a new combination of probiotics, improves irritable bowel syndrome-related quality of life. *World J Gastroenterol.* 2014;20:8709–8716.

Mansueto P, Seidita A, D'Alcamo A, Carroccio A. Role of FODMAPs in patients with irritable bowel syndrome: A review. *Nutr Clin Pract.* Published online before print February 18, 2015, doi: 10.1177/0884533615569886.

Nahikian-Nelms M. Diseases of the lower gastrointestinal tract. In: Nelms M, Sucher K, Lacey K. *Nutrition Therapy and Pathophysiology.* 3rd ed. Belmont, CA: Cengage Learning; 2016:376–436.

Ong DK, Mitchell SB, Barrett JS, et al. Manipulation of dietary short chain carbohydrates alters the pattern of gas production and genesis of symptoms in irritable bowel syndrome. *J Gastroenterology and Hepatology.* 2010;25:1366–1373.

Ruepert L, Quartero AO, de Wit NJ, van der Heijden GJ, Muris JW. Bulking agents, antispasmodics and antidepressants for the treatment of irritable bowel syndrome. *Cochrane Database Syst Rev.* 2011;10:CD0003460.

Quigley EM, Abdel-Hamid H, Barbara G, et al. A global perspective on irritable bowel syndrome. A consensus statement of the World Gastroenterology Organisation Summit Task Force on irritable bowel syndrome. *J Clin Gastroenterol.* 2012;46:356–366.

Scarlata K. Successful low-FODMAP living: Experts discuss meal-planning strategies to help IBS clients better control GI distress. *Today's Dietitian.* 2012;14:36–38.

Shepherd SJ, Halmos E, Glance S. The role of FODMAPs in irritable bowel syndrome. *Curr Opin Clin Nutr Metab Care.* 2014;17:605–609.

Simren M. Diet as therapy for irritable bowel syndrome: Progress at last. *Gastroenterology.* 2014;146:10–12.

Staudacher HM, Irving PM, Lomer MC, Whelan K. Mechanisms and efficacy of dietary FODMAP restriction in IBS. *Nat Rev Gastroenterol Hepatol.* 2014;11:256–266.

Tuck CJ, Muir JG, Barrett JS, Gibson PR. Fermentable oligosaccharides, disaccharides, monosaccharides and polyols: Role in irritable bowel syndrome. *Expert Rev Gastroenterol Hepatol.* 2014;8(7):819–834.

Yoon JS, Sohn W, Lee OY, et al. Effect of multispecies probiotics on irritable bowel syndrome: A randomized, double-blind, placebo-controlled trial. *J Gastroenterol Hepatol.* 2014;29:52–59.

Webb AN, Kukuruzovic RH, Catto-Smith AG, Sawyer SM. Hypnotherapy for treatment of irritable bowel syndrome. *Cochrane Database Syst Rev.* 2006;(1):CD004116.

Internet Resources

AND Evidence Analysis Library: http://www.andeal.org

DrugBank: http://www.drugbank.ca/

Shepherd Works: Low FODMAP Diet: http://shepherd works.com.au/disease-information/low-fodmap-diet

International Foundation for Functional Gastrointestinal Disorders: http://www.aboutibs.org/

Lotronex: https://www.lotronex.com/

MedicineNet: http://www.medicinenet.com

Nutrition Care Manual: http://www.nutritioncaremanual .org

Rome Foundation: http://www.romecriteria.org/criteria/

WebMD: http://www.webmd.com/ibs /alternative-therapies

Inflammatory Bowel Disease: Crohn's Disease

Objectives

After completing this case, the student will be able to:

1. Apply knowledge of the pathophysiology of Crohn's disease to identify and explain common nutritional problems associated with this disease.
   a. Describe physiological changes resulting from Crohn's disease.
   b. Identify nutritional consequences of Crohn's disease.
   c. Identify nutritional consequences of surgical resection of the small intestine.
2. Describe current medical care for Crohn's disease.
3. Identify potential drug–nutrient interactions.
4. Analyze nutrition assessment data to evaluate nutritional status and identify specific nutrition problems.
5. Determine nutrition diagnoses and write appropriate PES statements.
6. Calculate parenteral nutrition formulations.
7. Evaluate a parenteral nutrition regimen.
8. Develop a nutrition care plan—with appropriate measurable goals, interventions, and strategies for monitoring and evaluation—that addresses the nutrition diagnoses of this case.

Mike Page was diagnosed with Crohn's disease 2½ years ago. He is now admitted with an acute exacerbation of that disease.

Page, Mike, Male, 35 y.o.
Allergies: Peanuts
Pt. Location: RM 1952

Code: FULL
Physician: D Tucker

Isolation: None
Admit Date: 12/15

Patient Summary: Mike Page was hospitalized this past September with an abscess and acute exacerbation of Crohn's disease.

History:

Onset of disease: Dx Crohn's disease 2½ years ago
Medical history: Initial diagnostic workup indicated acute disease within last 5–7 cm of jejunum and first 5 cm of ileum. Regimens have included corticosteroids, mesalamine. Plans are to initiate Humira.
Surgical history: No surgeries
Medications at home: 6-mercaptopurine
Tobacco use: No
Alcohol use: No
Family history: Noncontributory

Demographics:

Marital status: Married—lives with wife, Mary and son, age 5; both are well.
Years education: Bachelor's degree
Language: English only
Occupation: High school math teacher
Hours of work: 8–4:30, some after-school meetings and responsibilities as advisor for school clubs
Ethnicity: Caucasian
Religious affiliation: Episcopalian

Admitting History/Physical:

Chief complaint: "I was diagnosed with inflammatory bowel disease almost 3 years ago. At first they thought I had ulcerative colitis but six months later it was identified as Crohn's disease. I was really sick at that time and was in the hospital for more than two weeks. I have done OK until school started this fall. I've noticed more diarrhea and abdominal pain, but I tried to keep going since school just started. I was here in September and we switched medicine. I was a little better and I went back to work. Now my abdominal pain is unbearable—I seem to have diarrhea constantly, and now I am running a fever."
General appearance: Thin, 35-year-old white male in apparent distress

Vital Signs: Temp: 101.5°F   Pulse: 81   Resp rate: 18
                    BP: 125/82   Height: 5'9"   Weight: 140 lbs

Heart: RRR without murmurs or gallops
HEENT: Eyes: PERRLA, normal fundi
          Ears: Noncontributory

Page, Mike, Male, 35 y.o.
Allergies: Peanuts
Pt. Location: RM 1952

Code: FULL
Physician: D Tucker

Isolation: None
Admit Date: 12/15

Nose: Noncontributory
Throat: Pharynx clear
Rectal: No evidence of perianal disease
Neurologic: Oriented × 4
Extremities: No edema; pulses full; no bruits; normal strength, sensation, and DT
Skin: Warm, dry
Chest/lungs: Lungs clear to auscultation and percussion
Peripheral vascular: WNL
Abdomen: Distension, extreme tenderness with rebound and guarding; minimal bowel sounds

Nursing Assessment	12/15
Abdominal appearance (concave, flat, rounded, obese, distended)	rounded
Palpation of abdomen (soft, rigid, firm, masses, tense)	soft
Bowel function (continent, incontinent, flatulence, no stool)	continent
Bowel sounds (P=present, AB=absent, hypo, hyper)	
RUQ	P
LUQ	P
RLQ	P
LLQ	P
Stool color	light brown
Stool consistency	soft to liquid
Tubes/ostomies	N/A
Genitourinary	
Urinary continence	catheter
Urine source	catheter
Appearance (clear, cloudy, yellow, amber, fluorescent, hematuria, orange, blue, tea)	clear, yellow
Integumentary	
Skin color	pale
Skin temperature (DI=diaphoretic, W=warm, dry, CL=cool, CLM=clammy, CD+=cold, M=moist, H=hot)	W
Skin turgor (good, fair, poor, TENT=tenting)	good
Skin condition (intact, EC=ecchymosis, A=abrasions, P=petechiae, R=rash, W=weeping, S=sloughing, D=dryness, EX=excoriated, T=tears, SE=subcutaneous emphysema, B=blisters, V=vesicles, N=necrosis)	intact

(Continued)

Page, Mike, Male, 35 y.o.
Allergies: Peanuts
Pt. Location: RM 1952

Code: FULL
Physician: D Tucker

Isolation: None
Admit Date: 12/15

Nursing Assessment *(Continued)*

Nursing Assessment	12/15
Mucous membranes (intact, EC=ecchymosis, A=abrasions, P=petechiae, R=rash, W=weeping, S=sloughing, D=dryness, EX=excoriated, T=tears, SE=subcutaneous emphysema, B=blisters, V=vesicles, N=necrosis)	intact
Other components of Braden score: special bed, sensory pressure, moisture, activity, friction/shear (>18=no risk, 15–16=low risk, 13–14=moderate risk, ≤12=high risk)	activity, 17

Orders:
R/O acute exacerbation of Crohn's disease vs. infection vs. small bowel obstruction.
CBC/Chem 24
ASCA
CT scan of abdomen and possible esophagogastroduodenoscopy
D5W NS @ 75 cc/hr;
Clear liquids
Surgical consult
Nutrition support consult

Nutrition:
General: Patient states he has been eating fairly normally for the last year. After hospitalization at initial diagnosis, he had lost almost 25 lbs, which he regained. He initially ate a low-fiber diet and worked hard to regain the weight he had lost. He drank Boost between meals for several months. His usual weight before his illness was 166–168 lbs. He was at his highest weight (168 lbs) about 6 months ago but now states he has lost most of what he regained and has even lost more since his last hospitalization when he was at 144 lbs.

Recent dietary intake:

AM:	Cereal, small amount of skim milk, toast or bagel; juice
AM snack:	Cola—sometimes crackers or pastry
Lunch:	Sandwich (ham or turkey) from home, fruit, chips, cola
Dinner:	Meat, pasta or rice, some type of bread; rarely eats vegetables
Bedtime snack:	Cheese and crackers, cookies, cola

24-hr recall: Clear liquids for past 24 hours since admission

Food allergies/intolerances/aversions: peanuts

Previous nutrition therapy? Yes. If yes, when: Last hospitalization.

Page, Mike, Male, 35 y.o.
Allergies: Peanuts
Pt. Location: RM 1952

Code: FULL
Physician: D Tucker

Isolation: None
Admit Date: 12/15

What? "The dietitian talked to me about ways to decrease my diarrhea—ways to keep from being dehydrated—and then we worked out a plan to help me regain weight. I know what to do—it is just that the pain and diarrhea make my appetite so bad. It is really hard for me to eat."
Food purchase/preparation: Self and spouse
Vit/min intake: Multivitamin daily

Intake/Output

Weight: 67.8 kg

Date		12/20 0701 – 12/21 0700			
Time		0701–1500	1501–2300	2301–0700	Daily total
IN	P.O.	**NPO**	**NPO**	**NPO**	
	I.V.	**600**	**600**	**600**	**1800**
	(mL/kg/hr)	(1.1)	(1.1)	(1.1)	(1.1)
	I.V. piggyback				
	TPN	**400**	**600**	**600**	**1600**
	Total intake	**1000**	**1200**	**1200**	**3400**
	(mL/kg)	(14.7)	(17.6)	(17.6)	(50.1)
OUT	Urine	**700**	**970**	**820**	**2490**
	(mL/kg/hr)	(1.29)	(1.79)	(1.51)	(1.53)
	Emesis output				
	Other				
	Stool				
	Total output	**700**	**970**	**820**	**2490**
	(mL/kg)	(10.3)	(14.3)	(12.1)	(36.7)
Net I/O		**+300**	**+230**	**+380**	**+910**
Net since admission (12/15)		**+2643**	**+2873**	**+3253**	**+3253**

Page, Mike, Male, 35 y.o.
Allergies: Peanuts
Pt. Location: RM 1952

Code: FULL
Physician: D Tucker

Isolation: None
Admit Date: 12/15

Laboratory Results

	Ref. Range	12/15 1522	12/19 0600	12/20 0600
Chemistry				
Sodium (mEq/L)	136–145	136	141	142
Potassium (mEq/L)	3.5–5.1	3.7	3.9	4.5
Chloride (mEq/L)	98–107	101	102	105
Carbon dioxide (CO_2, mEq/L)	23–29	26	24	27
Bicarbonate (mEq/L)	23–28	25	24	27
BUN (mg/dL)	6–20	17	18	16
Creatinine serum (mg/dL)	0.6–1.1 F 0.9–1.3 M	1.1	0.9	1.0
BUN/Crea ratio	10.0–20.0	15.45	20	16
Uric acid (mg/dL)	2.8–8.8 F 4.0–9.0 M	4.2		
Est GFR, non-Afr Amer (mL/min/1.73 m2)	>60	76	109	96
Glucose (mg/dL)	70–99	74	141 !↑	172 !↑
Phosphate, inorganic (mg/dL)	2.2–4.6	2.5	2.4	3.1
Magnesium (mg/dL)	1.5–2.4	1.8	1.9	1.8
Calcium (mg/dL)	8.6–10.2	9.1	9.2	9.7
Osmolality (mmol/kg/H_2O)	275–295	285	296 !↑	299 !↑
Bilirubin total (mg/dL)	≤1.2	0.3	0.4	0.3
Bilirubin, direct (mg/dL)	<0.3	0.2	0.25	0.29
Protein, total (g/dL)	6–7.8	6.1	6.7	7.1
Albumin (g/dL)	3.5–5.5	3.2 !↓	3.3 !↓	3.4 !↓
Prealbumin (mg/dL)	18–35	16 !↓	15 !↓	17 !↓
Ammonia (NH_3, µg/L)	6–47	7	11	18
Alkaline phosphatase (U/L)	30–120	119	85	110
ALT (U/L)	4–36	21	25	37 !↑
AST (U/L)	0–35	22	26	39 !↑
CPK (U/L)	30–135 F 55–170 M	161	152	145
C-reactive protein (mg/dL)	<1.0	22 !↑	35 !↑	15 !↑
Lactate dehydrogenase (U/L)	208–378	315	275	272
Cholesterol (mg/dL)	<200	149		
HDL-C (mg/dL)	>59 F, >50 M	38 !↓		
VLDL (mg/dL)	7–32	12		

Page, Mike, Male, 35 y.o.
Allergies: Peanuts
Pt. Location: RM 1952

Code: FULL
Physician: D Tucker

Isolation: None
Admit Date: 12/15

Laboratory Results *(Continued)*

	Ref. Range	12/15 1522	12/19 0600	12/20 0600
LDL (mg/dL)	<130	98		
LDL/HDL ratio	<3.22 F <3.55 M	2.57		
Triglycerides (mg/dL)	35–135 F 40–160 M	62		
Coagulation (Coag)				
PT (sec)	11–13	11.5	11.9	12.4
PTT (sec)	24–34	26	27	31
Hematology				
WBC (× 10³/mm³)	3.9–10.7	11.1 !↑	10.5	9.5
RBC (× 10⁶/mm³)	4.2–5.4 F 4.5–6.2 M	6.1		
Hemoglobin (Hgb, g/dL)	12–16 F 14–17 M	12.9 !↓		
Hematocrit (Hct, %)	37–47 F 41–51 M	38 !↓		
Mean cell volume (μm³)	80–96	71 !↓		
Mean cell Hgb (pg)	28–32	26 !↓		
Mean cell Hgb content (g/dL)	32–36	29 !↓		
RBC distribution (%)	11.6–16.5	16.9 !↑		
Platelet count (× 10³/mm³)	150–350	278		
Ferritin (ng/mL)	20–120 F 20–300 M	17 !↓		
Iron (μg/dL)	65–165 F 75–175 M	62 !↓		
Vitamin B₁₂ (ng/dL)	24.4–100	32		
Folate (ng/dL)	5–25	23		
Zinc, serum (μg/mL)	0.60–1.2	0.64		
Vitamin D, 25 hydroxy (ng/mL)	30–100	22.7 !↓		
Free retinol (vitamin A; μg/dL)	20–80	17.2 !↓		
Ascorbic acid (mg/dL)	0.2–2.0	<0.1 !↓		
Selenium (ng/mL)	70–150	123		

Note: Values and units of measurement listed in these tables are derived from several resources. Substantial variation exists in the ranges quoted as "normal" and these may vary depending on the assay used by different laboratories.

Case Questions

I.   Understanding the Disease and Pathophysiology

1. What is inflammatory bowel disease? What does current medical literature indicate regarding its etiology?

2. Mr. Page was initially diagnosed with ulcerative colitis and then diagnosed with Crohn's. How could this happen? What are the similarities and differences between Crohn's disease and ulcerative colitis?

3. What did you find in Mr. Page's history and physical that is consistent with his diagnosis of Crohn's? Explain.

4. Crohn's patients often have extraintestinal symptoms of the disease. What are some examples of these symptoms? Is there evidence of these in his history and physical?

5. Mr. Page has been treated previously with corticosteroids and mesalamine. His physician had planned to start Humira prior to this admission. Explain the mechanism for each of these medications in the treatment of Crohn's. Identify any drug–nutrient interactions for each.

6. What laboratory values are consistent with an exacerbation of his Crohn's disease? Identify and explain these values.

7. Is Mr. Page a likely candidate for short bowel syndrome? Define *short bowel syndrome*, and provide a rationale for your answer.

8. What type of adaptation can the small intestine make after surgical resection?

II.   Understanding the Nutrition Therapy

9.   Mr. Page underwent resection of 200 cm of jejunum and proximal ileum. The ileocecal valve was preserved. Mr. Page did not have an ileostomy, and his entire colon remains intact. How long is the small intestine, and how significant is this resection?

10.   What nutrients are normally digested and absorbed in the portion of the small intestine that has been resected?

11.   Are there nutrition recommendations that could impact the inflammatory mechanisms of Mr. Page's disease process? If so, what are they? How might these recommendations be different from those aimed at controlling symptoms of his Crohn's disease such as diarrhea, gas, or abdominal pain?

III.   Nutrition Assessment

12.   Evaluate Mr. Page's %UBW and BMI.

13.   Calculate Mr. Page's energy and protein requirements.

14.   Identify any significant and/or abnormal laboratory measurements from both his hematology and his chemistry labs. Explain possible mechanisms for the abnormal labs.

IV.   Nutrition Diagnosis

15.   Select two nutrition problems and complete the PES statement for each.

V.   Nutrition Intervention

16.   The surgeon notes Mr. Page probably will not resume eating by mouth for at least 7–10 days. Using ASPEN guidelines, what would be the recommendation for nutrition support for Mr. Page?

17. The members of the nutrition support team note his serum phosphorus and serum magnesium are at the low end of the normal range. Why might that be of concern?

18. What is refeeding syndrome? Is Mr. Page at risk for this syndrome? How can it be prevented?

19. Mr. Page was placed on parenteral nutrition support immediately postoperatively, and a nutrition support consult was ordered. Initially, he was prescribed to receive 200 g dextrose/L, 42.5 g amino acids/L, and 30 g lipid/L. His parenteral nutrition was initiated at 50 cc/hr with a goal rate of 85 cc/hr. Do you agree with the team's decision to initiate parenteral nutrition? Will this meet his estimated nutritional needs? Explain. Calculate: pro (g); CHO (g); lipid (g); and total kcal from his PN.

20. For each of the PES statements you have written, establish an ideal goal (based on the signs and symptoms) and an appropriate intervention (based on the etiology).

VI. Nutrition Monitoring and Evaluation

21. Would you make any changes to his prescribed nutrition support? What should be monitored to ensure adequacy of his nutrition support? Explain. What recommendations would you make to transition to enteral feeding?

22. What should the nutrition support team monitor daily while on PN? What should be monitored weekly? Explain your answers.

23. Mr. Page's serum glucose increased to 172 mg/dL. Why do you think this level is now abnormal? What should be done about it?

24. Evaluate the following 24-hour urine data: 24-hour urinary nitrogen for 12/20: 18.4 grams. By using the daily input/output record for 12/20 that records the amount of PN received, calculate Mr. Page's nitrogen balance on 12/20. How would you interpret this information? Should you be concerned? Are there problems with the accuracy of nitrogen balance studies? Explain.

25. On post-op day 7 (12/22), Mr. Page's team notes he has had bowel sounds for the previous 48 hours and had his first bowel movement. The nutrition support team recommends consideration of an oral diet. What should Mr. Page be allowed to try first? What would you monitor for tolerance? If successful, when can the parenteral nutrition be weaned?

26. What would be the primary nutrition concerns as Mr. Page prepares for rehabilitation after his discharge? Be sure to address his need for supplementation of any vitamins and minerals. Identify two nutritional outcomes with specific measures for evaluation.

Bibliography

Academy of Nutrition and Dietetics. Nutrition Care Manual. Inflammatory Bowel Disease. https://www.nutritioncaremanual.org/topic.cfm?ncm_toc_id=19449. Accessed February 14, 2015.

Donnellan CF, Yann LH, Lal S. Nutritional management of Crohn's disease. *Ther Adv Gastroenterol.* 2013;6:231–242.

Grunbaum A, Holcroft C, Heilpern D, et al. Dynamics of vitamin D in patients with mild or inactive inflammatory bowel disease and their families. *Nutr Journal.* 2013;12:145–168.

Jensen GL, Mirtallo J, Compher C, et al. Adult starvation and disease related malnutrition: A proposal for etiology-based diagnosis in the clinical practice setting from the International Consensus Guideline Committee. *Clinical Nutrition.* 2010;29:151–153.

Ko J, Auyeung K. Inflammatory Bowel Disease: Etiology, Pathogenesis and Current Therapy. *Current Pharmaceutical Design.* 2014;20:1082–1096.

Lashner BA. Crohn's Disease. The Cleveland Clinic Disease Management Project. Published January 2013. http://www.clevelandclinicmeded.com/medicalpubs/diseasemanagement/gastroenterology/crohns-disease/. Accessed 02/15/15.

Lee D, Albenberg L, Compher C, Baldassano R, Piccoli D, Lewis JD, Wu GD. Diet in the Pathogenesis and Treatment of Inflammatory Bowel Diseases. *Gastroenterology.* 2015. http://dx.doi.org/10.1053/j.gastro.2015.01.007.

Lee J, Allen R, Ashley S, et al. British Dietetic Association evidence-based guidelines for the dietary management of Crohn's disease in adults. *J Hum Nutr Diet.* 2014;27:207–218.

Massironi S, Rossi RE, Cavalcoli FA, et al. Nutrition deficiencies in inflammatory bowel disease: Therapeutic approaches. *Clin Nutr.* 2013;32:904–910.

Nelms MN. Diseases of the lower gastrointestinal tract. In: Nelms M, Sucher K, Lacey K. *Nutrition Therapy and Pathophysiology.* 3rd ed. Belmont, CA: Cengage Learning; 2016:379–435.

Nelms MN. Enteral and parenteral nutrition support. In: Nelms M, Sucher K, Lacey K. *Nutrition Therapy and Pathophysiology.* 3rd ed. Belmont, CA: Cengage Learning; 2016:88–114.

Nelms MN, Habash D. Nutrition assessment: Foundations of the nutrition care process. In: Nelms M, Sucher K, Lacey K. *Nutrition Therapy and Pathophysiology.* 3rd ed. Belmont, CA: Cengage Learning; 2016:36–71.

Nelms MN. Metabolic stress and the critically ill. In: Nelms M, Sucher K, Lacey K. *Nutrition Therapy and Pathophysiology.* 3rd ed. Belmont, CA: Cengage Learning; 2016:665–685.

Neuman MG, Nanau RM. Inflammatory bowel disease: Role of diet, microbiota, lifestyle. *Trans Res.* 2012;160:29–44.

Nguyen DL, Parekh N, Bechtold ML, Jamal MM. National Trends and In-Hospital Outcomes of Adult Patients With Inflammatory Bowel Disease Receiving Parenteral Nutrition Support. *J Parenter Enteral Nutr.* Published online before print March 31, 2014, doi: 10.1177/0148607114528715. Accessed 03/01/15.

Olendzki BS, Silberstein TD, Persuitte Gm, et al. An anti-inflammatory diet for inflammatory bowel disease: A case series report. *Nutrition Journal.* 2014;13:5–20.

Richman E, Rhodes JM. Review article: Evidence-based dietary advice for patients with inflammatory bowel disease. *Aliment Pharmacol Ther.* 2013;38:1156–1171.

Rowe W, Lichtenstein G. Inflammatory Bowel Disease, Medscape. Updated: Jan 7, 2015. http://emedicine.medscape.com/article/179037-overview#aw2aab6b2b3. Date Accessed 2/10/15.

Semrad CE. Use of parenteral nutrition in patients with inflammatory bowel disease. *Gastroenterol Hepatol.* 2012;8:393–395.

Viladomiu M, Hontecillas R, Yuan L, et al. Nutritional protective mechanisms against gut inflammation. *J Nutr Biochem.* 2013;24:929–939.

Wall R, Ross RP, Fitzgerald GF, Stanton C. Fatty acids from fish: The anti-inflammatory potential of long chain omega-3-fatty acids. *Nutr Rev.* 2012;68:280–289.

White JV, Guenter P, Jensen G, et al. Consensus statement: Academy of Nutrition and Dietetics and American Society for Parenteral and Enteral Nutrition: Characteristics recommended for the identification and documentation of adult malnutrition (undernutrition). *J Parenter Enteral Nutr.* 2012;36:275–283.

Internet Resources

Academy of Nutrition and Dietetics Nutrition Care Manual: http://www.nutritioncaremanual.org

Crohn's & Colitis Foundation of America: http://www.ccfa.org

Mayo Clinic: http://www.mayoclinic.org/diseases-conditions/crohns-disease/basics/definition/con-20032061

National Digestive Diseases Information Clearinghouse (NDDIC): http://www.niddk.nih.gov/health-information/health-topics/digestive-diseases/crohns-disease/Pages/ez.aspx

Case 13

Gastrointestinal Surgery with Ostomy

Objectives

After completing this case, the student will be able to:

1. Describe common postoperative nutrition care concerns and the rationale for postoperative nutritional support.
2. Describe the types of ostomies that may result from gastrointestinal surgery.
3. Explain the nutritional management of the patient with an ostomy.
4. Analyze nutrition assessment data to evaluate nutritional status and identify specific nutrition problems.
5. Determine nutrition diagnoses and write appropriate PES statements.
6. Develop a nutrition care plan—with appropriate measurable goals, interventions, and strategies for monitoring and evaluation—that addresses the nutrition diagnoses of this case.

Betty Watson was admitted through the ED for emergency gastrointestinal surgery secondary to acute obstruction of her colon.

Watson, Betty, Female, 61 y.o.
Allergies: Shellfish, Penicillin
Pt. Location: RM 2252

Code: FULL
Physician: D. Ellison

Isolation: None
Admit Date: 11/2

Patient Summary: 61-year-old female presented to ED with severe abdominal pain. After examination with subsequent testing, an acute bowel obstruction due to the presence of mass in the ascending colon was diagnosed. She was prepped and went emergently to surgery, where she underwent a partial colectomy with colostomy.

History:
Onset of disease: Dx acute bowel obstruction secondary to mass in ascending colon.
Medical history: Type 2 diabetes; hypertension, osteoarthritis
Surgical history: s/p appendectomy age 17; s/p R knee replacement 5 years ago
Medications at home: Metformin 500 mg twice daily, hydrochlorothiazide 25 mg once daily
Tobacco use: No
Alcohol use: No
Family history: Mother—diabetes, breast cancer; Father—hypertension, CAD

Demographics:
Marital status: Divorced, no children
Years education: Master's degree
Language: English only
Occupation: Respiratory therapist and administrator of department at local hospital
Hours of work: 8–4:30
Ethnicity: Caucasian
Religious affiliation: Baptist

Admitting History/Physical:
Chief complaint: "I have been having some alternating diarrhea and constipation but this morning I woke up with overwhelming belly pain. I knew something was not right so I came to the ED." She notes that she has lost approximately 10 lbs. She also describes increased fatigue but states that she attributed this to working longer hours recently.
General appearance: Well-nourished, 61-year-old white female in apparent distress

Vital Signs: Temp: 99°F   Pulse: 83   Resp rate: 22
                     BP: 130/89   Height: 5'4"   Weight: 165 lbs
Heart: RRR without murmurs or gallops
HEENT: Eyes: PERRLA, normal fundi
          Ears: Noncontributory
          Nose: Noncontributory
          Throat: Pharynx clear
Rectal: WNL
Neurologic: Oriented ×4
Extremities: No edema; pulses full; no bruits; normal strength, sensation, and DT
Skin: Warm, dry
Chest/lungs: Lungs clear to auscultation and percussion

Watson, Betty, Female, 61 y.o.
Allergies: Shellfish, Penicillin
Pt. Location: RM 2252

Code: FULL
Physician: D. Ellison

Isolation: None
Admit Date: 11/2

Peripheral vascular: WNL
Abdomen: Distension, extreme tenderness with rebound and guarding; no bowel sounds

Nursing Assessment	11/2
Abdominal appearance (concave, flat, rounded, obese, distended)	rounded, distended
Palpation of abdomen (soft, rigid, firm, masses, tense)	rigid
Bowel function (continent, incontinent, flatulence, no stool)	no stool
Bowel sounds (P=present, AB=absent, hypo, hyper)	
RUQ	AB
LUQ	AB
RLQ	AB
LLQ	AB
Stool color	N/A
Stool consistency	N/A
Tubes/ostomies	New colostomy in place—minimal output
Genitourinary	
Urinary continence	catheter
Urine source	catheter
Appearance (clear, cloudy, yellow, amber, fluorescent, hematuria, orange, blue, tea)	clear, yellow
Integumentary	
Skin color	pale
Skin temperature (DI=diaphoretic, W=warm, dry, CL=cool, CLM=clammy, CD+ = cold, M=moist, H=hot)	W
Skin turgor (good, fair, poor, TENT=tenting)	good
Skin condition (intact, EC=ecchymosis, A=abrasions, P=petechiae, R=rash, W=weeping, S=sloughing, D=dryness, EX=excoriated, T=tears, SE=subcutaneous emphysema, B=blisters, V=vesicles, N=necrosis)	intact
Mucous membranes (intact, EC=ecchymosis, A=abrasions, P=petechiae, R=rash, W=weeping, S=sloughing, D=dryness, EX=excoriated, T=tears, SE=subcutaneous emphysema, B=blisters, V=vesicles, N=necrosis)	intact
Other components of Braden score: special bed, sensory pressure, moisture, activity, friction/shear (>18=no risk, 15–16=low risk, 13–14=moderate risk, ≤12=high risk)	19

Watson, Betty, Female, 61 y.o.
Allergies: Shellfish, Penicillin
Pt. Location: RM 2252

Code: FULL
Physician: D. Ellison

Isolation: None
Admit Date: 11/2

MD Note 11/3 POD#1

s/p partial colectomy 3 × 3 × 4 cm mass removed. Approximately 80 cm ascending/transverse colon removed. Dx: adenocarcinoma of the colon Stage IIA T2N0M0.

General appearance: 61-year-old white female—pale

Physical exam:

Heart: Regular rate and rhythm, heart sounds normal

HEENT: Noncontributory

Neurologic: Oriented ×4

Extremities: Noncontributory

Skin: Warm and dry to touch

Chest/lungs: Rapid breath sounds, lungs clear

Peripheral vascular: Pulses full—no bruits

Abdomen: Tender with guarding, absent bowel sounds. New colostomy in place—surgical site without drainage.

24 hr. Vital Signs:

Temp: 99	Pulse: 78	Resp rate: 32
BP: 101/72	Height: 5'4"	Weight: 163 lbs

Assessment and Plan:

61 yo female POD#1 total colectomy secondary to acute obstruction now with newly diagnosed adenocarcinoma of the colon Stage IIA T2N0M0. Pain well controlled.

Plan:

NPO with ice chips

Continue D5.45NS@50 mL/hr. Switch to oral pain meds.

Oncology consult.

Begin PT for ambulation.

Nutrition consult.

Stoma care—begin teaching colostomy care for home.

D. Ellison, MD

Nutrition:

General: Patient states that her eating habits have not really changed over the past year—she tries to watch the amount of salt and carbohydrate in her diet. She lives by herself so she does not cook as often as she would like. Generally eats out for lunch at work and picks something up on her way home for dinner. Meets friends for dinner 1–2× per week.

Recent dietary intake:

AM:	Egg and toast or oatmeal with nuts and berries; coffee with Splenda
Lunch:	Soup or salad from cafeteria, diet cola
Dinner:	Will pick up dinner from grocery store salad bar or restaurant—pizza, fish, or chicken. Usually has 2–3 vegetables, potato or rice.
Bedtime snack:	Sometimes popcorn or ice cream

Watson, Betty, Female, 61 y.o.
Allergies: Shellfish, Penicillin
Pt. Location: RM 2252

Code: FULL
Physician: D. Ellison

Isolation: None
Admit Date: 11/2

24-hr recall: NPO
Food allergies/intolerances/aversions: Shellfish
Previous nutrition therapy? Yes. If yes, when? Has never met with RD but does limit added salt and tries to limit total amount of carbohydrate.
Food purchase/preparation: Self
Vit/min intake: Multivitamin daily

Intake/Output

Date		11/3 0701 – 11/4 0700			
Time		0701–1500	1501–2300	2301–0700	Daily total
IN	P.O.	NPO	NPO	NPO	
	I.V.	400	400	400	1200
	(mL/kg/hr)	(0.67)	(0.67)	(0.67)	(0.67)
	I.V. piggyback	200	200	200	600
	TPN				
	Total intake	600	600	600	1800
	(mL/kg)	(8.1)	(8.1)	(8.1)	(24.3)
OUT	Urine	400	320	640	1360
	(mL/kg/hr)	(0.67)	(0.54)	(1.08)	(0.76)
	Emesis output	0	0	0	0
	Other	0	0	0	0
	Stool	0	0	0	0
	Total output	400	320	640	1360
	(mL/kg)	(5.4)	(4.3)	(8.6)	(18.37)
Net I/O		+200	+280	−40	+440
Net since admission (12/15)		+2405	+2685	+2645	+2645

Watson, Betty, Female, 61 y.o.
Allergies: Shellfish, Penicillin
Pt. Location: RM 2252

Code: FULL
Physician: D. Ellison

Isolation: None
Admit Date: 11/2

Laboratory Results

	Ref. Range	11/2 1200	11/3 0600
Chemistry			
Sodium (mEq/L)	136–145	137	141
Potassium (mEq/L)	3.5–5.1	3.7	3.6
Chloride (mEq/L)	98–107	101	104
Carbon dioxide (CO_2, mEq/L)	23–29	24	26
Bicarbonate (mEq/L)	23–28	24	27
BUN (mg/dL)	6–20	12	15
Creatinine serum (mg/dL)	0.6–1.1 F 0.9–1.3 M	0.7	0.9
BUN/Crea ratio	10.0–20.0	17	16.6
Uric acid (mg/dL)	2.8–8.8 F 4.0–9.0 M	3.1	4.2
Est GFR, non-Afr Amer (mL/min/1.73 m²)	>60	103	77
Glucose (mg/dL)	70–99	151 !↑	163 !↑
Phosphate, inorganic (mg/dL)	2.2–4.6	3.2	3.5
Magnesium (mg/dL)	1.5–2.4	1.8	1.9
Calcium (mg/dL)	8.6–10.2	9.1	8.9
Osmolality (mmol/kg/H_2O)	275–295	286	296 !↑
Bilirubin total (mg/dL)	≤1.2	0.7	0.8
Bilirubin, direct (mg/dL)	<0.3	0.1	0.1
Protein, total (g/dL)	6–7.8	6.8	6.3
Albumin (g/dL)	3.5–5.5	3.9	3.6
Prealbumin (mg/dL)	18–35	29	22
Ammonia (NH_3, µg/L)	6–47	8	7
Alkaline phosphatase (U/L)	30–120	45	66
ALT (U/L)	4–36	17	15
AST (U/L)	0–35	11	17
CPK (U/L)	30–135 F 55–170 M	121	127
C-reactive protein (mg/dL)	<1.0	1.3 !↑	1.1 !↑
Lactate dehydrogenase (U/L)	208–378	210	
Cholesterol (mg/dL)	<200	235 !↑	
HDL-C (mg/dL)	>59 F, >50 M	64	

Watson, Betty, Female, 61 y.o.
Allergies: Shellfish, Penicillin
Pt. Location: RM 2252

Code: FULL
Physician: D. Ellison

Isolation: None
Admit Date: 11/2

Laboratory Results *(Continued)*

	Ref. Range	11/2 1200	11/3 0600
VLDL (mg/dL)	7–32	22	
LDL (mg/dL)	<130	149 !↑	
LDL/HDL ratio	<3.22 F <3.55 M	2.33	
Triglycerides (mg/dL)	35–135 F 40–160 M	110	
T_4 (µg/dL)	5–12	7.2	
T_3 (µg/dL)	75–98	81	
HbA_{1c} (%)	<5.7	6.5 !↑	
Coagulation (Coag)			
PT (sec)	11–13	12.1	
PTT (sec)	24–34	27	
Hematology			
WBC ($\times 10^3$/mm^3)	3.9–10.7	8.5	9.7
RBC ($\times 10^6$/mm^3)	4.2–5.4 F 4.5–6.2 M	4.4	4.9
Hemoglobin (Hgb, g/dL)	12–16 F 14–17 M	11.5 !↓	10.7 !↓
Hematocrit (Hct, %)	37–47 F 41–51 M	36 !↓	34 !↓
Platelet count ($\times 10^9$/mm^3)	150–350	273	318

Note: Values and units of measurement listed in these tables are derived from several resources. Substantial variation exists in the ranges quoted as "normal" and these may vary depending on the assay used by different laboratories.

Case Questions

I.   Understanding the Disease and Pathophysiology

1.   Describe the partial colectomy procedure. How does this change the function of the gastrointestinal tract?

2.   What is a colostomy? What kind of fecal output can Ms. Watson expect?

3.   The physician has ordered a consult for Ms. Watson for teaching regarding the care of her ostomy. What is an enterostomal therapist? Describe this specialist's training and what he or she will most likely teach Ms. Watson.

II.   Understanding the Nutrition Therapy

4.   What is the typical postoperative sequence for nutritional intake? How long will Ms. Watson be NPO?

5.   What are the nutrition therapy recommendations for someone with a colostomy? How would this be different if she had an ileostomy?

III.   Nutrition Assessment

6.   Evaluate Ms. Watson's %UBW and BMI.

7.   Calculate Ms. Watson's energy and protein requirements.

8.   Identify any significant and/or abnormal laboratory measurements for Ms. Watson. Explain possible mechanisms for the abnormal labs.

IV.   Nutrition Diagnosis

9.   Select two nutrition problems and complete the PES statement for each.

V.   Nutrition Intervention

10. The surgeon notes Ms. Watson probably will not resume eating by mouth for at least 3–5 days. Using ASPEN guidelines, what would be your recommendation for nutrition support for Ms. Watson?

11. For each of the PES statements you have written, establish an ideal goal (based on the signs and symptoms) and an appropriate intervention (based on the etiology).

VI.   Nutrition Monitoring and Evaluation

12. What would be the primary nutrition concerns as Ms. Watson prepares for rehabilitation after her discharge? Identify two nutritional outcomes and outline specific measures for evaluation.

Bibliography

Academy of Nutrition and Dietetics. Nutrition Care Manual. Nutrition Therapy for Colostomy. https://www.nutritioncaremanual.org/topic.cfm?ncm_toc_id=19449. Accessed 4/12/15.

Cronin E. Dietary advice for patients with a stoma. *Gastrointestinal Nursing*. 2013;11:14–24.

Klappenbach RF, Quintas FA, Rodriguez JA. Early oral feeding versus traditional postoperative care after abdominal emergency surgery: A randomized controlled trial. *World J Surg*. 2013;37:2293–2299.

Lee HS, Shim H, Jang JY, Lee, H, Lee JG. Early feeding is feasible after emergency gastrointestinal surgery. *Yonsei Med J*. 2014;55:395–402.

McDonough MR. A dietitian's guide to colostomies and ileostomies. *Support Line*. 2013;35:3–12.

Medlin S. Nutritional and fluid requirements: High output stomas. *Br J Nurs*. 2012;21:S22–S27.

Nelms MN. Diseases of the lower gastrointestinal tract. In: Nelms M, Sucher K, Lacey K. *Nutrition Therapy and Pathophysiology*. 3rd ed. Belmont, CA: Cengage Learning; 2016:379–435.

Nelms MN, Habash D. Nutrition assessment: Foundations of the nutrition care process. In: Nelms M, Sucher K, Lacey K. *Nutrition Therapy and Pathophysiology*. 3rd ed. Belmont, CA: Cengage Learning; 2016:36–71.

Nelms MN. Metabolic stress and the critically ill. In: Nelms M, Sucher K, Lacey K. *Nutrition Therapy and Pathophysiology*. 3rd ed. Belmont, CA: Cengage Learning; 2016:665–685.

Toth PE. Ostomy care and rehabilitation in colorectal cancer. *Semin Oncol Nurs*. 2006;22:174–177.

United Ostomy Association. Discharge planning for a patient with a new ostomy: Best practice for clinicians. http://www.ostomy.org/uploaded/files/ostomy_info/wocn_discharge_planning.pdf?direct=1. Accessed 04/15/15.

Willcutts K, Touger-Decker R. Nutritional management of ostomates. *Top Clin Nutr*. 2013;28:373–383.

Internet Resources

Academy of Nutrition and Dietetics Nutrition Care Manual: http://www.nutritioncaremanual.org

National Institute of Diabetes and Digestive and Kidney Diseases: Ostomy Surgery of the Bowel: http://www.niddk.nih.gov/health-information/health-topics/digestive-diseases/ostomy-surgery-bowel/Pages/ez.aspx

United Ostomy Associations of America, Inc.: http://www.ostomy.org

Unit Five

NUTRITION THERAPY FOR HEPATOBILIARY AND PANCREATIC DISORDERS

The liver and pancreas are often called ancillary organs of digestion; however, the term *ancillary* does little to describe their importance in digestion, absorption, and metabolism of carbohydrate, protein, and lipid. The cases in this section portray common conditions affecting these organs and outline their effects on nutritional status. The incidence of hepatobiliary disease has significantly increased over the last several decades, with cirrhosis being the most frequent diagnosis. The most common cause of cirrhosis is chronic alcohol ingestion; the second most common cause is viral hepatitis.

The incidence of malnutrition is very high in these disease states. Generalized symptoms of these diseases center around interruption of normal metabolism within these organs. Jaundice, anorexia, fatigue, abdominal pain, steatorrhea, and malabsorption are signs or symptoms of hepatobiliary disease. These symptoms may be responsive to nutrition therapy but also interfere with maintenance of an adequate nutritional status.

In Case 14, our patient is diagnosed with nonalcoholic fatty liver disease. The role of diet in treatment and etiology is the major focus of this case.

Case 15 focuses on the diagnosis of acute pancreatitis associated with chronic alcohol use. The use of nutrition support for acute pancreatitis has changed dramatically over the last decade, and this case allows for the application of new evidenced-based guidelines when planning the care for this patient.

Nonalcoholic Fatty Liver Disease (NAFLD)

Objectives

After completing this case, the student will be able to:

1. Describe the characteristics of nonalcoholic fatty liver disease (NAFLD).
2. Explain the potential etiology of NAFLD and the current epidemiology.
3. Summarize the potential components of nutrition therapy used to treat NAFLD.
4. Analyze nutrition assessment data to evaluate nutritional status and identify specific nutrition problems.
5. Determine nutrition diagnoses and write appropriate PES statements.
6. Develop a nutrition care plan—with appropriate measurable goals, interventions, and strategies for monitoring and evaluation—that addresses the nutrition diagnoses of this case.

Mr. Kim is a 38-year-old male who is at the outpatient gastroenterology clinic after being referred by his primary care physician. Mr. Kim had a physical for his current job and the primary care physician noted an enlarged liver and elevated liver enzymes. Mr. Kim is subsequently diagnosed with nonalcoholic fatty liver disease; this diagnosis is confirmed by ultrasound and supported by the results of physical examination and biochemical tests.

Kim, Myung, Male, 38 y.o.
Allergies: NKA
Pt. Location: RM 2252

Code: FULL
Physician: L. Reyes

Isolation: None
Admit Date: 9/26

Patient Summary: 38-year-old male presented to outpatient gastroenterology clinic after being referred by his primary care physician. Mr. Kim had a physical for his current job and the primary care physician noted an enlarged liver and elevated liver enzymes. He is referred to Dr. Reyes for an evaluation.

History:
Onset of disease: Asymptomatic—hepatomegaly and elevated ALT, AST documented in physical 6 weeks ago.
Medical history: No significant medical history
Surgical history: No previous surgeries
Medications at home: None
Tobacco use: Yes
Alcohol use: Only occasionally
Family history: Mother—diabetes; Father—hypertension, CAD

Demographics:
Marital status: Married, 3 children
Years education: High school and 2 years at community college
Language: Korean/English
Occupation: Production supervisor—automotive manufacturer
Hours of work: 7 am–3 pm or 3 pm–11 pm
Ethnicity: Korean
Religious affiliation: Methodist

Physical:
Chief complaint: "I recently had my physical for work—the doctor there said my liver was bigger than it should be and that there were changes in my blood tests."
General appearance: Overweight, 38-year-old Korean male in no apparent distress

Vital Signs: Temp: 98.7°F   Pulse: 77   Resp rate: 12
                  BP: 142/86   Height: 5'8"   Weight: 205 lbs

Heart: RRR without murmurs or gallops
HEENT: Normocephalic, negative for scleral icterus, normal-appearing oropharynx without any appreciable cervical lymphadenopathy
Rectal: No hemorrhoids, no skin tags, no rectal discomfort, normal tone
Neurologic: Oriented × 4
Extremities: Pulses full; no bruits; normal strength, sensation; trace LE edema
Skin: Warm, dry, no jaundice
Chest/lungs: Lungs clear to auscultation and percussion
Peripheral vascular: WNL
Abdomen: Firm liver, prominent left lobe + spleen tip. No ascites, masses, or tenderness.

Kim, Myung, Male, 38 y.o.
Allergies: NKA
Pt. Location: RM 2252

Code: FULL
Physician: L. Reyes

Isolation: None
Admit Date: 9/26

Ultrasound Results (8/15):

Liver: The liver parenchyma has increased echogenicity with loss of internal architecture. There is no overt nodularity. There is no evidence of an intrahepatic mass or biliary ductal dilation. Doppler ultrasound demonstrates hepatopetal flow in the main portal vein. Flow velocity is 42 cm/sec, which is normal.

Biliary/Gallbladder: The gallbladder is normal without evidence of radiopaque stones. The biliary tree is nondilated.

Spleen: Spleen is enlarged, measuring 14.8 cm in craniocaudal dimension. No focal lesions.
Pancreas: Pancreas is normal. There is no evidence of pancreatic mass or peripancreatic fluid.
Impression: No overt morphological changes of cirrhosis. No focal mass lesions. Increased echogenicity of the liver likely reflects steatosis. Hepatosplenomegaly and hepatic steatosis.

Assessment and Plan:

Dx: Hepatosplenomegaly; hepatic steatosis—NAFLD. Hyperlipidemia and hyperglycemia noted.

Medical Tx plan: Repeat labs and ultrasound in six months. Referred to outpatient nutrition for weight loss and nutrition interventions for NAFLD. Explained in detail his diagnosis, potential complications, and steps to treat. Refer back to primary care MD for treatment of hyperlipidemia and hyperglycemia. F/U six months.

.... L. Reyes, MD

Nutrition:

General: Patient states his appetite is good and he has no problems chewing or swallowing. He reports no diarrhea or constipation. Patient reports that he likes all meats, rice, or noodles. Likes fruit. Eats whatever vegetables his wife cooks but does not choose these on his own. Says he has a "sweet tooth" and often will buy candy and cookies as his snacks between meals. He does not drink alcohol regularly but states that he will on special occasions or when he is watching soccer or football on TV. His meals do change if he is working a different shift; he is currently on days, which means he works 7:00 am–3:00 pm. When he works the afternoon shift, his big meal is in the middle of the day prior to going to work at 3:00 pm.

Usual dietary intake:

AM:	Coffee with sugar and milk
At work:	Doughnuts or some type of pastry from vending machines
Lunch:	Sub sandwich or burger, chips or fries, slice of pie or cookies from work cafeteria, soda
Dinner:	Wife prepares evening meal—meat, 1–2 c short-grain rice, vegetables, kimchi, and usually some type of fruit
Bedtime snack:	Chips, cookies, popcorn

Kim, Myung, Male, 38 y.o.
Allergies: NKA
Pt. Location: RM 2252

Code: FULL
Physician: L. Reyes

Isolation: None
Admit Date: 9/26

Food allergies/intolerances/aversions: NKFA
Previous nutrition therapy? No
Food purchase/preparation: Wife
Vit/min intake: None

Laboratory Results

	Ref. Range	9/26 0600
Chemistry		
Sodium (mEq/L)	136–145	137
Potassium (mEq/L)	3.5–5.1	4.1
Chloride (mEq/L)	98–107	99
Carbon dioxide (CO_2, mEq/L)	23–29	25
Bicarbonate (mEq/L)	23–28	25
BUN (mg/dL)	6–20	13
Creatinine serum (mg/dL)	0.6–1.1 F 0.9–1.3 M	1.05
BUN/Crea ratio	10.0–20.0	12
Uric acid (mg/dL)	2.8–8.8 F 4.0–9.0 M	5.9
Est GFR, non-Afr Amer (mL/min/1.73 m^2)	>60	>60
Glucose (mg/dL)	70–99	121 !↑
Phosphate, inorganic (mg/dL)	2.2–4.6	3.8
Magnesium (mg/dL)	1.5–2.4	1.9
Calcium (mg/dL)	8.6–10.2	8.7
Osmolality (mmol/kg/H_2O)	275–295	285
Bilirubin total (mg/dL)	≤1.2	1.1
Bilirubin, direct (mg/dL)	<0.3	0.25
Protein, total (g/dL)	6–7.8	6.9
Albumin (g/dL)	3.5–5.5	4.8
Prealbumin (mg/dL)	18–35	28
Ammonia (NH_3, µg/L)	6–47	32
Alkaline phosphatase (U/L)	30–120	114
ALT (U/L)	4–36	54 !↑
AST (U/L)	0–35	42 !↑
CPK (U/L)	30–135 F 55–170 M	101

Kim, Myung, Male, 38 y.o.
Allergies: NKA
Pt. Location: RM 2252

Code: FULL
Physician: L. Reyes

Isolation: None
Admit Date: 9/26

Laboratory Results (Continued)

	Ref. Range	9/26 0600
Lactate dehydrogenase (U/L)	208–378	302
Cholesterol (mg/dL)	<200	285 !↑
HDL-C (mg/dL)	>59 F, >50 M	43 !↓
VLDL (mg/dL)	7–32	70 !↑
LDL (mg/dL)	<130	189 !↑
LDL/HDL ratio	<3.22 F <3.55 M	4.39 !↑
Triglycerides (mg/dL)	35–135 F 40–160 M	350 !↑
T_4 (µg/dL)	5–12	10.1
T_3 (µg/dL)	75–98	82
HbA_{1C} (%)	<5.7	6.1 !↑
Coagulation (Coag)		
PT (sec)	11–13	11.9
INR	0.9–1.1	0.95
PTT (sec)	24–34	25
Hematology		
WBC ($\times 10^3$/mm^3)	3.9–10.7	8.1
RBC ($\times 10^6$/mm^3)	4.2–5.4 F 4.5–6.2 M	6.11
Hemoglobin (Hgb, g/dL)	12–16 F 14–17 M	16.8
Hematocrit (Hct, %)	37–47 F 41–51 M	48
Hematology, Manual Diff		
Neutrophil (%)	40–70	63.4
Lymphocyte (%)	22–44	27.1
Monocyte (%)	0–7	6.7
Eosinophil (%)	0–5	1.2
Basophil (%)	0–2	0.6
Blasts (%)	3–10	3
Urinalysis		
Collection method	—	Clean catch

(Continued)

Kim, Myung, Male, 38 y.o.
Allergies: NKA
Pt. Location: RM 2252

Code: FULL
Physician: L. Reyes

Isolation: None
Admit Date: 9/26

Laboratory Results *(Continued)*

	Ref. Range	9/26 0600
Color	—	Yellow
Appearance	—	Cear
Specific gravity	1.001–1.035	1.004
pH	5–7	6.1
Protein (mg/dL)	Neg	Neg
Glucose (mg/dL)	Neg	Neg
Ketones	Neg	Neg
Blood	Neg	Neg
Bilirubin	Neg	Neg
Nitrites	Neg	Neg
Urobilinogen (EU/dL)	<1.0	0.1
Leukocyte esterase	Neg	Neg
Prot chk	Neg	Neg
WBCs (/HPF)	0–5	0
RBCs (/HPF)	0–2	0
Bact	0	0
Mucus	0	0
Crys	0	0
Casts (/LPF)	0	0
Yeast	0	0

Note: Values and units of measurement listed in these tables are derived from several resources. Substantial variation exists in the ranges quoted as "normal" and these may vary depending on the assay used by different laboratories.

Case Questions

I.   Understanding the Disease and Pathophysiology

1.   Define *nonalcoholic fatty liver disease* and *nonalcoholic steatohepatitis.*

2.   What is the potential etiology(ies) of nonalcoholic fatty liver disease (NAFLD)? Does the research indicate that there are any genetic contributions to this condition?

3.   In regard to the epidemiology of this condition, are individuals of specific ethnicities or of either gender at higher risk for the development of NAFLD?

4.   How is this condition typically diagnosed? Are there common presenting signs and symptoms for NAFLD? How might the markers of metabolic syndrome be related to NAFLD?

5.   Explain the potential role of diet in the development of NAFLD. Specifically address the roles of simple sugars, fructose, refined carbohydrates, and saturated fat.

6.   What are the long-term consequences of NAFLD if the condition progresses?

II.   Understanding the Nutrition Therapy

7.   Explain the rationale for prescribing a low-carbohydrate diet in the treatment of NAFLD.

8.   Describe the Mediterranean diet and how this eating pattern may support the nutritional goals of treatment of NAFLD.

9.   Is there a role for supplementation of antioxidants in the treatment of individuals with NAFLD?

10. Mr. Kim asks you about an article he recently read about the benefits of coffee consumption in fatty liver disease. What recommendations might you give him?

III.   Nutrition Assessment

11. Evaluate Mr. Kim's weight status.

12. Calculate Mr. Kim's energy and protein requirements for weight maintenance and for weight loss.

13. What other anthropometric measurements, if any, may be helpful in fully assessing Mr. Kim's nutritional status and disease risk?

14. Identify any significant and/or abnormal laboratory measurements for Mr. Kim. Explain possible mechanisms for the abnormal labs.

15. Assess Mr. Kim's typical diet for total energy intake and % carbohydrate, protein, and fat. How does his estimated energy intake compare to his recommended requirements for weight loss that you calculated in question 12? Identify the most important factors that may impact his NAFLD.

16. How will you assess Mr. Kim's physical activity level? List three questions that you would use in your interview to support your understanding of his daily and recreational activity.

IV.   Nutrition Diagnosis

17. Select two nutrition problems and complete the PES statement for each using the nutrition diagnostic terminology.

V.   Nutrition Intervention

18. What culturally appropriate nutrition therapy recommendations will you make for Mr. Kim?

19. Identify the nutrition education materials and tools you may use in your nutrition education.

20. What steps might you use to assess Mr. Kim's readiness for dietary and behavior change?

21. Are there Korean traditional health practices that you would want to address?

22. Does Mr. Kim meet the criteria for metabolic syndrome? Explain how the nutrition interventions for NAFLD will help with the components of this condition.

VI.   Nutrition Monitoring and Evaluation

23. What topics might you want to address with Mr. Kim in follow-up nutrition appointments?

24. What outcomes will you monitor to evaluate the effectiveness of your nutrition intervention?

Bibliography

Academy of Nutrition and Dietetics. Nutrition Care Manual. Diseases and conditions of the liver, gallbladder and pancreas. https://www.nutritioncaremanual.org/topic.cfm?ncm_category_id=1&lv1=5522&lv2=145224&ncm_toc_id=18609&ncm_heading=Nutrition%20Care. Accessed 4/19/15.

Aller R, De Luis DA, Izaola O, et al. Effect of a high monounsaturated vs high polyunsaturated fat hypocaloric diets in nonalcoholic fatty liver disease. *Eur Rev Med Pharma Sci.* 2014;18:1041–1047.

Al-Shaalan R, Aljiffry M, Al-Busafi S, et al. Nonalcoholic fatty liver disease: Noninvasive methods of diagnosing hepatic steatosis. *The Saudi Journal of Gastroenterology.* 2015;21:64–72.

Berlanga A, Guiu-Jurado E, Porras JA, Auguet T. Molecular pathways in non-alcoholic fatty liver disease. *Clin Exp Gastroenterol.* 2014;7:221–239.

Bettermann K, Hohensee T, Haybaeck J. Steatosis and steatohepatitis: Complex disorders. *Int J Mol Sci.* 2014;15:9924–9944.

Chiu S, Sievenpiper JL, de Souza RJ, et al. Effect of fructose on markers of non-alcoholic fatty liver disease (NAFLD): A systematic review and meta-analysis of controlled feeding trials. *Eur J Clin Nutr.* 2014;68:416–423.

Dongiovanni P, Anstee Q, Valenti L. Genetic Predisposition in NAFLD and NASH: Impact on Severity of Liver Disease and Response to Treatment. *Curr Pham Des.* 2013;19:5219–5238.

Hashemi Kani A, Alavian S, Haghighatdoost F, Azadbakht L. Diet macronutrients composition in nonalcoholic fatty liver disease: A review on the related documents. *Hepat Mon.* 2014;14:e10939.

Kim NH, Kim YJ, Yoo HJ, et al. Clinical and metabolic factors associated with development and regression of nonalcoholic fatty liver disease in nonobese subjects. *Liver Intl.* 2014;34:604–611.

Kontogianni MD, Tileli N, Margariti A, et al. Adherence to the Mediterranean diet is associated with the severity of non-alcoholic fatty liver disease. *Clin Nutr.* 2014;33:678–683.

Nelms MN, Habash D. Nutrition assessment: Foundations of the nutrition care process. In: Nelms M, Sucher K, Lacey K. *Nutrition Therapy and Pathophysiology.* 3rd ed. Belmont, CA: Cengage Learning; 2016:36–71.

Saab S, Mallam D, Cox G, Tong MJ. Impact of coffee on liver disease: A systematic review. *Liver Intl.* 2014;34:495–504.

Sucher K, Mattfeldt-Beman M. Diseases of the liver, gallbladder, and exocrine pancreas. In: Nelms M, Sucher K, Lacey K. *Nutrition Therapy and Pathophysiology.* 3rd ed. Belmont, CA: Cengage Learning; 2016:436–468.

Takaki A, Kawai D, Yamamoto K. Molecular mechanisms and new treatment strategies for non-alcoholic steatohepatitis (NASH). *Int J Mol Sci.* 2014;15:7352–7379.

Velasco N, Contreras A, Grassi B. The Mediterranean diet, hepatic steatosis and nonalcoholic fatty liver disease. *Curr Opin Clin Nutr Metabl Care.* 2014;17:453–457.

Internet Resources

Academy of Nutrition and Dietetics Nutrition Care Manual: http://www.nutritioncaremanual.org

American College of Gastroenterology: Non-alcoholic Fatty Liver Disease (NAFLD): http://patients.gi.org/topics/fatty-liver-disease-nafld/

American Liver Foundation: NAFLD: http://www.liverfoundation.org/abouttheliver/info/nafld/

National Institute of Diabetes and Digestive and Kidney Diseases: Nonalcoholic Steatohepatitis: http://www.niddk.nih.gov/health-information/health-topics/liver-disease/nonalcoholic-steatohepatitis/Pages/facts.aspx

Case 15

Acute Pancreatitis

Objectives

After completing this case, the student will be able to:

1. Understand the physiological role of the pancreas.
2. Determine the etiology of acute versus chronic pancreatitis.
3. Evaluate the signs and symptoms consistent with pancreatitis.
4. Evaluate the current literature regarding nutrition support for acute pancreatitis.
5. Develop a nutrition care plan—with appropriate measurable goals, interventions, and strategies for monitoring and evaluation—that addresses the nutrition diagnoses for this case.

Mr. Mahon is a 29-year-old graduate student who has been suffering from nausea, vomiting, and acute abdominal pain for several days. He is now admitted after a worsening of symptoms with a diagnosis of acute pancreatitis, which is most likely related to chronic alcohol intake.

Mahon, Jon, Male, 29 y.o.
Allergies: NKA
Pt. Location: MICU Bed 5

Code: FULL
Physician: C. Conrad

Isolation: None
Admit Date: 4/21

Patient Summary: Patient is 29-year-old white male who presented to the ED 48 hours ago with increasing abdominal pain. Patient returned to the ED when abdominal pain continued to get worse and is now admitted to MICU.

History:

Onset of disease: Patient is a graduate student who began experiencing acute abdominal pain, N, V several days ago. Assumed it was a viral illness but when symptoms continued he was brought to the ER by neighbor and friend. When questioned about alcohol intake, patient states that he didn't realize how much he had been drinking. States he was trying to stop his antidepressant medications and guesses he steadily increased his alcohol intake.

Medical history: Depression
Surgical history: s/p appendectomy age 12
Medications at home: None
Tobacco use: None
Alcohol use: 6 pack beer, 4–5 shots bourbon daily; weekends: wine and other mixed drinks
Family history: Mother—breast cancer; father—hypertension

Demographics:

Marital status: Single
Years education: 16+
Language: English only
Occupation: PhD student in English
Hours of work: In school full-time; works as research assistant in department
Household members: Lives with roommate
Ethnicity: Caucasian
Religious affiliation: Jewish

Admitting History/Physical:

Chief complaint: "My stomach pain is so bad—I just can't stand it. I can't seem to quit vomiting and cannot keep anything down."
General appearance: Pale, obese male in obvious distress

Vital Signs: Temp: 101.7   Pulse: 108   Resp rate: 27
              BP: 132/96   Height: 5'11"   Weight: 245 lbs

Heart: RRR, unremarkable
HEENT: Head: WNL
        Eyes: PERRLA
        Ears: Clear

Mahon, Jon, Male, 29 y.o.
Allergies: NKA
Pt. Location: MICU Bed 5

Code: FULL
Physician: C. Conrad

Isolation: None
Admit Date: 4/21

Nose: Dry mucous membranes
Throat: Dry mucous membranes
Genitalia: Deferred
Neurologic: Alert and oriented
Extremities: WNL
Skin: Clammy
Chest/lungs: Respirations are rapid but clear to auscultation and percussion
Peripheral vascular: Diminished pulses bilaterally
Abdomen: Hypoactive bowel sounds ×4; extreme tenderness, rebound and guarding

Nursing Assessment	4/22
Abdominal appearance (concave, flat, rounded, obese, distended)	obese
Palpation of abdomen (soft, rigid, firm, masses, tense)	tense
Bowel function (continent, incontinent, flatulence, no stool)	continent
Bowel sounds (P=present, AB=absent, hypo, hyper)	
RUQ	P, hypo
LUQ	P, hypo
RLQ	P, hypo
LLQ	P, hypo
Stool color	none
Stool consistency	
Tubes/ostomies	NA
Genitourinary	
Urinary continence	catheter
Urine source	catheter
Appearance (clear, cloudy, yellow, amber, fluorescent, hematuria, orange, blue, tea)	cloudy, amber
Integumentary	
Skin color	pale
Skin temperature (DI=diaphoretic, W=warm, dry, CL=cool, CLM=clammy, CD1=cold, M=moist, H=hot)	W
Skin turgor (good, fair, poor, TENT=tenting)	TENT
Skin condition (intact, EC=ecchymosis, A=abrasions, P=petechiae, R=rash, W=weeping, S=sloughing, D=dryness, EX=excoriated, T=tears, SE=subcutaneous emphysema, B=blisters, V=vesicles, N=necrosis)	intact, D

(Continued)

Mahon, Jon, Male, 29 y.o.
Allergies: NKA   **Code:** FULL   **Isolation:** None
Pt. Location: MICU Bed 5   **Physician:** C. Conrad   **Admit Date:** 4/21

Nursing Assessment *(Continued)*

Nursing Assessment	4/22
Mucous membranes (intact, EC=ecchymosis, A=abrasions, P=petechiae, R=rash, W=weeping, S=sloughing, D=dryness, EX=excoriated, T=tears, SE=subcutaneous emphysema, B=blisters, V=vesicles, N=necrosis)	intact, D
Other components of Braden score: special bed, sensory pressure, moisture, activity, friction/shear (>18=no risk, 15–16=low risk, 13–14=moderate risk, ≤12=high risk)	19

Admission Orders:
Laboratory: CBC, CMP, Amylase, Lipase, and Mg
Repeat CBC, Amylase, Lipase in 12 hrs
Repeat Chem 7 every 6 hrs

Radiology:
Abdominal series: pancreatitis, rule out small bowel obstruction
CT abdomen/pelvis: pancreatitis, rule out pseudo cyst
Abdominal U/S: pancreatitis, rule out pseudo cyst, biliary tract disease
Vital Signs: Every 4 hrs
I & O recorded every 8 hrs
NG tube to low intermittent suction (if persistent vomiting, obstruction, severe ileus)
Notify MD for fever >101, WBC >16,000, Calcium <8 mg/dL, unstable vital signs or worsening condition
Diet: NPO
Activity: Bed rest
IVF: D_5W 40 MEq KCl 125 mL/hr

Scheduled Medications:
Imipenem 1000 mg every 6 hrs
Pepcid 20 mg IVP every 12 hrs
Meperidine 50–150 mg IV every 3 hrs prn
Ondansetron 2–4 mg IV every 4–6 hrs prn
Colace (docusate) 100 mg po two times daily prn; if no bowel movement
Milk of Magnesia (MOM) 30 mL po daily prn
Ativan 0.5–1 mg po every 8 hrs prn

Nutrition:
Meal type: NPO
Fluid requirement: 1900–2400 mL

Mahon, Jon, Male, 29 y.o.
Allergies: NKA
Pt. Location: MICU Bed 5

Code: FULL
Physician: C. Conrad

Isolation: None
Admit Date: 4/21

History: Patient states that he has gained weight over the last 5 years—almost 50 lbs. Eats out usually for dinner—drinks coffee at breakfast with a bagel or toast—lunch is usually a sub sandwich or pizza. Patient states that he has eaten very little over the past 3 days because of pain, nausea, and vomiting. When questioned about alcohol intake, patient states that he didn't realize how much he had been drinking but states he was trying to stop his antidepressant medications and guesses he increased his alcohol intake.

Intake/Output

Date		4/21 0701–4/22 0700			
Time		0701–1500	1501–2300	2301–0700	Daily total
IN	P.O.	0	0	0	0
	I.V. (mL/kg/hr)	1,000 (1.12)	1,000 (1.12)	1,000 (1.12)	3,000 (1.12)
	I.V. piggyback	500	500	500	1,500
	TPN				
	Total intake (mL/kg)	1,500 (13.5)	1,500 (13.5)	1,500 (13.5)	4,500 (40.4)
OUT	Urine (mL/kg/hr)	1,312 (1.47)	1,410 (1.58)	1,622 (1.82)	4,344 (1.63)
	Emesis output				
	Other: NG tube to suction	100	120	115	335
	Stool	200	0	0	200
	Total output (mL/kg)	1,612 (14.5)	1,530 (13.7)	1,737 (15.6)	4,879 (43.8)
Net I/O		−112	−30	−237	−379
Net since admission (4/21)		−112	−142	−379	−379

MD Progress Note:

4/22 0840
Subjective: Jon Mahon's previous 24 hours reviewed
Vitals: Temp: 101.5 Pulse: 82 Resp rate: 25 BP: 122/78
Urine Output: 4344 mL (39 mL/kg)

Physical Exam
General: Well-developed, alert and oriented to person, place, and time. Continues with acute abdominal pain. APACHE Score 4.
HEENT: WNL
Neck: WNL

Mahon, Jon, Male, 29 y.o.
Allergies: NKA
Pt. Location: MICU Bed 5

Code: FULL
Physician: C. Conrad

Isolation: None
Admit Date: 4/21

Heart: WNL
Lungs: Clear to auscultation
Abdomen: Hypoactive bowel sounds, abdominal tenderness, rebound, guarding, N, V
Assessment/Plan: Results from abdominal ultrasound: inflammation, peripancreatic stranding, and fluid collection. Elevated lipase, amylase, and CRP.

Dx: Acute Pancreatitis

Plan: Continue D5W 40 MEq KCl 125 mL/hr with current medications. Monitor urine output to ensure >40 mL/kg. Nutrition consult for nutrition support recommendations.
.... C. Conrad, MD

Laboratory Results

	Ref. Range	11/29 1522
Chemistry		
Sodium (mEq/L)	136–145	138
Potassium (mEq/L)	3.5–5.1	3.5
Chloride (mEq/L)	98–107	98
Carbon dioxide (CO_2, mEq/L)	23–29	29
Bicarbonate (mEq/L)	23–28	24
BUN (mg/dL)	6–20	30 !↑
Creatinine serum (mg/dL)	0.6–1.1 F 0.9–1.3 M	1.6 !↑
BUN/Crea ratio	10.0–20.0	18
Uric acid (mg/dL)	2.8–8.8 F 4.0–9.0 M	5.2
Est GFR, non-Afr Amer (mL/min/1.73 m^2)	>60	101
Glucose (mg/dL)	70–99	142 !↑
Phosphate, inorganic (mg/dL)	2.2–4.6	3.4
Magnesium (mg/dL)	1.5–2.4	1.9
Calcium (mg/dL)	8.6–10.2	10.2
Anion gap (mmol/L)	10–20	18
Osmolality (mmol/kg/H_2O)	275–295	294.6
Bilirubin total (mg/dL)	≤1.2	1.9 !↑
Bilirubin, direct (mg/dL)	<0.3	0.9 !↑
Protein, total (g/dL)	6–7.8	6.8

Mahon, Jon, Male, 29 y.o.
Allergies: NKA
Pt. Location: MICU Bed 5

Code: FULL
Physician: C. Conrad

Isolation: None
Admit Date: 4/21

Laboratory Results *(Continued)*

	Ref. Range	11/29 1522
Albumin (g/dL)	3.5–5.5	3.3 !↓
Prealbumin (mg/dL)	18–35	22
Ammonia (NH$_3$, µg/L)	6–47	25
Alkaline phosphatase (U/L)	30–120	256 !↑
ALT (U/L)	4–36	42 !↑
AST (U/L)	0–35	56 !↑
CPK (U/L)	30–135 F 55–170 M	219 !↑
Lactate dehydrogenase (U/L)	208–378	402 !↑
Lipase (U/L)	0–110	980 !↑
Amylase (U/L)	25–125	543 !↑
CRP (mg/dL)	<1	141 !↑
Cholesterol (mg/dL)	<200	210 !↑
HDL-C (mg/dL)	>59 F, >50 M	54
VLDL (mg/dL)	7–32	29
LDL (mg/dL)	<130	127
LDL/HDL ratio	<3.22 F <3.55 M	2.35
Triglycerides (mg/dL)	35–135 F 40–160 M	585 !↑
HbA$_{1C}$ (%)	<5.7	5.3
Coagulation (Coag)		
PT (sec)	11–13	13
INR	0.9–1.1	0.97
PTT (sec)	24–34	27
Hematology		
WBC (×10^3/mm^3)	3.9–10.7	19.8 !↑
RBC (×10^6/mm^3)	4.2–5.4 F 4.5–6.2 M	5.2
Hemoglobin (Hgb, g/dL)	12–16 F 14–17 M	15.8
Hematocrit (Hct, %)	37–47 F 41–51 M	49

(Continued)

Mahon, Jon, Male, 29 y.o.
Allergies: NKA
Pt. Location: MICU Bed 5

Code: FULL
Physician: C. Conrad

Isolation: None
Admit Date: 4/21

Laboratory Results *(Continued)*

	Ref. Range	11/29 1522
Hematology, Manual Diff		
Neutrophil (%)	40–70	90 !↑
Lymphocyte (%)	22–44	32
Monocyte (%)	0–7	5
Eosinophil (%)	0–5	1
Basophil (%)	0–2	2
Blasts (%)	3–10	3
Segs (%) *WBC*	0–60	74 !↑
Bands (%) *immature*	0–10	16 !↑
Urinalysis		
Collection method	—	Cath
Color	—	Dark, amber
Appearance	—	Cloudy
Specific gravity	1.001–1.035	1.029
pH	5–7	5.1
Protein (mg/dL)	Neg	+ !↑
Glucose (mg/dL)	Neg	Neg
Ketones	Neg	+ !↑
Blood	Neg	Neg
Bilirubin	Neg	+ !↑
Nitrites	Neg	Neg
Urobilinogen (EU/dL)	<1.0	1.2 !↑
Leukocyte esterase	Neg	Neg
Prot chk	Neg	+ !↑
WBCs (/HPF)	0–5	2
RBCs (/HPF)	0–2	0
Bact	0	0
Mucus	0	0
Crys	0	0
Casts (/LPF)	0	0
Yeast	0	0
Arterial Blood Gases (ABGs)		
pH	7.35–7.45	7.40

Mahon, Jon, Male, 29 y.o.
Allergies: NKA
Pt. Location: MICU Bed 5

Code: FULL
Physician: C. Conrad

Isolation: None
Admit Date: 4/21

Laboratory Results *(Continued)*

	Ref. Range	11/29 1522
pCO$_2$ (mm Hg)	35–45	40
SO$_2$ (%)	≥95	97
CO$_2$ content (mmol/L)	25–30	29
O$_2$ content (%)	15–22	18
pO$_2$ (mm Hg)	≥80	95
HCO$_3^-$ (mEq/L)	21–28	24

Note: Values and units of measurement listed in these tables are derived from several resources. Substantial variation exists in the ranges quoted as "normal" and these may vary depending on the assay used by different laboratories.

Case Questions

I.   Understanding the Diagnosis and Pathophysiology

1.   Describe the normal exocrine and endocrine functions of the pancreas.

2.   Determine the potential etiology of both acute and chronic pancreatitis. What information provided in the physical assessment supports the diagnosis of acute pancreatitis?

3.   What laboratory values or other tests support this diagnosis? List all abnormal values and explain the likely cause for each abnormal value.

4.   The physician lists an APACHE score in his note. What factors are used to determine this score? What does this mean? Ranson's Criteria and the Atlanta Criteria are also used to determine the severity of pancreatitis. Define each of these sets of criteria.

5.   What are the potential complications of acute pancreatitis?

II.   Understanding the Nutrition Therapy

6.   Historically, the patient with acute pancreatitis was made NPO. Why?

7.   The physician has written an order for a nutrition consult. Using the most current literature and ASPEN guidelines, explain the role of enteral feeding in acute pancreatitis. Do you agree with the initiation of enteral feeding? Why or why not?

8.   Does this patient's case indicate the use of an immune-modulating formula?

III.   Nutrition Assessment

9.   Assess Mr. Mahon's height and weight. Calculate his BMI and % usual body weight.

10.   Evaluate Mr. Mahon's initial nursing assessment. What important factors noted in his nutrition assessment will affect your nutrition recommendations?

11. Determine Mr. Mahon's energy and protein requirements. Explain the rationale for the method you used to calculate these requirements.

12. Determine Mr. Mahon's fluid requirements. Compare this with the information on the intake/output record.

13. From the nutrition history, assess Mr. Mahon's alcohol intake. What is his average caloric intake from alcohol each day using the information that he provided to you?

14. List all medications that Mr. Mahon is receiving. Determine the action of each medication and identify any drug–nutrient interactions that you should monitor.

IV. Nutrition Diagnosis
15. Identify the pertinent nutrition problems and the corresponding nutrition diagnoses.

16. Write your PES statement for each nutrition problem.

V. Nutrition Intervention
17. Determine your enteral feeding recommendations for Mr. Mahon. Provide a formula choice, goal rate, and instructions for initiation and advancement.

18. What recommendations can you make to the patient's critical care team to help improve tolerance to the enteral feeding?

VI. Nutrition Monitoring and Evaluation
19. List factors that you would monitor to assess tolerance and adequacy of nutrition support.

20. If this patient's acute pancreatitis resolves, what will be the recommendations for him regarding nutrition and his alcohol intake when he is discharged?

21. Write an ADIME note that provides your initial nutrition assessment and enteral feeding recommendations.

Bibliography

Bakker OJ, van Brunschot S, Farre A, et al. Timing of enteral nutrition in acute pancreatitis: Meta-analysis of individuals using a single-arm of randomized trials. *Pancreatology*. 2014;14:340–346.

Bankhead R, Boullata J, Brantley S, et al. Enteral nutrition practice recommendations. *JPEN J Parenter Enteral Nutr*. 2009;33:122–167.

Banks PA, Bollen TL, Dervenis C, et al. Classification of acute pancreatitis-2012: Revision of the Atlanta classification and definitions by international consensus. *Gut*. 2013;62:102–111.

Krenitsky J, Makola D, Parrish CR. Pancreatitis part II—Revenge of the cyst: A practical guide to jejunal feeding. *Pract Gastroenterol*. 2007;31:54.

Krenitsky J, Makola D, Parrish CR. Parenteral nutrition in pancreatitis is passe: But are we ready for gastric feeding? *Pract Gastroenterol*. 2007;31:92.

Parrish CR, Krenitsky J, McClave SA. Pancreatitis. In: *The ASPEN Adult Nutrition Support Core Curriculum*. 2nd ed. Silver Spring, MD: American Society for Enteral and Parenteral Nutrition; 2012;472–490.

McClave SA, Heyland DK. The physiologic response and associated clinical benefits from provision of early enteral nutrition. *Nutr Clin Prac*. 2009;24:305–315.

McClave SA, Martindale RG, Vanek VW, et al. Guidelines for the provision and assessment of nutrition support therapy in the adult critically ill patient: Society of Critical Care Medicine (SCCM) and American Society for Parenteral and Enteral Nutrition (ASPEN). *J Parenter Enteral Nutr*. 2009;33:277–316.

Meier R. Enteral fish oil in acute pancreatitis. *Clin Nutr*. 2005;24(2):169–171.

Mirtallo J. et al. for the International Consensus Guideline Committee for Pancreatitis Task Force. International consensus guidelines for nutrition therapy in pancreatitis. *J Parenter Enteral Nutr*. 2012;36:284–291.

Moraes JM, Felga GE, Chebli LA, et al. A full solid diet as the initial meal in mild acute pancreatitis is safe and results in a shorter length of hospitalization. *J Clin Gastroenterol*. Jan 5, 2010;44(7):517–522.

Nahikian-Nelms M. Metabolic stress and the critically ill. In: Nelms M, Sucher K, Lacey K. *Nutrition Therapy and Pathophysiology*. 3rd ed. Belmont, CA: Cengage Learning; 2016:665–685.

Nahikian-Nelms M, Habash D. Nutrition assessment: Foundation of the nutrition care process. In: Nelms M, Sucher K, Lacey K. *Nutrition Therapy and Pathophysiology*. 3rd ed. Belmont, CA: Cengage Learning; 2016:36–71.

Nally DM, Kelly EG, Clarke M, Ridgway P. Nasogastric nutrition is efficacious in severe acute pancreatitis: A systematic review and meta-analysis. *Br J Nutr*. 2014;112:1769–1778.

Petrov MS, Loveday BPT, Pylypchuk RD, McIlroy K, Phillips ARJ, Windsor JA. Systematic review and meta-analysis of enteral nutrition formulations in acute pancreatitis. *Br J Surg*. 2009;96:1243–1252.

Rajkumar N, Karthikeyan VS, Ali SM, Sistia SC, Kate V. Clear liquid diet vs soft diet as the initial meal in patients with mild acute pancreatitis: A randomized interventional trial. *Nutr Clin Pract*. 2013;28:365–370.

Sathiaraj E, Murthy S, Mansard MJ, Rao GV, Mahukar S, Reddy DN. Clinical trial: Oral feeding with a soft diet compared with clear liquid diet as initial meal in mild acute pancreatitis. *Aliment Pharmacol Ther*. 2008;28:777–781.

Sucher K, Mattfeldt-Beman M. Diseases of the liver, gallbladder and exocrine pancreas. In: Nahikian-Nelms M, Sucher K, Lacey K, Roth S. *Nutrition Therapy and Pathophysiology*. 3rd ed. Belmont, CA: Cengage Learning; 2016:436–468.

Tenner S, Baillie J, DeWitt J, Vege SS. American College of Gastroenterology guideline: Management of acute pancreatitis. *Am J Gastroenterol*. 2013;108:1400–1416.

Thomson A. Enteral versus parenteral nutritional support in acute pancreatitis: A clinical review. *J Gastroenterol Hepatol*. 2006;21:22–25.

Uomo G. Pancreatic rest or not? The debate on the nutrition in acute pancreatitis continues. *J Pancreas*. 2013;14:216–217.

Internet Resources

AND Evidence Analysis Library: http://www.andeal.org/

American Gastroenterology Association: http://www.gastro.org/patient-care/conditions-diseases/pancreatitis

Cleveland Clinic: http://www.clevelandclinicmeded.com/medicalpubs/diseasemanagement/gastroenterology/acute-pancreatitis/Default.htm

Drug Bank: http://www.drugbank.ca/drugs/

National Pancreatitis Foundation: http://www.pancreasfoundation.org/patient-information/acute-pancreatitis/

National Institute of Diabetes and Digestive and Kidney Diseases: http://www.niddk.nih.gov/health-information/health-topics/digestive-diseases/pancreatitis/Pages/facts.aspx

Nutrition Care Manual: http://www.nutritioncaremanual.org

NUTRITION THERAPY FOR ENDOCRINE DISORDERS

The most common of all endocrine disorders is diabetes mellitus, a currently incurable chronic disease. Diabetes mellitus is actually a group of diseases characterized by hyperglycemia resulting from cessation of insulin production, impairment in insulin secretion, and/or impairment in insulin action. Type 1 and Type 2 diabetes are the major classifications for this disorder. The three cases in this section provide examples of patients at all stages of treatment and diagnosis. The first two focus on newly diagnosed type 1 diabetes—not only the typical presentation in a pediatric patient but also the atypical presentation in an adult. Case 18 describes untreated T2DM complicated by the admission diagnosis of hyperosmolar hyperglycemic state.

Diabetes mellitus is a serious public health problem in the United States. New diagnoses of diabetes have more than tripled in the last 20 years. In 2014, this chronic disease was known to affect 29.1 million Americans, and it was estimated that at least 8.1 million more were undiagnosed (available from: http://www.diabetes.org/diabetes-basics/statistics/).

Diabetes affects men and women equally, but minorities (especially American Indians and Alaska Natives) are almost twice as likely as non-Hispanic whites to develop diabetes in their lifetime. In addition, diabetes is one of the most costly health problems in the United States. In 2012, health care and other direct medical costs combined with indirect costs (such as loss of productivity) totaled approximately $245 billion. (available from: http://www.diabetes.org/advocacy/news-events/cost-of-diabetes.html). Diabetes is the seventh leading cause of death in the United States. Each year, more than 200,000 people die as a result of diabetes and its complications. Diabetes is also the leading cause of both new-onset blindness and kidney failure requiring dialysis or organ transplant for survival in the United States.

Medical nutrition therapy is integral to total diabetes care and management. The Diabetes Control and Complications Trial (DCCT) corroborated the significance of integrating nutrition and blood glucose self-management education in achieving and maintaining target blood glucose levels. Nutrition and meal planning are among the most challenging aspects of diabetes care for the person with diabetes and for the health care team. The major components of successful nutrition management are learning about nutrition therapy, altering eating habits, implementing new behaviors, participating in exercise, evaluating changes, and integrating this information into diabetes care. Observance of meal-planning principles requires people with diabetes to make demanding lifestyle changes. To be effective, the registered dietitian must be able to customize his or her approach to the personal lifestyle and diabetes management goals of the individual with diabetes. Cases 16–18 allow you to put these guidelines into practice.

Pediatric Type 1 Diabetes Mellitus

Objectives

After completing this case, the student will be able to:

1. Describe the pathophysiology of type 1 diabetes mellitus.
2. Develop a nutrition care plan—with appropriate measurable goals, interventions, and strategies for monitoring and evaluation—that addresses the nutrition diagnoses for this case.
3. Integrate an insulin regimen with nutrition therapy and provide appropriate recommendations for carbohydrate-to-insulin ratios and correction dosages.
4. Interpret laboratory parameters to assess fluid, electrolyte, and acid-base balance.
5. Prioritize teaching and educational requirements for a newly diagnosed type 1 diabetic.

Rachel Roberts is a 12-year-old 7th grader previously in good health who is admitted through the ED with a new diagnosis of acute hyperglycemia—R/O diabetes mellitus.

Roberts, Rachel, Female, 12 y.o.
Allergies: NKA
Pt. Location: RM 744

Code: FULL
Physician: M. Cho

Isolation: None
Admit Date: 5/4

Patient Summary: Rachel Roberts is a 12-year-old female admitted with acute-onset hyperglycemia.

History:

Onset of disease: Patient presented to ED after fainting at soccer practice. During ED assessment, patient was noted to have serum glucose of 724 mg/dL.
Medical history: None—recently had strep throat
Surgical history: None
Medications at home: None
Tobacco use: Nonsmoker
Alcohol use: None
Family history: Father—HTN; Mother—hyperthyroidism; Sister—celiac disease

Demographics:

Marital status: Single 7th-grade female
Years education: 7 years
Language: English only
Occupation: Student
Hours of work: N/A
Household members: Mother, sister age 8 and brother age 4—parents divorced. Father lives in city and shares custody.
Ethnicity: Caucasian
Religious affiliation: Catholic

Admitting History/Physical:

Chief complaint: "I have just gotten over strep throat a few days ago. I felt like I was well enough to go to soccer practice today but after playing about 15 minutes, I just felt horrible. I sat down and they tell me I fainted. . . . I have been really thirsty—thirstier than I have ever been in my whole life and then I have had to use the bathroom a lot. . . . I even have to get up at night to go to the bathroom."
General appearance: Slim, healthy-appearing, 12-year-old female

Vital Signs: Temp: 98.6   Pulse: 101   Resp rate: 22
               BP: 122/77   Height: 5'   Weight: 82 lbs

Heart: Regular rate and rhythm
HEENT: Head: WNL
          Eyes: PERRLA
          Ears: Clear
          Nose: Clear
          Throat: Dry mucous membranes without exudates or lesions
Genitalia: Deferred
Neurologic: Alert but slightly confused. Glasgow Coma Scale: 15.

Roberts, Rachel, Female, 12 y.o.
Allergies: NKA   **Code:** FULL   **Isolation:** None
Pt. Location: RM 744   **Physician:** M. Cho   **Admit Date:** 5/4

Extremities: Noncontributory
Skin: Warm and dry
Chest/lungs: Respirations are rapid—clear to auscultation and percussion
Peripheral vascular: Pulse 41 bilaterally, warm, no edema
Abdomen: Active bowel sounds ×4; tender, nondistended

Orders:

1. Regular insulin 1 unit/mL NS 40 mEq KCl/liter @ 135 mL/hr. Begin infusion at 0.1 unit/kg/hr=3.7 units/hr and increase to 5 units/hr. Flush new IV tubing with 50 mL of insulin drip solution prior to connecting to patient and starting insulin infusion.

2. Labs: BMP Stat
    Phos Stat
    Calcium Stat
    UA with culture if indicated Stat Clean catch
    Bedside glucose Stat
    Bedside I-Stat: EG7 Stat
    Islet cell autoantibodies screen
    Thyroid peroxidase antibodies
    TSH
    Comp metabolic panel (CMP)
    Thyroglobulin antibodies
    C-peptide
    Immunoglobulin A level
    Hemoglobin A_{1c}
    IgA-tTG; IgG-tTG

3. NPO except for ice chips and medications. After 12 hours, clear liquids if stable. Then, advance to consistent carbohydrate diet order—70–80 g breakfast and lunch; 85–95 g dinner; 3–15 gram snacks.

5. Consult diabetes education team for self-management training for patient and parents to begin education after stabilized.

Nursing Assessment	5/4
Abdominal appearance (concave, flat, rounded, obese, distended)	flat
Palpation of abdomen (soft, rigid, firm, masses, tense)	soft
Bowel function (continent, incontinent, flatulence, no stool)	continent
Bowel sounds (P=present, AB=absent, hypo, hyper)	
RUQ	P

(Continued)

Roberts, Rachel, Female, 12 y.o.
Allergies: NKA
Pt. Location: RM 744

Code: FULL
Physician: M. Cho

Isolation: None
Admit Date: 5/4

Nursing Assessment *(Continued)*

Nursing Assessment	5/4
LUQ	P
RLQ	P
LLQ	P
Stool color	light brown
Stool consistency	soft
Tubes/ostomies	NA
Genitourinary	
Urinary continence	yes
Urine source	clean specimen
Appearance (clear, cloudy, yellow, amber, fluorescent, hematuria, orange, blue, tea)	cloudy, amber
Integumentary	
Skin color	pale
Skin temperature (DI=diaphoretic, W=warm, dry, CL=cool, CLM=clammy, CD +=cold, M=moist, H=hot)	DI
Skin turgor (good, fair, poor, TENT=tenting)	good
Skin condition (intact, EC=ecchymosis, A=abrasions, P=petechiae, R=rash, W=weeping, S=sloughing, D=dryness, EX=excoriated, T=tears, SE=subcutaneous emphysema, B=blisters, V=vesicles, N=necrosis)	intact
Mucous membranes (intact, EC=ecchymosis, A=abrasions, P=petechiae, R=rash, W=weeping, S=sloughing, D=dryness, EX=excoriated, T=tears, SE=subcutaneous emphysema, B=blisters, V=vesicles, N=necrosis)	intact
Other components of Braden score: special bed, sensory pressure, moisture, activity, friction/shear (>18=no risk, 15–16=low risk, 13–14=moderate risk, ≤12=high risk)	21

Nutrition:

Meal type: NPO then progress to clear liquids and then consistent carbohydrate-controlled diet

Fluid requirement: 1840 mL

History: Parents present—patient states that she thinks she has lost weight recently: "My clothes are a little loose but I don't usually weigh myself." Mom states that the last weight she remembers was when they went to fast-care clinic for strep throat and that she weighed about 90 lbs. Patient confirms that that is what she usually weighs. Appetite has been normal—if anything patient states she has been more hungry than usual—but thought it was probably due to starting soccer season and exercising more. Relates history of increased thirst and increased urination.

Roberts, Rachel, Female, 12 y.o.
Allergies: NKA   **Code:** FULL   **Isolation:** None
Pt. Location: RM 744   **Physician:** M. Cho   **Admit Date:** 5/4

Usual intake (for past several months): Mom and Dad state that Rachel is kind of a picky eater. She eats only chicken and fish—eats salad, broccoli, carrots, tomatoes, and asparagus as her only vegetables. Breakfast—cereal and milk or Pop-Tart® with milk; packs lunch for school—peanut butter and jelly or turkey and cheese sandwich, chips, carrots, and usually drinks water. Has a cereal or granola bar before soccer practice—drinks water throughout practice. Dinner is usually prepared by Mom when she is at her house—always some salad, meat, and pasta, potato, or rice. Dad states that when the kids are with him he doesn't cook very often and they usually order in pizza or Chinese food. Snacks include cereal, ice cream, yogurt, some fruits (apples, bananas), popcorn, chips, or cookies.

MD Progress Note:
5/5 0820
Subjective: Rachel Roberts's previous 24 hours reviewed
Vitals: Temp: 99.5, Pulse: 82, Resp rate: 25, BP: 101/78
Urine Output: 2660 mL (71.8 mL/kg)

<u>Physical Exam</u>
General: Alert and oriented to person, place, and time
HEENT: WNL
Neck: WNL
Heart: WNL
Lungs: Clear to auscultation
Abdomen: Active bowel sounds
Assessment/Plan: Results: +ICA, GADA, IAA consistent with type 1 DM. Negative tTG.

Dx: New Diagnosis Type 1 Diabetes Mellitus

Plan: Change IVF to D_5.45NS with 40MEq K @ 135 mL/hr. Begin Apidra 0.5 u every 2 hours until glucose is 150–200 mg/dL. Tonight begin glargine 6 u at 9 pm. Progress Apidra using ICR 1:15. Continue bedside glucose checks hourly. Notify MD if blood glucose >200 or <80.

....M Cho, MD

Roberts, Rachel, Female, 12 y.o.
Allergies: NKA   **Code:** FULL   **Isolation:** None
Pt. Location: RM 744   **Physician:** M. Cho   **Admit Date:** 5/4

Intake/Output

Date		5/4 0701–5/5 0700			
Time		0701–1500	1501–2300	2301–0700	Daily total
IN	P.O.	**NPO**	**NPO**	**320**	**320**
	I.V.	**1,080**	**1,080**	**1,080**	**3,240**
	(mL/kg/hr)	(3.6)	(3.6)	(3.6)	(3.6)
	I.V. piggyback				
	TPN				
	Total intake	**1,080**	**1,080**	**1,400**	**3,560**
	(mL/kg)	(29.0)	(29.0)	(37.6)	(95.5)
OUT	Urine	**600**	**480**	**1,580**	**2,660**
	(mL/kg/hr)	(2.01)	(1.61)	(5.30)	(2.97)
	Emesis output				
	Other				
	Stool				
	Total output	**600**	**480**	**1,580**	**2,660**
	(mL/kg)	(16.1)	(12.9)	(42.4)	(71.4)
Net I/O		**+480**	**+600**	**−180**	**+900**
Net since admission (5/4)		**+480**	**+1,080**	**+900**	**+900**

Roberts, Rachel, Female, 12 y.o.
Allergies: NKA
Pt. Location: RM 744

Code: FULL
Physician: M. Cho

Isolation: None
Admit Date: 5/4

Laboratory Results

	Ref. Range	5/4 1780	5/5 0600
Chemistry			
Sodium, 1014 yo (mEq/L)	136–145	126 !↓	131 !↓
Potassium, 10–14 yo (mEq/L)	3.5–5.0	4.3	4.0
Chloride, 10–14 yo (mEq/L)	98–108	99	98
Carbon dioxide, 10–14 yo (CO_2, mEq/L)	22–30	27	28
Bicarbonate, 10–14 yo (mEq/L)	22–26	23	24
BUN, 10–14 yo (mg/dL)	5–18	15	12
Creatinine serum, 10–14 yo (mg/dL)	≤1.2	0.9	0.8
BUN/Crea ratio	10.0–20.0	16.6	15
Uric acid, 10–14 yo (mg/dL)	2.5–5.5	2.9	2.8
Est GFR, non-Afr Amer (mL/min/1.73 m²)	>60	98	113
Glucose, 10–14 yo (mg/dL)	70–99	683 !↑	250 !↑
Phosphate, inorganic, 10–14 yo (mg/dL)	2.2–4.6	1.9 !↓	2.1 !↓
Magnesium, 10–14 yo (mg/dL)	1.6–2.6	1.7	2.0
Calcium, 10–14 yo (mg/dL)	8.6–10.5	10	9.8
Anion gap (mmol/L)	10–20	4.0 !↓	9.0 !↓
Osmolality, 10–14 yo (mmol/kg/H_2O)	275–295	295.3 !↑	280
Bilirubin total, 10–14 yo (mg/dL)	≤1.2	0.8	
Bilirubin, direct, 10–14 yo (mg/dL)	<0.3	0.009	
Protein, total, 10–14 yo (g/dL)	6–7.8	6.1	
Albumin, 10–14 yo (g/dL)	3.5–5.5	3.7	
Prealbumin, 10–14 yo (mg/dL)	17–39	17	
Ammonia, 10–14 yo (NH_3, μg/L)	40–80	41	
Alkaline phosphatase, 10–14 yo (U/L)	<500	102	
ALT, 10–14 yo (U/L)	3–28	7.1	
AST, 10–14 yo (U/L)	19–28	21	
CPK, 10–14 yo (U/L)	0–70	31	

(Continued)

Roberts, Rachel, Female, 12 y.o.
Allergies: NKA
Pt. Location: RM 744

Code: FULL
Physician: M. Cho

Isolation: None
Admit Date: 5/4

Laboratory Results *(Continued)*

	Ref. Range	5/4 1780	5/5 0600
Lactate dehydrogenase, 10–14 yo (U/L)	208–378	208	
Cholesterol, 10–14 yo (mg/dL)	124–201 F 119–202 M	124	
Triglycerides, 10–14 yo (mg/dL)	10–103	55	
T_4, 10–14 yo (μg/dL)	5.6–11.7	8.1	
T_3, 10–14 yo (μg/dL)	83–213	85	
HbA$_{1C}$, 10–14 yo (%)	3.9–5.2	14.6 !↑	
C-peptide (ng/mL)	0.51–2.72	0.10 !↓	
ICA	—	+ !↑	
GADA	—	+ !↑	
IA-2A	—	+ !↑	
IAA	—	+ !↑	
tTg IgA antibody (U/mL)	<4	2	
tTg IgG antibody (U/mL)	<6	1	
Hematology			
WBC, 10–14 yo ($\times 10^3$/mm^3)	4.0–13.5	9.6	
RBC, 10–14 yo ($\times 10^6$/mm^3)	3.7–5.3	4.8	
Hemoglobin, 10–14 yo (Hgb, g/dL)	11–16	12.5	
Hematocrit, 10–14 yo (Hct, %)	31–43	37	
Hematology, Manual Diff			
Neutrophil, 10–14 yo (%)	36–38	37	
Lymphocyte, 10–14 yo (%)	25–33	28	
Monocyte, 10–14 yo (%)	0–7	4	
Eosinophil, 10–14 yo (%)	0–5	0	
Basophil, 10–14 yo (%)	0–2	1	
Blasts, 10–14 yo (%)	3–10	3	
Urinalysis			
Collection method	—	Clean catch	
Color	—	yellow	
Appearance	—	clear	

Roberts, Rachel, Female, 12 y.o.
Allergies: NKA   **Code:** FULL   **Isolation:** None
Pt. Location: RM 744   **Physician:** M. Cho   **Admit Date:** 5/4

Laboratory Results *(Continued)*

	Ref. Range	5/4 1780	5/5 0600
Specific gravity, 10–14 yo	1.001–1.035	1.036 !↑	
pH, 10–14 yo	5–7	4.9 !↓	
Protein (mg/dL)	Neg	+4 !↑	
Glucose (mg/dL)	Neg	+3 !↑	
Ketones	Neg	1 !↑	
Blood	Neg	Neg	
Bilirubin	Neg	Neg	
Nitrites	Neg	Neg	
Urobilinogen, 10–14 yo (EU/dL)	<1.0	0.01	
Leukocyte esterase	Neg	Neg	
Prot chk	Neg	+4 !↑	
WBCs, 10–14 yo (/HPF)	0–5	3–4	
RBCs, 10–14 yo (/HPF)	0–2	0	
Bact	0	0	
Mucus	0	0	
Crys	0	0	
Casts (/LPF)	0	0	
Yeast	0	0	

Case Questions

I. **Understanding the Diagnosis and Pathophysiology**

1. What are the current thoughts regarding the etiology of type 1 diabetes mellitus (T1DM)? No one else in Rachel's family has diabetes—is this unusual? Are there any other findings in her family medical history that would be important to note?

2. What are the standard diagnostic criteria for T1DM? Which are found in Rachel's medical record?

3. Dr. Cho requested these labs be drawn: Islet cell autoantibodies screen; TSH; thyroglobulin antibodies; C-peptide; immunoglobulin A level; hemoglobin A_{1c}; and tissue transglutaminase antibodies. Describe how each is related to the diagnosis of type 1 diabetes.

4. Using the information from Rachel's medical record, identify the factors that would allow the physician to distinguish between T1DM and T2DM.

5. Describe the metabolic events that led to Rachel's symptoms and subsequent admission to the ED (polyuria, polydipsia, polyphagia, fatigue, and weight loss), integrating the pathophysiology of T1DM into your discussion.

6. Describe the metabolic events that result in the signs and symptoms associated with DKA. Was Rachel in this state when she was admitted? What precipitating factors may lead to DKA?

7. Rachel will be started on a combination of Apidra prior to meals and snacks, with glargine given in the a.m. and p.m. Describe the onset, peak, and duration for each of these types of insulin. Her discharge dosages are as follows: 7 u glargine with Apidra prior to each meal or snack—1:15 insulin:carbohydrate ratio. Rachel's parents want to know why she cannot take oral medications for her diabetes like some of their friends do. What would you tell them?

8. Rachel's physician explains to Rachel and her parents that Rachel's insulin dose may change due to something called a honeymoon phase. Explain what this is and how it might affect her insulin requirements.

9. How does physical activity affect blood glucose levels? Rachel is a soccer player and usually plays daily. What recommendations will you make to Rachel to assist with managing her glucose during exercise and athletic events?

10. At a follow-up visit, Rachel's blood glucose records indicate that her levels have been consistently high when she wakes in the morning before breakfast. Describe the dawn phenomenon. Is Rachel experiencing this? How might it be prevented?

II.   Understanding the Nutrition Therapy

11. The MD ordered a carbohydrate-controlled diet for when Rachel begins to eat. Explain the rationale for monitoring carbohydrate in diabetes nutrition therapy.

12. Outline the basic principles for Rachel's nutrition therapy to assist in control of her T1DM.

III.   Nutrition Assessment

13. Assess Rachel's ht/age; wt/age; ht/wt; and BMI. What is her desirable weight?

14. Identify any abnormal laboratory values measured upon her admission. Explain how they may be related to her newly diagnosed T1DM.

15. Determine Rachel's energy and protein requirements. Be sure to explain what standards you used to make this estimation.

IV.   Nutrition Diagnosis

16. Prioritize two nutrition problems and complete the PES statement for each.

V.   Nutrition Intervention

17. Determine Rachel's initial nutrition prescription using her usual intake at home as a guideline, as well as your assessment of her energy requirements.

18. What is an insulin:CHO ratio (ICR)? Rachel's physician ordered her ICR to start at 1:15. If her usual breakfast is 2 Pop-Tarts and 8 oz skim milk, how much Apidra should she take to cover the carbohydrate in this meal?

19. Dr. Cho set Rachel's fasting blood glucose goal at 90–180 mg/dL. If her total daily insulin dose is 33 u and her fasting a.m. blood glucose is 240 mg/dL, what would her correction dose be?

VI.   Nutrition Monitoring and Evaluation

20. Write an ADIME note for your initial nutrition assessment.

21. When Rachel comes back to the clinic, she brings the following food and blood glucose record with her.

   a.   Determine the amount of carbohydrates she is consuming at each meal.

   b.   Determine whether she is taking adequate amounts of Apidra for each meal according to her record.

Time	Diet	Grams of CHO	Exercise	BG (mg/dL)	Insulin dosages	
					What patient took	What you would recommend
7:30 a.m.	2 Pop-Tarts 1 banana 16 oz skim milk with Ovaltine (2 tbsp)			(Pre) 150	5 u Apidra	
10:30 a.m.						
12 noon	2 slices of pepperoni pizza 2 chocolate chip cookies Water			(Pre) 180	6 u Apidra	
2 p.m.	Granola bar		PE class—30 minutes			

(Continued)

Time	Diet	Grams of CHO	Exercise	BG (mg/dL)	Insulin dosages	
					What patient took	What you would recommend
4:30 p.m.	Apple 6 saltines with 2 tbsp peanut butter			(Pre) 110		
5–6:30 p.m.	16 oz Gatorade		Soccer practice—1.5 hours	(Pre) 140		
6:30 p.m.	Chicken with broccoli stir-fry (1 c fried rice, 2 oz chicken, ½ c broccoli) Egg roll—1 2 c skim milk			(Pre) 80	5 u Apidra	
8:30 p.m.	2 c ice cream With 2 tbsp peanuts			(Pre) 150	4 u Apidra	
10:30 p.m.	Bed					

Bibliography

American Diabetes Association. Standards of medical care in diabetes—2015. *Diabetes Care*. 2015;38:S1–S94.

Atkinson MA, Eisenbarth GS, Michels AW. Type 1 diabetes. *Lancet*. 2014;383:69–82.

Chiang JL, Kirkman MS, Laffel LM, Peters AL. Type 1 diabetes through the life span: A position statement of the American Diabetes Association. *Diabetes Care*. 2014;37:2034–2054.

Hanas R, Donaghue KC, Klingensmith G, Swift PGF. ISPAD Clinical Practice Consensus Guidelines. *Pediatric Diabetes*. 2009;10:S1–S210.

Haas L, Maryniuk M, Beck J, et al. National standards for diabetes self-management education and support. *Diabetes Educ*. 2012;38:619–629.

Lawrence JM, Imperatore G, Dabelea D, et al. Trends in incidence of type 1 diabetes among non-hispanic white youth in the U.S., 2002–2009. *Diabetes*. 2014;63:3938–3945.

Nahikian-Nelms M. Diseases of the endocrine system. In: Nelms M, Sucher K, Lacey K. *Nutrition Therapy and Pathophysiology*. 3rd ed. Belmont, CA: Cengage Learning; 2016:469–520.

Stephens E. Insulin therapy in type 1 diabetes. *Med Clin North Am*. 2015;99:145–156.

Umpierrez G, Latif K, Murphy M, et al. Thyroid dysfunction in patients with Type 1 diabetes. *Diabetes Care*. 2003;26:1181–1185.

Internet Resources

AND Evidence Analysis Library: http://www.andeal.org

American Diabetes Association: http://www.diabetes.org/

International Society for Pediatric and Adolescent Diabetes: http://www.ispad.org/

JDRF Kids: http://jdrf.org/hello-jdrf-kids -online-community/

Pediatric Nutrition Care Manual: http://www .nutritioncaremanual.org

Type One Nation: http://typeonenation.org/

Case 17

Type 1 Diabetes Mellitus in the Adult

Objectives

After completing this case, the student will be able to:

1. Describe the pathophysiology of type 1, type 2, and latent autoimmune diabetes mellitus.
2. Discuss diagnostic criteria for type 1, type 2, and latent autoimmune diabetes mellitus.
3. Understand the acute complications of hyperglycemia and assess the appropriate medical and nutritional care for both HHS and DKA.
4. Develop a nutrition care plan—with appropriate measurable goals, interventions, and strategies for monitoring and evaluation—that addresses the nutrition diagnoses for this case.

5. Integrate an insulin regimen with nutrition therapy and provide appropriate recommendations for carbohydrate-to-insulin ratios and correction dosages.
6. Interpret laboratory parameters to assess fluid, electrolyte, and acid-base balance.
7. Prioritize survival skills and educational requirements for a newly diagnosed type 1 adult diabetic.

Matias Gutierrez is a 32-year-old male admitted from the ED to the endocrinology service with acute uncontrolled hyperglycemia.

Gutierrez, Matias, Male, 32 y.o.
Allergies: NKA   **Code:** FULL   **Isolation:** None
Pt. Location: 848   **Physician:** C. Harris   **Admit Date:** 7/1

Patient Summary: Matias Gutierrez is a 32-year-old male admitted from the ER to the endocrinology service.

History:
Onset of disease: Patient transported to ED when found ill in his apartment by a friend. During ED assessment, patient was noted to have serum glucose of 610 mg/dL. Mr. Gutierrez was diagnosed with T2DM one year ago and has been on metformin since that diagnosis. He does not take the medication regularly as he felt it really wasn't necessary.
Medical history: None
Surgical history: None
Medications at home: None
Tobacco use: Smoker 1 ppd × 10 years
Alcohol use: Daily
Family history: Father—MI; Mother—ovarian cancer, T2DM

Demographics:
Marital status: Divorced
Years education: 16
Language: English/Spanish
Occupation: Computer software engineer
Hours of work: 8–7 M–F, some weekends
Ethnicity: Hispanic
Religious affiliation: none

Admitting History/Physical:
Chief complaint: Friend states that Mr. Gutierrez had not been feeling well at work the previous day. He thought he was fighting off a virus. He did note that for the last few days Mr. Gutierrez had noticed increased thirst and increased frequency in urination. Mr. Gutierrez had mentioned this over coffee earlier in the week. When he didn't show up for work or answer his cell phone this morning, his friend went to check on him and found him groggy and almost unconscious at his apartment. He called 911 and patient was transported to University Hospital.
General appearance: Slim, Hispanic male, in obvious distress

Vital Signs: Temp: 99.6   Pulse: 100   Resp rate: 24
                    BP: 78/100   Height: 5'11"   Weight: 165 lbs

Heart: tachycardia
HEENT: Head: WNL
          Eyes: PERRLA
          Ears: Clear
          Nose: Clear
          Throat: Dry mucous membranes without exudates or lesions
Genitalia: Deferred
Neurologic: Lethargic but able to arouse. Follows commands appropriately. Glasgow Coma Scale: 13.

Gutierrez, Matias, Male, 32 y.o.
Allergies: NKA
Pt. Location: 848

Code: FULL
Physician: C. Harris

Isolation: None
Admit Date: 7/1

Extremities: +4 ROM; DTR 2+
Skin: Warm and dry
Chest/lungs: Respirations are rapid—clear to auscultation and percussion
Peripheral vascular: Pulse 4+ bilaterally, warm, no edema
Abdomen: Active bowel sounds ×4; tender, nondistended

Orders:

1. Regular insulin 1 unit/mL NS 40 mEq KCl/liter @ 300 mL/hr. Begin 6 units/hr and adjust according to the following: BG >360 6 u/h; 330–359 4 u/h; 240–299 3 u/h; 180–239 2 u; 120–179 1.5 u; 110–119 0.5 u; 70–109 0.2 u; <70 off. Flush new IV tubing with 50 mL of insulin drip solution prior to connecting to patient and starting insulin infusion.

2. Labs: BMP Stat
    Phos Stat
    Calcium Stat
    UA with culture if indicated Stat Clean catch
    Bedside glucose Stat
    Bedside I-Stat: EG7 Stat
    Islet cell autoantibodies screen (ICA)
    GADA
    TSH
    Comp metabolic panel (CMP)
    Thyroglobulin antibodies
    C-peptide
    Immunoglobulin A level
    Hemoglobin A$_{1c}$
    IgA-tTG; IgG-tTG

3. NPO except for ice chips and medications. After 12 hours, clear liquids when stable. Then, advance to carbohydrate-controlled diet—70–80 g breakfast and lunch; 85–95 g dinner; 30-gram snack pm and HS.

4. Consult diabetes education team for self-management training for patient to begin education after stabilized.

Nursing Assessment	7/1
Abdominal appearance (concave, flat, rounded, obese, distended)	flat
Palpation of abdomen (soft, rigid, firm, masses, tense)	tense with guarding
Bowel function (continent, incontinent, flatulence, no stool)	continent
Bowel sounds (P=present, AB=absent, hypo, hyper)	
RUQ	P
LUQ	P
RLQ	P

(Continued)

Gutierrez, Matias, Male, 32 y.o.
Allergies: NKA
Pt. Location: 848

Code: FULL
Physician: C. Harris

Isolation: None
Admit Date: 7/1

Nursing Assessment *(Continued)*

Nursing Assessment	7/1
LLQ	P
Stool color	light brown
Stool consistency	soft
Tubes/ostomies	NA
Genitourinary	
Urinary continence	catheter in place
Urine source	clean specimen
Appearance (clear, cloudy, yellow, amber, fluorescent, hematuria, orange, blue, tea)	cloudy, amber
Integumentary	
Skin color	pale
Skin temperature (DI=diaphoretic, W=warm, dry, CL=cool, CLM=clammy, CD+=cold, M=moist, H=hot)	DI; CLM
Skin turgor (good, fair, poor, TENT=tenting)	fair
Skin condition (intact, EC=ecchymosis, A=abrasions, P=petechiae, R=rash, W=weeping, S=sloughing, D=dryness, EX=excoriated, T=tears, SE=subcutaneous emphysema, B=blisters, V=vesicles, N=necrosis)	intact, D
Mucous membranes (intact, EC=ecchymosis, A=abrasions, P=petechiae, R=rash, W=weeping, S=sloughing, D=dryness, EX=excoriated, T=tears, SE=subcutaneous emphysema, B=blisters, V=vesicles, N=necrosis)	intact, D
Other components of Braden score: special bed, sensory pressure, moisture, activity, friction/shear (>18=no risk, 15–16=low risk, 13–14=moderate risk, ≤12=high risk)	21

Nutrition:

Meal type: NPO then progress to clear liquids and then consistent carbohydrate-controlled diet
Fluid requirement: 2200 mL
History: Usual intake (for past several months):
AM: Toast, jelly, coffee, and scrambled egg
Lunch: Subway sandwich, chips, diet soda
Dinner: Usually cooks pasta, rice, vegetables, and some type of meat; eats out 3–4 times per week at dinner.

MD Progress Note:

7/1 0700
Subjective: Matias Guiterrez previous 24 hours reviewed. Previously diagnosed with T2DM; treated with metformin but appears to not have taken it regularly.

Gutierrez, Matias, Male, 32 y.o.
Allergies: NKA
Pt. Location: 848

Code: FULL
Physician: C. Harris

Isolation: None
Admit Date: 7/1

Vitals: Temp: 99.5, Pulse: 82, Resp rate: 25, BP: 101/78
Urine output: 2660 mL (35.5 mL/kg)

Physical Exam
General: Alert and oriented to person, place, and time
HEENT: WNL
Neck: WNL
Heart: WNL
Lungs: Clear to auscultation
Abdomen: Active bowel sounds

Assessment/Plan: Results: +ICA, GADA, IAA consistent with type 1 DM vs LADA. Low C-peptide.

Dx: Suspect Type 1 Diabetes Mellitus vs latent autoimmune diabetes of adult (LADA)

Plan: Change IVF to D$_5$.45NS with 40 mEq K @ 135 mL/hr. Begin Novolog 0.5 u every 2 hours until glucose is 150–200 mg/dL. Tonight begin glargine 15 u at 9 pm. Progress Novolog using ICR 1:15. Continue bedside glucose checks hourly. Notify MD if blood glucose >200 or <80.
.... C. Harris, MD

Intake/Output

Date		7/1 0701–7/2 0700			
Time		0701–1500	1501–2300	2301–0700	Daily total
IN	P.O.	NPO	NPO	720	720
	I.V.	2,400	2,400	2,400	7,200
	(mL/kg/hr)	(4.0)	(4.0)	(4.0)	(4.0)
	I.V. piggyback				
	TPN				
	Total intake	2,400	2,400	3,120	7,920
	(mL/kg)	(32.0)	(32.0)	(41.6)	(105.6)
OUT	Urine	2,150	2,671	3,000	7,821
	(mL/kg/hr)	(3.58)	(4.45)	(5.00)	(4.34)
	Emesis output	150	0	0	150
	Other				
	Stool	0	×1	0	×1
	Total output	2,300	2,671	3,000	7,971
	(mL/kg)	(30.7)	(35.6)	(40.0)	(106.3)
Net I/O		+100	−271	+120	−51
Net since admission (7/1)		+100	−171	−51	−51

Gutierrez, Matias, Male, 32 y.o.
Allergies: NKA
Pt. Location: 848

Code: FULL
Physician: C. Harris

Isolation: None
Admit Date: 7/1

Laboratory Results

	Ref. Range	7/1 1780
Chemistry		
Sodium (mEq/L)	136–145	130 !↓
Potassium (mEq/L)	3.5–5.1	3.6
Chloride (mEq/L)	98–107	99
Carbon dioxide (CO_2, mEq/L)	23–29	31 !↑
Bicarbonate (mEq/L)	23–28	29 !↑
BUN (mg/dL)	6–20	18
Creatinine serum (mg/dL)	0.6–1.1 F 0.9–1.3 M	1.1
BUN/Crea ratio	10.0–20.0	16.3
Uric acid (mg/dL)	2.8–8.8 F 4.0–9.0 M	5.2
Est GFR, non-Afr Amer (mL/min/1.73 m^2)	>60	88
Glucose (mg/dL)	70–99	550 !↑
Phosphate, inorganic (mg/dL)	2.2–4.6	2.1 !↓
Magnesium (mg/dL)	1.5–2.4	1.9
Calcium (mg/dL)	8.6–10.2	10
Anion gap (mmol/L)	10–20	2.0 !↓
Osmolality (mmol/kg/H_2O)	275–295	304.4 !↑
Bilirubin total (mg/dL)	≤1.2	0.2
Bilirubin, direct (mg/dL)	<0.3	0.01
Protein, total (g/dL)	6–7.8	6.9
Albumin (g/dL)	3.5–5.5	4.4
Prealbumin (mg/dL)	18–35	32
Ammonia (NH_3, µg/L)	6–47	9
Alkaline phosphatase (U/L)	30–120	110
ALT (U/L)	4–36	6.2
AST (U/L)	0–35	21
CPK (U/L)	30–135 F 55–170 M	61
Lactate dehydrogenase (U/L)	208–378	229
Cholesterol (mg/dL)	<200	210 !↑

Gutierrez, Matias, Male, 32 y.o.
Allergies: NKA
Pt. Location: 848

Code: FULL
Physician: C. Harris

Isolation: None
Admit Date: 7/1

Laboratory Results *(Continued)*

	Ref. Range	7/1 1780
HDL-C (mg/dL)	>59 F, >50 M	38 !↓
VLDL (mg/dL)	7–32	35 !↑
LDL (mg/dL)	<130	137 !↑
LDL/HDL ratio	<3.22 F <3.55 M	3.6 !↑
Triglycerides (mg/dL)	35–135 F 40–160 M	175 !↑
T_4 (µg/dL)	5–12	7.2
T_3 (µg/dL)	75–98	81
HbA$_{1c}$ (%)	<5.7	10.2 !↑
C-peptide (ng/mL)	0.51–2.72	0.09 !↓
ICA	—	+ !↑
GADA	—	+ !↑
IA-2A	—	−
IAA	—	+ !↑
tTg IgA antibody (U/mL)	<4	1.2
tTg IgG antibody (U/mL)	<6	3.1
Hematology		
WBC (×10^3/mm^3)	3.9–10.7	10.6
RBC (×10^6/mm^3)	4.2–5.4 F 4.5–6.2 M	5.8
Urinalysis		
Collection method	—	catheter
Color	—	yellow
Appearance	—	clear
Specific gravity	1.001–1.035	1.008
pH	5–7	4.9 !↓
Protein (mg/dL)	Neg	+1 !↑
Glucose (mg/dL)	Neg	+3 !↑
Ketones	Neg	+4 !↑
Blood	Neg	Neg
Bilirubin	Neg	Neg
Nitrites	Neg	Neg

(Continued)

Gutierrez, Matias, Male, 32 y.o.
Allergies: NKA
Pt. Location: 848

Code: FULL
Physician: C. Harris

Isolation: None
Admit Date: 7/1

Laboratory Results *(Continued)*

	Ref. Range	7/1 1780
Urobilinogen (EU/dL)	<1.0	0.003
Leukocyte esterase	Neg	Neg
Prot chk	Neg	+1
WBCs (/HPF)	0–5	2
RBCs (/HPF)	0–2	1
Bact	0	0
Mucus	0	0
Crys	0	0
Casts (/LPF)	0	0
Yeast	0	0
Arterial Blood Gases (ABGs)		
pH	7.35–7.45	7.31 !↓
pCO_2 (mm Hg)	35–45	35
SO_2 (%)	≥95	97
CO_2 content (mmol/L)	25–30	28
O_2 content (%)	15–22	21
pO_2 (mm Hg)	≥80	93
HCO_3^- (mEq/L)	21–28	20 !↓
COHb (%)	<2	1.1

Note: Values and units of measurement listed in these tables are derived from several resources. Substantial variation exists in the ranges quoted as "normal" and these may vary depending on the assay used by different laboratories.

Case Questions

I.   Understanding the Diagnosis and Pathophysiology

1. What are the differences among T1DM, T2DM, and LADA?

2. What are the standard diagnostic criteria for each of these diagnoses?

3. Why do you think Matias was originally diagnosed with T2DM? Why does the MD now suspect he may actually have T1DM or LADA?

4. Describe the metabolic events that led to Matias's symptoms and subsequent admission to the ED (polyuria, polydipsia, polyphagia, fatigue, and weight loss), integrating the pathophysiology of T1DM into your discussion.

5. Describe the metabolic events that result in the signs and symptoms associated with DKA. Was Matias in this state when he was admitted? What precipitating factors may lead to DKA?

6. Matias will be started on a combination of Novolog prior to meals and snacks with glargine given in the p.m. Describe the onset, peak, and duration for each of these types of insulin.

7. Using his current weight of 165 lbs, determine the discharge dose of glargine as well as an appropriate ICR for Matias to start with.

8. Intensive insulin therapy requires frequent blood glucose self-monitoring. What are some of the barriers to success for patients who begin this type of therapy? Give suggestions on how you might work with Matias to support his compliance.

9. Matias tells you that he is very frightened of having his blood sugar drop too low. What is hypoglycemia? What are the symptoms? What information would you give to Matias to make sure he is well prepared to prevent or treat hypoglycemia?

10. Matias's mother has T2DM. She is currently having problems with vision and burning in her feet. What is she most likely experiencing? Describe the pathophysiology of these complications. You can tell that Matias is worried not only about his mother but also about his own health. Explain, using the results of the Diabetes Control and Complications Trial (DCCT) as well as any other pertinent research data, how he can prevent these complications.

II.   Understanding the Nutrition Therapy

11. Outline the basic principles for Matias's nutrition therapy to assist in control of his DM.

III.   Nutrition Assessment

12. Assess Matias's height and weight. Calculate his BMI.

13. Identify any abnormal laboratory values measured upon his admission. Explain how they may be related to his newly diagnosed DM.

14. Determine Matias's energy and protein requirements. Be sure to explain what standards you used to make this estimation. Would you recommend that he either gain or lose weight in the future?

IV.   Nutrition Diagnosis

15. Prioritize two nutrition problems and complete the PES statement for each.

V.   Nutrition Intervention

16. Determine Matias's initial CHO prescription using his usual intake at home as a guideline, as well as your assessment of his energy requirements. What nutrition education material would you use to teach Matias CHO counting?

17. Matias's usual breakfast consists of 2 slices of toast, butter, 2 tbsp jelly, 2 scrambled eggs, and orange juice (~1 c). Using the ICR that you calculated in question #7, how much Novolog should he take to cover the carbohydrate in this meal?

18. Using the ADA guidelines, what would be appropriate fasting and postprandial target glucose levels for Matias?

VI.   Nutrition Monitoring and Evaluation

19. Write an ADIME note for your initial nutrition assessment.

20. Matias comes back to the clinic 2 weeks after his diagnosis. List the key questions you will ask him in order to plan the next steps for providing any additional education that he needs.

21. Matias states that he would like to start exercising again as he is feeling better. He is used to playing tennis several times per week as well as cycling at least 2 days per week for over 20 miles each time. Again, he expresses his concern regarding low blood sugar. How would you counsel Matias regarding physical activity, his diet, and his blood glucose monitoring?

22. Matias states that one of his friends has talked about using the glycemic index as a way to manage his diabetes. He says that he has also seen some television commercials advertising food products as being "low glycemic index." Explain glycemic index, glycemic load, and how he might use this information within his nutrition therapy plans.

Bibliography

Academy of Nutrition and Dietetics Nutrition Care Manual. Type 1 Diabetes Mellitus. https://www.nutritioncaremanual.org/topic.cfm?ncm_category_id=1&lv1=5517&lv2=18399&ncm_toc_id=18399&ncm_heading=Nutrition%20Care. Accessed 5/5/15.

American Diabetes Association. Standards of medical care in diabetes—2015. *Diabetes Care*. 2015;38:S1–S94.

Barclay AW, Brand-Miller JC, Wolever TMS. Glycemic index, glycemic load, and glycemic response are not the same. *Diabetes Care*. 2005;28:1839–1840.

Craig J. Carbohydrate counting, glycemic index, and glycemic load. Putting them all together. *Diabetes Self Manag*. 2012;29:41–50.

Davidson N, Moreland P. Overcoming barriers to self-monitoring of blood glucose. *Mayo Clin Patient Care Health Info*. 2009. ttp://www.mayoclinic.org/diseases-conditions/diabetes/expert-blog/blood-glucose/bgp-20056587. Accessed 5/5/15.

Diabetes Complication and Control Trial Study Research Group. Intensive diabetes treatment and cardiovascular disease in patients with type 1 diabetes. *NEJM*. 2005;353:2643–2653.

Esfahani A, Wong JM, Mirrahimi A, et al. The application of the glycemic index and glycemic load in weight loss: A review of the clinical evidence. *IUBMB Life*. 2011;63:7–13.

Evert AB, Boucher JL, Cypress M, et al. Nutrition therapy recommendations for the management of adults with diabetes. *Diabetes Care*. 2013;36:3821–3842.

Haas L, Maryniuk M, Beck J, et al. National standards for diabetes self-management education and support. *Diabetes Educ*. 2012;38:619–629.

Hayes C, Kriska A. Role of physical activity in diabetes management and prevention. *J Am Diet Assoc*. 2008;108:S19–S23.

Hortensius K, Kars MC, Wierenga WS, et al. Perspectives of patients with type 1 or insulin-treated type 2 diabetes on self-monitoring of blood glucose: A qualitative study. *BMC Public Health*. 2012;12:167–179.

Lachin JM, White NH, Hainsworth DP, et al. Effect of intensive diabetes therapy on the progression of diabetic retinopathy in patients with type 1 diabetes: 18 years of follow-up in the DCCT/EDIC. *Diabetes*. 2015;64:631–642.

Laugesen E, Ostergaard J, Leslie R. Latent autoimmune diabetes of the adult: Current knowledge and uncertainty. *Diabet Med*. 2015;37:843–852.

Liao Y, Xiang Y, Zhou H. Diagnostic criteria of latent autoimmune diabetes in adults (LADA): A review and reflection. *Front Med*. 2012;6:243–247.

Malanda UL, Welschen LM, Riphagen II, et al. Self-monitoring of blood glucose in patients with type 2 diabetes mellitus who are not using insulin. *Cochrane Database Syst Rev*. 2012;1:AN:CD004060; PMID:22258959.

McNaughton CD, Self WH, Slovis C. Diabetes in the emergency department: Acute care of diabetes patients. *Clin Diabetes*. 2011;29:51–59.

Medeiros D, Wildman R. *Advanced Human Nutrition*. 3rd ed. Burlington, MA: Jones and Bartlett Learning. 2015.

Nelms MN. Diseases of the endocrine system. In: Nelms M, Sucher K, Lacey K, Roth SL. *Nutrition Therapy and Pathophysiology*. 3rd ed. Belmont, CA: Cengage Learning; 2016:469–520.

Ong WM, Chua SS, Ng CJ. Barriers and facilitators to self-monitoring of blood glucose in people with type 2 diabetes using insulin: A qualitative study. *Patient Prefer Adherence*. 2014;8:237–246.

Stenstr P G, Gottsotts A, Bakhtadze E, Berger B, Sundkvist G. Latent autoimmune diabetes in adults definition, prevalence, cell function, and treatment. *Diabetes*. 2005;54(suppl 2):S68–S72.

Internet Resources

American Diabetes Association: http://www.diabetes.org/
AND Evidence Analysis Library: http://www.andeal.org

Nutrition Care Manual: http://www.nutritioncaremanual.org

Adult Type 1 Blogs and Social Media

A Sweet Life: asweetlife.org
Close Concerns: www.closeconcerns.com
Diabetes Daily: www.diabetesdaily.com

Adult Type 2 Diabetes Mellitus: Transition to Insulin

Objectives

After completing this case, the student will be able to:

1. Describe the pathophysiology of type 2 diabetes mellitus and hyperglycemic hyperosmolar state.
2. Explain the pharmacology of oral medications for type 2 DM.
3. Integrate an insulin regimen with nutrition therapy and provide appropriate recommendations for carbohydrate-to-insulin ratios and correction dosages.
4. Develop a nutrition care plan—with appropriate measurable goals, interventions, and strategies for monitoring and evaluation—that addresses the nutrition diagnoses for this case.
5. Explain the appropriate use and interpretation of self-monitoring of blood glucose to adjust rapid-acting insulin.

Mr. Fagan is a 53-year-old with type 2 diabetes mellitus who has a history of noncompliance. He is admitted through the ED with severe hyperglycemia and dehydration.

Fagan, Mitchell, Male, 53 y.o.
Allergies: NKA
Pt. Location: MICU Bed #5

Code: FULL
Physician: R. Petersen

Isolation: None
Admit Date: 4/12

Patient Summary: Mitchell Fagan is a 53-year-old male admitted with acute hyperglycemia and probable HHS.

History:

Onset of disease: Patient's coworker became concerned when patient did not report to work or answer his phone when called. Coworker went to patient's home and found him drowsy and confused. Took patient to ED, where patient was noted to have serum glucose of 855 mg/dL.
Medical history: Type 2 DM × 1 year—prescribed glyburide and metformin but admits that he has not taken the medications regularly; HTN; hyperlipidemia; gout
Surgical history: ORIF R ulna; hernia repair
Medications at home: Glyburide 20 mg daily; 500 mg metformin twice daily; Dyazide once daily (25 mg hydrochlorothiazide and 37.5 mg triamterene); Lipitor 20 mg daily
Tobacco use: 1 ppd ×20 years—now quit
Alcohol use: 3–4 drinks per week
Family history: Father—HTN, CAD; mother—type 2 DM

Demographics:

Marital status: Single
Years education: 16
Language: English only
Occupation: Retired military—now works as consultant to military equipment company
Hours of work: 8–5 daily
Household members: NA—lives alone
Ethnicity: Caucasian
Religious affiliation: NA

Admitting History/Physical:

Chief complaint: "I had a lot of vomiting that I thought at first was food poisoning but I just kept getting worse." When questioned about medications, patient admits that he has not taken medications for the diabetes regularly—"I hate how they make me feel but I almost always take my other medications for blood pressure and cholesterol."
General appearance: Obese, 53-year-old male.

Vital Signs: Temp: 100.5   Pulse: 105   Resp rate: 26
                   BP: 90/70   Height: 5'9"   Weight: 214 lbs

Heart: Regular rate and rhythm
HEENT: Head: WNL
          Eyes: PERRLA
          Ears: Clear
          Nose: Clear
          Throat: Dry mucous membranes without exudates or lesions
Genitalia: Deferred
Neurologic: Alert but previously drowsy with mild confusion

Fagan, Mitchell, Male, 53 y.o.
Allergies: NKA   **Code:** FULL   **Isolation:** None
Pt. Location: MICU Bed #5   **Physician:** R. Petersen   **Admit Date:** 4/12

Extremities: Noncontributory
Skin: Warm and dry; poor turgor
Chest/lungs: Respirations are rapid—clear to auscultation and percussion
Peripheral vascular: Pulse 4 + bilaterally, warm, no edema
Abdomen: Active bowel sounds ×4; tender, nondistended

Orders:

1. Replace 1 L NS stat. Then begin regular insulin. 1 unit/kg/hr in NS 40 mEq KCl/liter @ 500 mL/ hr ×3 hours. Then regular insulin 1 unit/mL NS 10 mEq KCl/liter @135 mL/hr. Flush new IV tubing with 50 mL of insulin drip solution prior to connecting to patient and starting insulin infusion.

2. Labs: BMP, Phos, Calcium
   UA with culture Stat Clean catch
   Bedside glucose Stat
   Bedside I-Stat: EG7 Stat
   Islet cell autoantibodies screen
   Thyroid peroxidase antibodies; TSH; Thyroglobulin antibodies
   Comp metabolic panel (CMP); Hematology panel
   C-peptide
   Hemoglobin A_{1c}
   Tissue transglutaminase antibodies

3. NPO except for ice chips and medications. After 12 hours, clear liquids if stable. Then, advance to consistent-carbohydrate diet. Consult dietitian for advancement, total carbohydrate Rx, and distribution.

4. Consult diabetes education team for self-management training for patient after stabilized and when transferred to floor.

Nursing Assessment	4/12
Abdominal appearance (concave, flat, rounded, obese, distended)	obese
Palpation of abdomen (soft, rigid, firm, masses, tense)	tense
Bowel function (continent, incontinent, flatulence, no stool)	continent
Bowel sounds (P=present, AB=absent, hypo, hyper)	
RUQ	P
LUQ	P
RLQ	P
LLQ	P
Stool color	light brown
Stool consistency	soft
Tubes/ostomies	NA

(Continued)

Fagan, Mitchell, Male, 53 y.o.
Allergies: NKA
Pt. Location: MICU Bed #5

Code: FULL
Physician: R. Petersen

Isolation: None
Admit Date: 4/12

Nursing Assessment *(Continued)*

Nursing Assessment	4/12
Genitourinary	
Urinary continence	yes
Urine source	clean specimen
Appearance (clear, cloudy, yellow, amber, fluorescent, hematuria, orange, blue, tea)	cloudy, amber
Integumentary	
Skin color	pale
Skin temperature (DI=diaphoretic, W=warm, dry, CL=cool, CLM=clammy, CD+=cold, M=moist, H=hot)	DI
Skin turgor (good, fair, poor, TENT=tenting)	poor
Skin condition (intact, EC=ecchymosis, A=abrasions, P=petechiae, R=rash, W=weeping, S=sloughing, D=dryness, EX=excoriated, T=tears, SE=subcutaneous emphysema, B=blisters, V=vesicles, N=necrosis)	intact
Mucous membranes (intact, EC=ecchymosis, A=abrasions, P=petechiae, R=rash, W=weeping, S=sloughing, D=dryness, EX=excoriated, T=tears, SE=subcutaneous emphysema, B=blisters, V=vesicles, N=necrosis)	intact
Other components of Braden score: special bed, sensory pressure, moisture, activity, friction/shear (>18=no risk, 15–16=low risk, 13–14=moderate risk, ≤12=high risk)	20

Nutrition:

Meal type: NPO, then progress to clear liquids and then consistent carbohydrate-controlled diet
Fluid requirement: 2000–2500 mL after rehydration
History: Patient states that he really doesn't follow any strict diet except for not adding salt—tries to avoid high-cholesterol foods and stays away from high-sugar desserts. Most recently he had experienced vomiting for approximately 12–24 hours and so had not eaten anything and only had sips of water. He has never seen anyone for diabetes teaching, beyond what his physician has told him.
Usual intake (for past several months):

AM:	Coffee with half and half
Midmorning:	Bagel with cream cheese, 2–3 c of coffee
Lunch:	Out at restaurant—usually Jimmy John's or fast-food sandwich, chips, and diet soda
Dinner:	Cooks sometimes at home—this would be grilled chicken or beef, salad, and potatoes or rice. Often will meet friends for dinner—likes all foods and especially likes to try different ethnic foods such as Chinese, Mexican, Indian, or Thai.

MD Progress Note:

4/13 0750
Subjective: Mitchell Fagan's previous 24 hours reviewed
Vitals: Temp: 99.6, Pulse: 83, Resp rate: 25, BP: 129/92

Fagan, Mitchell, Male, 53 y.o.
Allergies: NKA
Pt. Location: MICU Bed #5

Code: FULL
Physician: R. Petersen

Isolation: None
Admit Date: 4/12

Physical Exam
General: Alert and oriented to person, place, and time
Neck: WNL
Heart: WNL
Lungs: Clear to auscultation
Abdomen: Active bowel sounds

Assessment/Plan:

Results: Negative ICA, GADA, IAA, negative tTg, +C-peptide with insulin level indicating T2DM—now requiring insulin at home

Dx: Type 2 DM uncontrolled with HHS

Plan: Change IVF to $D_5.45NS$ with 20MEq K @ 135 mL/hr. Begin Lispro 0.5 u every 2 hours until glucose is 150–200 mg/dL. Tonight begin glargine 19 u at 9 pm. Progress Lispro using ICR 1:15. Continue bedside glucose checks hourly. Notify MD if blood glucose >200 or <80.
.... R. Peterson, MD

Intake/Output

Date		4/12 0701–4/13 0700			
Time		0701–1500	1501–2300	2301–0700	Daily total
IN	P.O.	**NPO**	NPO	NPO	
	I.V.	**2,175**	**1,080**	**1,080**	**4,335**
	(mL/kg/hr)	(2.80)	(1.39)	(1.39)	(1.86)
	I.V. piggyback	**0**	**0**	**0**	**0**
	TPN	**0**	**0**	**0**	**0**
	Total intake	**2,175**	**1,080**	**1,080**	**4,335**
	(mL/kg)	(22.4)	(11.1)	(11.1)	(44.6)
OUT	Urine	**1,100**	**450**	**525**	**2,075**
	(mL/kg/hr)	(1.41)	(0.58)	(0.67)	(0.89)
	Emesis output	**120**	**0**	**0**	**120**
	Other	**0**	**0**	**0**	**0**
	Stool	**0**	×1	**0**	
	Total output	**1,220**	**450**	**525**	**2,195**
	(mL/kg)	(12.5)	(4.6)	(5.4)	(22.6)
Net I/O		**+955**	**+630**	**+555**	**+2,140**
Net since admission (4/12)		**+955**	**+1,585**	**+2,140**	**+2,140**

Fagan, Mitchell, Male, 53 y.o.
Allergies: NKA
Pt. Location: MICU Bed #5

Code: FULL
Physician: R. Petersen

Isolation: None
Admit Date: 4/12

Laboratory Results

	Ref. Range	4/12 1780	4/13 1522
Chemistry			
Sodium (mEq/L)	136–145	132 !↓	135 !↓
Potassium (mEq/L)	3.5–5.1	3.9	4.0
Chloride (mEq/L)	98–107	101	100
Carbon dioxide (CO_2, mEq/L)	23–29	27	28
Bicarbonate (mEq/L)	23–28	25	24
BUN (mg/dL)	6–20	31 !↑	20
Creatinine serum (mg/dL)	0.6–1.1 F 0.9–1.3 M	1.9 !↑	1.3
BUN/Crea ratio	10.0–20.0	16	15.3
Uric acid (mg/dL)	2.8–8.8 F 4.0–9.0 M	5.3	5.9
Est GFR, non-Afr Amer (mL/min/1.73 m^2)	>60	39 !↓	62
Glucose (mg/dL)	70–99	855 !↑	475 !↑
Phosphate, inorganic (mg/dL)	2.2–4.6	1.8 !↓	2.1 !↓
Magnesium (mg/dL)	1.5–2.4	1.9	2.1
Calcium (mg/dL)	8.6–10.2	10	9.8
Anion gap (mmol/L)	10–20	6.0 !↓	11
Osmolality (mmol/kg/H_2O)	275–295	322.6 !↑	303.5 !↑
Bilirubin total (mg/dL)	≤1.2	0.9	
Bilirubin, direct (mg/dL)	< 0.3	0.019	
Protein, total (g/dL)	6–7.8	7.1	
Albumin (g/dL)	3.5–5.5	4.9	
Prealbumin (mg/dL)	18–35	33	
Ammonia (NH_3, µg/L)	6–47	15	
Alkaline phosphatase (U/L)	30–120	112	
ALT (U/L)	4–36	21	
AST (U/L)	0–35	17	
CPK (U/L)	30–135 F 55–170 M	145	
Lactate dehydrogenase (U/L)	208–378	275	
Cholesterol (mg/dL)	<200	205 !↑	
HDL-C (mg/dL)	>59 F, >50 M	55	

Fagan, Mitchell, Male, 53 y.o.
Allergies: NKA
Pt. Location: MICU Bed #5

Code: FULL
Physician: R. Petersen

Isolation: None
Admit Date: 4/12

Laboratory Results (Continued)

	Ref. Range	4/12 1780	4/13 1522
VLDL (mg/dL)	7–32	37 !↑	
LDL (mg/dL)	<130	123	
LDL/HDL ratio	<3.22 F <3.55 M	2.24	
Triglycerides (mg/dL)	35–135 F 40–160 M	185 !↑	
T_4 (μg/dL)	5–12	12	
T_3 (μg/dL)	75–98	77	
HbA$_{1C}$ (%)	<5.7	11.5 !↑	
C-peptide (ng/mL)	0.51–2.72	1.10	
ICA	—	Neg	
GADA	—	Neg	
IA-2A	—	Neg	
IAA	—	Neg	
tTg IgA antibody (U/mL)	<4	2	
tTg IgG antibody (U/mL)	<6	1	
Hematology			
WBC (×10^3/mm^3)	3.9–10.7	13.5 !↑	
RBC (×10^6/mm^3)	4.2–5.4 F 4.5–6.2 M	6.1	
Hemoglobin (Hgb, g/dL)	12–16 F 14–17 M	14.5	
Hematocrit (Hct, %)	37–47 F 41–51 M	57 !↑	
Urinalysis			
Collection method	—	Clean catch	
Color	—	Amber	
Appearance	—	Cloudy	
Specific gravity	1.001–1.035	1.045 !↑	
pH	5–7	5.1	
Protein	Neg	10 !↑	
Glucose	Neg	+3 !↑	
Ketones	Neg	+1 !↑	

(Continued)

Fagan, Mitchell, Male, 53 y.o.
Allergies: NKA
Pt. Location: MICU Bed #5

Code: Full
Physician: R. Petersen

Isolation: None
Admit Date: 4/12

Laboratory Results *(Continued)*

	Ref. Range	4/12 1780	4/13 1522
Blood	Neg	Neg	
Bilirubin	Neg	Neg	
Nitrites	Neg	Neg	
Urobilinogen (EU/dL)	<1.0	0.01	
Leukocyte esterase	Neg	Neg	
Prot chk	Neg	+	
WBCs (/HPF)	0–5	3	
RBCs (/HPF)	0–2	1	
Bact	0	0	
Mucus	0	0	
Crys	0	0	
Casts (/LPF)	0	0	
Yeast	0	0	

Note: Values and units of measurement listed in these tables are derived from several resources. Substantial variation exists in the ranges quoted as "normal" and these may vary depending on the assay used by different laboratories.

Case Questions

I.   Understanding the Diagnosis and Pathophysiology

1. What are the standard diagnostic criteria for T2DM? Identify those found in Mitch's medical record.

2. Mitch was previously diagnosed with T2DM. He admits that he often does not take his medications. What types of medications are metformin and glyburide? Describe their mechanisms as well as their potential side effects/drug–nutrient interactions.

3. What other medications does Mitch take? List their mechanisms and potential side effects/drug–nutrient interactions.

4. Describe the metabolic events that led to Mitch's symptoms and subsequent admission to the ER with the diagnosis of uncontrolled T2DM with HHS (be sure to include the information in Mitch's chart that supports his diagnosis. Compare and contrast HHS with the other common clinical emergency condition of diabetes—diabetic ketoacidosis (DKA).

5. HHS is often associated with dehydration. After reading Mitch's chart, list the data that are consistent with dehydration. What factors in Mitch's history may have contributed to his dehydration?

6. Assess Mitch's intake/output record for the first 24 hours of his admission. What does this tell you? Assuming that Mitch tells you that his usual weight is 228 lbs, can you estimate the volume of his dehydration?

7. Mitch was started on normal saline with potassium as well as an insulin drip. Why are these fluids a component of his rehydration and correction of the HHS?

8. Describe the insulin therapy that was started for Mitch. What is Lispro? What is glargine? How likely is it that Mitch will need to continue insulin therapy?

II.   Understanding the Nutrition Therapy

9.Mitch was NPO when admitted to the hospital. What does this mean? What are the signs that will alert the RD and physician that Mitch may be ready to eat?

10. Outline the basic principles for Mitch's nutrition therapy to assist in control of his DM.

III.   Nutrition Assessment

11. Assess Mitch's weight and BMI. What would be a healthy weight range for Mitch?

12. Identify and discuss any abnormal laboratory values measured upon his admission. How did they change after hydration and initial treatment of his HHS?

13. Determine Mitch's energy and protein requirements for weight maintenance. What energy and protein intakes would you recommend to assist with weight loss?

IV.   Nutrition Diagnosis

14. Prioritize two nutrition problems and complete the PES statement for each.

V.   Nutrition Intervention

15. Determine Mitch's initial CHO prescription using his diet history as well as your assessment of his energy requirements.

16. Identify two initial nutrition goals to assist with weight loss.

17. Mitch also has hypertension and high cholesterol levels. Describe how your nutrition interventions for diabetes can include nutrition therapy for his other conditions.

VI.   Nutrition Monitoring and Evaluation

18. Write an ADIME note for your initial nutrition assessment.

Bibliography

Academy of Nutrition and Dietetics Nutrition Care Manual. Type 2 Diabetes Mellitus. https://www.nutritioncaremanual.org/topic.cfm?ncm_category_id=1&lv1=5517&lv2=18469&ncm_toc_id=18469&ncm_heading=Nutrition20Care. Accessed 05/06/15.

American Diabetes Association. Standards of medical care in diabetes—2015. *Diabetes Care.* 2015;38:S1–S94.

Chaithongdi N, Subauste JS, Koch CA, Geraci SA. Diagnosis and management of hyperglycemic emergencies. *Hormones.* 2011;10:250–260.

Corwell B, Knight B, Olivieri L, Willis GC. Current diagnosis and treatment of hyperglycemic emergencies. *Emergency Medicine Clinics of North America.* 2014;32:437–452.

Hemphill R.R. Hyperosmolar hyperglycemic state. Available from: http://emedicine.medscape.com/article/1914705-overview. Accessed 05/06/15.

Kitabchi AE, Umpierrex GE, Fisher JN, Murph Stentz FB. Thirty years of personal experience in hyperglycemic crises: Diabetic ketoacidosis and hyperglycemic hyperosmolar state. *J Clin Endocrinol Metab.* 2008;93:1541–1552.

Mayo Clinic. Dehydration symptoms. *Mayo Clinic Patient Care Health Info.* 2014. http://www.mayoclinic.org/diseases-conditions/dehydration/basics/symptoms/con-20030056. Accessed 05/06/15.

McNaughten CD, Self WH, Slovis C. Diabetes in the emergency department: Acute care of diabetes patients. *Clinical Diabetes.* 2011;29:51–59.

Nahikian-Nelms M. Diseases of the endocrine system. In: Nelms MN, Sucher K, Lacey K. *Nutrition Therapy and Pathophysiology.* 3rd ed. Belmont, CA: Cengage; 2016:469–520.

Nyenwe EA, Kitabchi AE. Evidence-based management of hyperglycemic emergencies in diabetes mellitus. *Diabetes Res Clin Prac.* 2011;94:340–351.

Pasquel FJ, Umpierrez GE. Hyperosmolar hyperglycemic state: A historic review of the clinical presentation, diagnosis, and treatment. *Diabetes Care.* 2014;37:3124–3131.

Umpierrez G, Murphy M, Kitabchi A. Diabetic ketoacidosis and hyperglycemic hyperosmolar syndrome. *Diabetes Spectrum.* 2002;15:28–36.

Internet Resources

American Diabetes Association: http://www.diabetes.org/

AND Evidence Analysis Library: http://www.andeal.org

The Metabolomics Innovation Centre (TMIC): Drug Bank: http://www.drugbank.ca/

Unit Seven

NUTRITION THERAPY FOR RENAL DISORDERS

There has been a noticeable growth in the field of medical nutrition therapy for patients with chronic kidney disease (CKD). The importance of nutrition in the care of patients with CKD is illustrated by the fact that indicators of nutritional status effectively predict morbidity and mortality in these patients. In 2011, over 20 million Americans had clinical evidence of kidney disease. Of this number, more than 85,000 Americans die each year because of kidney disease, and more than 485,000 suffer from advanced CKD and need renal replacement therapy to remain alive. Kidney disease is one of the costliest illnesses. In 2011, more than $42.5 billion was spent on renal replacement therapy (available at: http://www.niddk.nih.gov/health-information/health-statistics/Pages/kidney-disease-statistics-united-states.aspx, accessed May 10, 2015).

The primary cause of CKD is diabetes mellitus, which accounts for about 44 percent of all new cases each year. Uncontrolled hypertension is the second leading cause of CKD in the United States.

Cases 19 and 20 represent the progression of renal disease and the most common forms of renal replacement therapy—hemodialysis and peritoneal dialysis. Integrated into each case are factors that predispose an individual to CKD, such as diabetes mellitus and ethnicity. Incidence in African Americans is three times the rate seen in Caucasians. Researchers from the National Institutes of Health have established that CKD caused by diabetes mellitus is anywhere from 10 to 75 times more prevalent in Native Americans than in Caucasians, and the prevalence differs among tribes; 50 percent of Pima Indians age 35 years and over have type 2 diabetes mellitus—the highest rate in the world. Fundamental principles such as modification of nutrient composition in impaired renal function, CKD, and renal replacement therapy are included within these cases. Case 21 focuses on acute kidney injury (AKI). There are a large number of critically ill patients who experience AKI as a complication of their illness. You will use nutrition support and evidenced-based guidelines to determine the appropriate nutritional care for this patient.

Case 19

Chronic Kidney Disease (CKD) Treated with Dialysis

Objectives

After completing this case, the student will be able to:

1. Describe the pathophysiology of chronic kidney disease (CKD).
2. Describe the stages of CKD.
3. Differentiate between the mechanisms of peritoneal dialysis and hemodialysis.
4. Identify and explain common nutritional problems associated with CKD.
5. Interpret laboratory parameters for nutritional implications and significance.
6. Analyze nutrition assessment data to evaluate nutritional status and identify specific nutrition problems.
7. Determine nutrition diagnoses and write appropriate PES statements.
8. Develop a nutrition care plan—with appropriate measurable goals, interventions, and strategies for monitoring and evaluation—that addresses the nutrition diagnoses of this case.
9. Integrate sociocultural and ethnic food consumption issues within a nutrition care plan.
10. Make appropriate documentation in the medical record.

Enez Joaquin is a 24-year-old Pima Indian who has had type 2 diabetes mellitus since age 13. Mrs. Joaquin has experienced a declining glomerular filtration rate for the past two years. She is being admitted in preparation for kidney replacement therapy.

Joaquin, Enez, Female, 24 y.o.
Allergies: NKA
Pt. Location: RM 207

Code: FULL
Physician: L. Nila

Isolation: None
Admit Date: 3/5

Patient Summary: Mrs. Joaquin is a 24-year-old Native American woman who was diagnosed with type 2 DM when she was 13 years old and has been poorly compliant with prescribed treatment.

History:

Onset of disease: Diagnosed with Stage 3 chronic kidney disease 2 years ago. Her acute symptoms have developed over the last 2 weeks.

Medical history: Gravida 1/ para 1. Infant weighed 10 lbs at birth 7 years ago. Pt admits she recently stopped taking a prescribed hypoglycemic agent, and she has never filled her prescription for anti-hypertensive medication. Progressive decompensation of kidney function has been documented by declining GFR, increasing creatinine and urea concentrations, elevated serum phosphate, and normochromic, normocytic anemia. She is being admitted for preparation for kidney-replacement therapy.

Surgical history: No surgeries

Medications at home: Glucophage (metformin), 850 mg twice daily

Tobacco use: No

Alcohol use: Yes, 1–2 12-oz beers daily

Family history: What? T2DM. Who? Parents.

Demographics:

Marital status: Married—lives with husband and daughter; *Spouse name:* Eddie

Number of children: 1

Years education: High school

Language: English and Akimel O'odham (Pima)

Occupation: Secretary

Hours of work: 9–5

Ethnicity: Pima Indian

Religious affiliation: Catholic

5' 170 lb

Admitting History/Physical:

Chief complaint: Pt complains of anorexia; N/V; 4-kg weight gain in the past 2 weeks; edema in extremities, face, and eyes; malaise; progressive SOB with 3-pillow orthopnea; pruritus; muscle cramps; and inability to urinate

General appearance: Overweight Native American female who appears her age; lethargic, complaining of N/V.

Vital Signs: Temp: 98.6   Pulse: 86   Resp rate: 25
                   BP: 220/80   Height: 5'0" 152 4   Weight: 170 lbs 77.3 kg

Heart: S4, S1, and S2, regular rate and rhythm. I/VI systolic ejection murmur, upper-left sternal border.
HEENT: Head: Normocephalic, equal carotid pulses, neck supple, no bruits
          Eyes: PERRLA
          Ears: Noncontributory

BMI: 33.5

2, 3?

152.5
adjusted
BW

100 #

Joaquin, Enez, Female, 24 y.o.
Allergies: NKA
Pt. Location: RM 207

Code: FULL
Physician: L. Nila

Isolation: None
Admit Date: 3/5

Nose: Noncontributory
Throat: Noncontributory
Genitalia: Normal female
Neurologic: Oriented to person, place, and time; intact, mild asterixis
Extremities: Muscle weakness; 3+ pitting edema to the knees, no cyanosis
Skin: Dry and yellowish-brown
Chest/lungs: Generalized rhonchi with rales that are mild at the bases (Pt breathes with poor effort)
Peripheral vascular: Normal pulse (3+) bilaterally L
Abdomen: Bowel sounds positive, soft; generalized mild tenderness; no rebound

Nursing Assessment	3/5
Abdominal appearance (concave, flat, rounded, obese, distended)	rounded, obese
Palpation of abdomen (soft, rigid, firm, masses, tense)	soft
Bowel function (continent, incontinent, flatulence, no stool)	continent
Bowel sounds (P=present, AB=absent, hypo, hyper)	
RUQ	P
LUQ	P
RLQ	P
LLQ	P
Stool color	brown
Stool consistency	formed
Tubes/ostomies	N/A
Genitourinary	
Urinary continence	N/A
Urine source	N/A
Appearance (clear, cloudy, yellow, amber, fluorescent, hematuria, orange, blue, tea)	N/A
Integumentary	
Skin color	light brown
Skin temperature (DI=diaphoretic, W=warm, dry, CL=cool, CLM=clammy, CD += cold, M=moist, H=hot)	W
Skin turgor (good, fair, poor, TENT=tenting)	good
Skin condition (intact, EC=ecchymosis, A=abrasions, P=petechiae, R=rash, W=weeping, S=sloughing, D=dryness, EX=excoriated, T=tears, SE=subcutaneous emphysema, B=blisters, V=vesicles, N=necrosis)	intact, A
Mucous membranes (intact, EC=ecchymosis, A=abrasions, P=petechiae, R=rash, W=weeping, S=sloughing, D=dryness, EX=excoriated, T=tears, SE=subcutaneous emphysema, B=blisters, V=vesicles, N= necrosis)	intact

(Continued)

Joaquin, Enez, Female, 24 y.o.
Allergies: NKA   **Code:** FULL   **Isolation:** None
Pt. Location: RM 207   **Physician:** L. Nila   **Admit Date:** 3/5

Nursing Assessment *(Continued)*

Nursing Assessment	3/5
Other components of Braden score: special bed, sensory pressure, moisture, activity, friction/shear (>18=no risk, 15–16=low risk, 13–14= moderate risk, <12=high risk)	activity, 16

Orders:
Evaluate for kidney replacement therapy
Capoten/captopril 25 mg twice daily
Erythropoietin (r-HuEPO) 30 units/kg
Sodium bicarbonate 2 g daily
Renal caps—1 daily
Renvela—three times daily with each meal
Hectorol 2.5 pg four times daily 3 times/week
Glucophage (metformin) 850 mg twice daily
35 kcal/kg, 1.2 g protein/kg, 2 g K, 1 g phosphorus, 2 g Na, 1000 mL fluid + urine output per day
CBC, chemistry
Stool softener
Occult fecal blood
Nutrition consult

Nutrition:
History: Intake has been poor due to anorexia, N&V. Patient states that she tried to follow the diet that she was taught two years ago. "It went pretty well for a while, but it was hard to keep up with."
Usual dietary intake:
Breakfast: Cold cereal
                Bread or fried potatoes
                Fried egg (occasionally)
                Coffee
Lunch: Bologna sandwich
                Potato chips
                Coke
Dinner: Chili con carne
                Indian fry bread
                Iced tea
Snacks: Crackers and peanut butter
Food allergies/intolerances/aversions: None
Previous nutrition therapy? Yes. *If yes, when:* 2 years ago when Pt Dx with Stage 3 chronic kidney disease. Where? Reservation Health Service.
Current diet: Low simple sugar, 0.8 g protein/kg, 2–3 g Na

Joaquin, Enez, Female, 24 y.o.
Allergies: NKA
Pt. Location: RM 207

Code: FULL
Physician: L. Nila

Isolation: None
Admit Date: 3/5

Food purchase/preparation: Self
Vit/min intake: None

Intake/Output

Date		3/5 0701–3/6 0700				3/6 0701–3/7 0700			
Time		0701–1500	1501–2300	2301–0700	Daily total	0701–1500	1501–2300	2301–0700	Daily total
IN	P.O.	0	50	0	50	NPO	NPO	NPO	NPO
	I.V. (mL/kg/hr)								
	I.V. piggyback								
	TPN								
	Total intake (mL/kg)	0 (0)	50 (0.65)	0 (0)	50 (0.65)	0 (0)	0 (0)	0 (0)	0 (0)
OUT	Urine (mL/kg/hr)	0 (0)	100 (0.16)	0 (0)	100 (0.05)	200 (0.32)	800 (1.29)	0 (0)	1000 (0.54)
	Emesis output	0	50	0	50	0	100	50	150
	Other								
	Stool						×1		
	Total output (mL/kg)	0 (0)	150 (1.94)	0 (0)	150 (1.94)	200 (2.59)	900 (11.65)	50 (0.65)	1150 (14.88)
Net I/O		0	−100	0	−100	−200	−900	−50	−1150
Net since admission (3/5)		0	−100	−100	−100	−300	−1200	−1250	−1250

Joaquin, Enez, Female, 24 y.o.
Allergies: NKA   **Code:** FULL   **Isolation:** None
Pt. Location: RM 207   **Physician:** L. Nila   **Admit Date:** 3/5

Laboratory Results

	Ref. Range	3/5 0700
Chemistry		
Sodium (mEq/L)	136–145	130 !↓
Potassium (mEq/L)	3.5–5.1	5.8 !↑
Chloride (mEq/L)	98–107	91 !↓
Carbon dioxide (CO_2, mEq/L)	23–29	32 !↑
Bicarbonate (mEq/L)	23–28	22 !↓
BUN (mg/dL)	6–20	69 !↑
Creatinine serum (mg/dL)	0.6–1.1 F 0.9–1.3 M	12.0 !↑
BUN/Crea ratio	10.0–20.0	5.75 !↓
Uric acid (mg/dL)	2.8–8.8 F 4.0–9.0 M	5.1
Est GFR, non-Afr Amer (mL/min/1.73 m^2)	>60	4 !↓
Glucose (mg/dL)	70–99	282 !↑
Phosphate, inorganic (mg/dL)	2.2–4.6	6.4 !↑
Magnesium (mg/dL)	1.5–2.4	2.1
Calcium (mg/dL)	8.6–10.2	8.2 !↓
Anion gap (mmol/L)	10–20	17
Osmolality (mmol/kg/H_2O)	275–295	300.3 !↑
Bilirubin total (mg/dL)	≤1.2	0.9
Bilirubin, direct (mg/dL)	<0.3	0.2
Protein, total (g/dL)	6–7.8	5.9 !↓
Albumin (g/dL)	3.5–5.5	3.3 !↓
Prealbumin (mg/dL)	18–35	27
Ammonia (NH_3, μg/L)	6–47	8
Alkaline phosphatase (U/L)	30–120	44
ALT (U/L)	4–36	21
AST (U/L)	0–35	16
CPK (U/L)	30–135 F 55–170 M	119
Lactate dehydrogenase (U/L)	208–378	265
Cholesterol (mg/dL)	<200	220 !↑
HDL-C (mg/dL)	>59 F, >50 M	72

Joaquin, Enez, Female, 24 y.o.
Allergies: NKA
Pt. Location: RM 207

Code: FULL
Physician: L. Nila

Isolation: None
Admit Date: 3/5

Laboratory Results *(Continued)*

	Ref. Range	3/5 0700
VLDL (mg/dL)	7–32	36 !↑
LDL (mg/dL)	<130	111
LDL/HDL ratio	<3.22 F <3.55 M	1.54
Triglycerides (mg/dL)	35–135 F 40–160 M	182 !↑
T_4 (µg/dL)	5–12	6.1
T_3 (µg/dL)	75–98	81
HbA_{1C} (%)	<5.7	9.2 !↑
Coagulation (Coag)		
PT (sec)	11–13	12.1
INR	0.9–1.1	0.95
PTT (sec)	24–34	27
Hematology		
WBC ($\times$ 10³/mm³)	3.9–10.7	4.1
RBC ($\times$ 10⁶/mm³)	4.2–5.4 F 4.5–6.2 M	3.1 !↓
Hemoglobin (Hgb, g/dL)	12–16 F 14–17 M	10.5 !↓
Hematocrit (Hct, %)	37–47 F 41–51 M	33 !↓
Urinalysis		
Collection method	—	Random specimen
Color	—	Straw
Appearance	—	Hazy
Specific gravity	1.001–1.035	1.001
pH	5–7	7.9 !↑
Protein (mg/dL)	Neg	+2 !↑
Glucose (mg/dL)	Neg	+1 !↑
Ketones	Neg	+1 !↑
Blood	Neg	Neg
Bilirubin	Nog	Neg
Nitrites	Neg	Neg

(Continued)

Joaquin, Enez, Female, 24 y.o.
Allergies: NKA   **Code:** FULL   **Isolation:** None
Pt. Location: RM 207   **Physician:** L. Nila   **Admit Date:** 3/5

Laboratory Results *(Continued)*

	Ref. Range	**3/5 0700**
Urobilinogen (EU/dL)	<1.0	0.03
Leukocyte esterase	Neg	Neg
Prot chk	Neg	+2
WBCs (/HPF)	0–5	1
RBCs (/HPF)	0–2	1
Bact	0	0
Mucus	0	0
Crys	0	0
Casts (/LPF)	0	0
Yeast	0	0
Arterial Blood Gases (ABGs)		
pH	7.35–7.45	7.44
pCO_2 (mm Hg)	35–45	33 !↓
SO_2 (%)	≥95	97
CO_2 content (mmol/L)	25–30	29
O_2 content (%)	15–22	21
pO_2 (mm Hg)	≥80	91
HCO_3^- (mEq/L)	21–28	20 !↓

Note: Values and units of measurement listed in these tables are derived from several resources. Substantial variation exists in the ranges quoted as "normal" and these may vary depending on the assay used by different laboratories.

Case Questions

I.   Understanding the Disease and Pathophysiology

1.   Describe the basic physiological functions of the kidneys.

2.   List the diseases/conditions that most commonly lead to chronic kidney disease (CKD). Explain the role of diabetes in the development of CKD.

3.   Outline the stages of CKD, including the distinguishing signs and symptoms.

4.   From your reading of Mrs. Joaquin's history and physical, what signs and symptoms did she have that correlate with her chronic kidney disease?

5.   What are the three treatment options for Stage 5 CKD? Explain the differences between hemodialysis and peritoneal dialysis.

II.   Understanding the Nutrition Therapy

6.   Explain the reasons for the following components of Mrs. Joaquin's medical nutrition therapy.

35 kcal/kg:

1.2 g protein/kg:

2 g K:

1 g phosphorus:

2 g Na:

1000 mL fluid + urine output:

7.   Calculate and interpret Mrs. Joaquin's BMI. How does edema affect your interpretation?

8.   What is edema-free weight? Calculate Mrs. Joaquin's edema-free weight.

9.   What are the energy requirements for CKD?

10. Calculate what Mrs. Joaquin's energy and protein needs will be once she begins hemodialysis.

11. What are the differences in protein requirements among stages 1 and 2 CKD, stages 3 and 4 CKD, hemodialysis, and peritoneal dialysis patients? What is the rationale for these differences?

12. Mrs. Joaquin has a PO_4 restriction. Why? List the foods that have the highest levels of phosphorus.

13. Mrs. Joaquin tells you that one of her friends can drink only certain amounts of liquids and wants to know if that is the case for her. What foods are considered to be fluids? What fluid restriction is generally recommended for someone on hemodialysis? Is there a standard guideline for maximum fluid gain between dialysis visits? If a patient must follow a fluid restriction, what can be done to help assure adherence and reduce his or her thirst?

14. Several biochemical indices are used to diagnose chronic kidney disease. One is glomerular filtration rate (GFR). What does GFR measure? What is a normal GFR? Interpret her value.

15. Evaluate Mrs. Joaquin's chemistry report. What labs are altered due to her diagnosis of Stage 5 CKD?

16. Which of Mrs. Joaquin's symptoms would you expect to begin to improve when she starts dialysis?

17. The following medications were prescribed for Mrs. Joaquin. Explain why each was prescribed (the indications/mechanism) and describe any nutritional concerns and dietary recommendations related to the medication.

    Capoten/captopril:

    Erythropoietin:

    Sodium bicarbonate:

    Renal caps:

    Renvela:

Hectorol:

Glucophage:

18. List the nutrition-related health problems that have been identified in the Pima Indians through epidemiological data. Are the Pima at higher risk for complications of diabetes? Explain. What is meant by the "thrifty gene" theory?

III. Nutrition Diagnosis

19. Choose two high-priority nutrition problems and complete a PES statement for each.

IV. Nutrition Intervention

20. For each PES statement, establish an ideal goal (based on the signs and symptoms) and appropriate intervention (based on the etiology).

21. Why is it recommended that patients obtain at least 50% of their protein from sources that have high biological value?

22. What resources and counseling techniques would you use to teach Mrs. Joaquin about her diet?

23. **A.** Based on Mrs. Joaquin's energy needs, calculate her carbohydrate, protein, and fat needs. Using the Renal Exchange list, plan a 1-day diet that meets her energy needs and complies with her diet orders (see question 6).

B. Using Mrs. Joaquin's typical intake and the prescribed meal plan above, write a sample menu. Justify your changes; why did you make the change to comply with her nutrition prescription?

Diet PTA		Sample Menu
Breakfast:	Cold cereal (2 c unsweetened)	
	Bread (2 slices) or fried potatoes (1 medium potato)	
	1 fried egg (occasionally)	
	2 cups coffee	

(Continued)

(Continued)

Diet PTA		Sample Menu
Lunch:	Bologna sandwich (2 slices white bread, 2 slices bologna, mustard)	
	Potato chips (1 oz)	
	1 can Coke	
Dinner:	Chili con carne (3 oz beef)	
	Indian fry bread (1 slice, 6" diameter)	
	Iced tea with sugar (16 oz)	
HS Snack:	Crackers (6 saltines) and peanut butter (2 tbsp)	

24. Write an initial ADIME note for your consultation with Mrs. Joaquin.

Bibliography

Academy of Nutrition and Dietetics Evidence Analysis Library. Chronic Kidney Disease. Executive summary of recommendations (2010). http://www.andeal.org /topic.cfm?menu=5303&cat=3929. Accessed 03/30/15.

Academy of Nutrition and Dietetics Nutrition Care Manual. Chronic Kidney Disease (CKD) Stage 5 Dialysis. https://www.nutritioncaremanual.org/topic.cfm?ncm _category_id=1&lv1=5537&lv2=255347&ncm_toc _id=255666&ncm_heading=Nutrition%20Care. Accessed 03/30/15.

Ash S, Campbell KL, Bogard J, Millichamp A. Nutrition prescription to achieve positive outcomes in chronic kidney disease: A systematic review. *Nutrients.* 2014;6:416–451.

Beto JA, Ramirez WE, Bansal VK. Medical nutrition therapy in adults with chronic kidney disease: Integrating evidence and consensus into practice for the generalist registered dietitian nutritionist. *J Acad Nutr Diet.* 2014;114:1077–1087.

Brown TL. Ethnic populations. In: Ross TA, Boucher JL, O'Connell BS. *American Dietetic Association Guide to Diabetes Medical Nutrition Therapy and Education.* Chicago, IL: American Dietetic Association; 2005:227–238.

DeMouy J. *The Pima Indians: Pathfinders for Health.* http:// diabetes.niddk.nih.gov/dm/pubs/pima/pathfind /pathfind.htm. Accessed 05/10/15.

Hanson RL, Muller YL, Kobes S, et al. A genome-wide association study in American Indians implicates DNER as a susceptibility locus for type 2 diabetes. *Diabetes.* 2014;63:369–376.

Inker LA, Astor BC, Fox CH, et al. KDOQI US commentary on the 2012 KDIGO clinical practice guideline for the evaluation and management of CKD. *Am J Kidney Dis.* 2014;63:713–735.

Lacey K, Nahikian-Nelms M. Diseases of the renal system. In: Nelms M, Sucher K, Lacey K. *Nutrition Therapy and Pathophysiology.* 3rd ed. Belmont, CA: Cengage Learning; 2016:521–561.

National Institute of Diabetes and Digestive and Kidney Diseases (NIDDK). Diabetes in American Indians and Alaska Natives. http://diabetes.niddk.nih.gov/dm /pubs/americanindian/. Accessed 05/10/15.

National Kidney Foundation. K/DOQI Clinical practice guidelines for Chronic Kidney Disease: Evaluation, classification and stratification. *Am J Kidney Dis.* 2002 (Suppl 1):39:S1–S266.

Nelms MN, Habash D. Nutrition assessment: Foundations of the nutrition care process. In: Nelms M, Sucher K, Lacey K. *Nutrition Therapy and Pathophysiology.* 3rd ed. Belmont, CA: Cengage Learning; 2016:36–71.

Nelson RG, Bennett PH, Beck GJ, et al. Development and progression of renal disease in Pima Indians with non-insulin dependent diabetes mellitus. *N Engl J Med.* 1996;335:1636–1642.

Pronsky ZM. *Food-Medication Interactions.* 18th ed. Birchrunville, PA: Food-Medication Interactions; 2015.

Urquidez-Romero R, Esparza-Romero J, Chaudhari LS, et al. Study design of the Maycoba Project: Obesity and diabetes in Mexican Pimas. *Am J Health Behav.* 2014;38:370–378.

Internet Resources

American Association of Kidney Patients: http://www .aakp.org/

Cook's Thesaurus: http://www.foodsubs.com/

Culinary Kidney Cooks: http://www.culinarykidneycooks .com/

eMedicineHealth: http://www.emedicinehealth.com /chronic_kidney_disease/article_em.htm

Kidney School: http://kidneyschool.org/

National Institute of Diabetes and Digestive and Kidney Diseases (NIDDK): http://www2.niddk.nih.gov/

National Kidney Foundation Council on Renal Nutrition: http://www.kidney.org/

National Kidney Foundation KDOQI Guidelines: http:// www.kidney.org/professionals/kdoqi/guidelines_ckd /toc.htm

The Nephron Information Center: http://www.nephron .com/

Renal Dialysis … A Team Effort: http://www.nufs.sjsu.edu /renaldial/index.html

Renal Web: http://www.renalweb.com/

United States Renal Data System (USRDS): http://www .usrds.org/

Chronic Kidney Disease: Peritoneal Dialysis

Dawn B. Scheiderer, RD, LD—Davita Kidney Care
Columbus OH

Objectives

After completing this case, the student will be able to:

1. Describe the pathophysiology of chronic kidney disease (CKD).
2. Describe the basic concepts of kidney transplant.
3. Differentiate the physiology of peritoneal dialysis and hemodialysis.
4. Identify and explain common nutritional problems associated with CKD.
5. Interpret laboratory parameters for nutritional implications and significance.
6. Analyze nutrition assessment data to evaluate nutritional status, identify specific nutrition problems, and document corresponding PES statements.
7. Develop a nutrition care plan—with appropriate measurable goals, interventions, and strategies for monitoring and evaluation—that addresses the nutrition diagnoses of this case.

Mrs. Caldwell is a 49-year-old female who has a history of membranoproliferative glomerulonephritis. She has a history of kidney transplant $\times 2$ and is now experiencing acute rejection with chronic allograft nephropathy. Her creatinine level has been rising with worsening of fluid overload. She is admitted to the hospital for further evaluation.

Caldwell, Mona, Female, 49 y.o.
Allergies: Fish
Pt. Location: 789

Code: FULL
Physician: K. Wolf

Isolation: None
Admit Date: 1/21

Patient Summary: Patient is a 49-year-old female who has history of membranoproliferative glomerulonephritis resulting in kidney transplant ×2 and is now experiencing acute rejection with chronic allograft nephropathy. She has previously been treated with both hemodialysis and peritoneal dialysis before and between transplants. She is requesting to restart peritoneal dialysis as she would like to continue to work at the U.S. Postal Service. She is admitted for insertion of PD catheter and plans to use cycler at night so that she can continue to work.

History:

Onset of disease: Diagnosed with glomerulonephritis 15 years ago with resulting end-stage renal disease. Initiated hemodialysis at that time and received first transplant 1 year later. Acute rejection resulted in initiation of peritoneal dialysis. She received second transplant 2 years ago.

Medical history: Membranoproliferative glomerulonephritis; allograft transplant ×2; hypertension; dyslipidemia; anemia of chronic kidney disease

Surgical history: s/p unilateral oophorectomy; allograft kidney transplant ×2; umbilical hernia repair

Medications at home: Procardia, carvedilol, Catapres (clonidine), CellCept, fish oil, Lasix, prednisone, Gengraf, Prinivil, sodium bicarbonate, calcitriol, renal caps, Renvela

Tobacco use: 1 pack per day, 20 years of use; stopped tobacco use 5–6 years ago

Alcohol use: None

Family history: Mother—cervical cancer; father—lung cancer

Demographics:

Marital status: Married
Years education: 14+
Language: English only
Occupation: Postal clerk
Hours of work: 8–5
Household members: Lives with husband
Ethnicity: Caucasian
Religious affiliation: None

Admitting History/Physical:

Chief complaint: "They tell me that my transplant is failing—I am very short of breath and I have a lot of fluid—I am here to have a catheter placed so I can start dialysis again."

General appearance: Well-developed female in no acute distress; alert and oriented ×3.

Vital Signs: Temp: 98.4   Pulse: 62   Resp rate: 12
                  BP: 161/92   Height: 157.4 cm Weight: 77.1 kg   UBW: ~74 kg

Heart: RRR. No clicks, rubs, murmurs, or gallops noted.
HEENT: Head: WNL
          Eyes: PERRLA
          Ears: Clear

Caldwell, Mona, Female, 49 y.o.
Allergies: Fish   **Code:** FULL   **Isolation:** None
Pt. Location: 789   **Physician:** K. Wolf   **Admit Date:** 1/21

Nose: Dry mucous membranes
Throat: Dry mucous membranes
Genitalia: Deferred
Neurologic: Alert and oriented
Extremities: WNL
Skin: Warm and dry
Chest/lungs: Respirations are rapid but clear to auscultation and percussion
Peripheral vascular: No peripheral edema noted
Abdomen: Soft—no incisional hernias; signs of prior kidney transplants and umbilical hernia repair noted

Nursing Assessment	1/22
Abdominal appearance (concave, flat, rounded, obese, distended)	rounded
Palpation of abdomen (soft, rigid, firm, masses, tense)	soft
Bowel function (continent, incontinent, flatulence, no stool)	continent
Bowel sounds (P=present, AB=absent, hypo, hyper)	
RUQ	P
LUQ	P
RLQ	P
LLQ	P
Stool color	none
Stool consistency	NA
Tubes/ostomies	NA
Genitourinary	
Urinary continence	yes
Urine source	clean catch
Appearance (clear, cloudy, yellow, amber, fluorescent, hematuria, orange, blue, tea)	cloudy, amber
Integumentary	
Skin color	pale
Skin temperature (DI=diaphoretic, W=warm, dry, CL=cool, CLM=clammy, CD +=cold, M=moist, H=hot)	W
Skin turgor (good, fair, poor, TENT=tenting)	good
Skin condition (intact, EC=ecchymosis, A=abrasions, P=petechiae, R=rash, W=weeping, S=sloughing, D=dryness, EX=excoriated, T=tears, SE=subcutaneous emphysema, B=blisters, V=vesicles, N=necrosis)	intact
Mucous membranes (intact, EC=ecchymosis, A=abrasions, P=petechiae, R=rash, W=weeping, S=sloughing, D=dryness, EX=excoriated, T=tears, SE=subcutaneous emphysema, B=blisters, V=vesicles, N=necrosis)	intact, D

(Continued)

Caldwell, Mona, Female, 49 y.o.
Allergies: Fish   **Code:** FULL   **Isolation:** None
Pt. Location: 789   **Physician:** K. Wolf   **Admit Date:** 1/21

Nursing Assessment *(Continued)*

Nursing Assessment	1/22
Other components of Braden score: special bed, sensory pressure, moisture, activity, friction/shear (>18=no risk, 15–16=low risk, 13–14=moderate risk, ≤12=high risk)	20

Admission Orders:

Laboratory: CBC, Chemistry
Vital Signs: Every 4 hrs
I & O: Recorded every 8 hrs
Diet: 1500 kcal, 75 g pro, 3000 mg Na, 3500 mg K, 1000 mg P, 2000 cc fluid
Activity: Bed rest

Nutrition:

Meal type: 1500 kcal, 75 g pro, 3000 mg Na, 3500 mg K, 1000 mg P, 2000 cc fluid
History: Patient states she has noticed her appetite has not been as good lately. Describes mild nausea but no vomiting. Relates that food has a bad taste. Since her transplant she has only monitored her salt intake—no other restrictions.

24-hour recall:

AM:	Egg McMuffin™, 6 oz orange juice, coffee
Lunch:	Cheeseburger, fries, apple pie, and 12 oz Coke
Dinner:	6 oz roast beef au jus, 3 small oven-browned potatoes, ¼ c broccoli, iced tea, roll with butter

Laboratory Results

	Ref. Range	1/22 0700
Chemistry		
Sodium (mEq/L)	136–145	130 !↓
Potassium (mEq/L)	3.5–5.1	3.8
Chloride (mEq/L)	98–107	99
Carbon dioxide (CO_2, mEq/L)	23–29	26
Bicarbonate (mEq/L)	23–28	25
BUN (mg/dL)	6–20	124 !↑
Creatinine serum (mg/dL)	0.6–1.1 F 0.9–1.3 M	6.8 !↑
BUN/Crea ratio	10.0–20.0	18.2
Uric acid (mg/dL)	2.8–8.8 F 4.0–9.0 M	5.3

Caldwell, Mona, Female, 49 y.o.
Allergies: Fish
Pt. Location: 789

Code: FULL
Physician: K. Wolf

Isolation: None
Admit Date: 1/21

Laboratory Results *(Continued)*

	Ref. Range	1/22 0700
Est GFR, Afr-Amer (mL/min/1.73 m²)	>60	8 !↓
Glucose (mg/dL)	70–99	80
Phosphate, inorganic (mg/dL)	2.2–4.6	11.9 !↑
Magnesium (mg/dL)	1.5–2.4	1.9
Calcium (mg/dL)	8.6–10.2	8.3 !↓
Anion gap (mmol/L)	10–20	6.0 !↓
Osmolality (mmol/kg/H₂O)	275–295	308 !↑
Bilirubin total (mg/dL)	≤1.2	0.8
Bilirubin, direct (mg/dL)	<0.3	0.1
Protein, total (g/dL)	6–7.8	5.9 !↓
Albumin (g/dL)	3.5–5.5	3.3 !↓
Prealbumin (mg/dL)	18–35	19
Ammonia (NH₃, µg/L)	6–47	7
Alkaline phosphatase (U/L)	30–120	106
ALT (U/L)	4–36	5
AST (U/L)	0–35	9
CPK (U/L)	30–135 F 55–170 M	35
Lactate dehydrogenase (U/L)	208–378	209
Cholesterol (mg/dL)	<200	154
HDL–C (mg/dL)	>59 F, >50 M	56 !↓
VLDL (mg/dL)	7–32	15
LDL (mg/dL)	<130	83
LDL/HDL ratio	<3.22 F <3.55 M	1.48
Triglycerides (mg/dL)	35–135 F 40–160 M	77
Coagulation (Coag)		
PT (sec)	11–13	16.9 !↑
INR	0.9–1.1	1.4 !↑
Hematology		
WBC (× 10³/mm³)	3.9–10.7	8.27
RBC (× 10⁶/mm³)	4.2–5.4 F 4.5–6.2 M	2.33 !↓

(Continued)

Caldwell, Mona, Female, 49 y.o.
Allergies: Fish
Pt. Location: 789

Code: FULL
Physician: K. Wolf

Isolation: None
Admit Date: 1/21

Laboratory Results *(Continued)*

	Ref. Range	1/22 0700
Hemoglobin (Hgb, g/dL)	12–16 F 14–17 M	6.6 !↓
Hematocrit (Hct, %)	37–47 F 41–51 M	19.0 !↓
Mean cell volume (μm³)	80–96	65.3 !↓
Mean cell Hgb (pg)	28–32	21.5 !↓
Mean cell Hgb content (g/dL)	32–36	19.5 !↓
RBC distribution (%)	11.6–16.5	16.8 !↑
Transferrin (mg/dL)	250–380 F 215–365 M	219 !↓
Ferritin (mg/mL)	20–120 F 20–300 M	5 !↓

Note: Values and units of measurement listed in these tables are derived from several resources. Substantial variation exists in the ranges quoted as "normal" and these may vary depending on the assay used by different laboratories.

Intake/Output

Date		1/22 0701–1/23 0700			
Time		0701–1500	1501–2300	2301–0700	Daily total
IN	P.O.	**650**	**400**	**750**	**1800**
	I.V. (mL/kg/hr)				
	IV. piggyback				
	TPN				
	Total intake (mL/kg)	**650** (8.43)	**400** (5.19)	**750** (9.73)	**1800** (23.35)
OUT	Urine (mL/kg/hr)	**812** (1.32)	**410** (0.66)	**310** (0.50)	**1532** (0.83)
	Emesis output				
	Other				
	Stool	×1	0	0	0
	Total output (mL/kg)	812 (10.53)	410 (5.32)	310 (4.02)	1532 (19.87)
Net I/O		−162	−10	+440	+268
Net since admission (1/21)		−162	−172	+268	+268

Case Questions

I.   Understanding the Diagnosis and Pathophysiology

1.   Describe the major exocrine and endocrine functions of the kidney.

2.   What is glomerulonephritis and how can it lead to kidney failure?

3.   What laboratory values or other tests support Mrs. Caldwell's diagnosis of chronic kidney disease? List all abnormal values and explain the likely cause for each abnormal value.

4.   This patient has had two previous kidney transplants. What are the potential sources for a donor kidney? How is rejection prevented after a kidney transplant? What does it mean when the physician states she is experiencing acute rejection?

5.   Based on the admitting history and physical, what signs and symptoms does this patient have that are consistent with acute rejection of the transplant?

6.   Mrs. Caldwell has requested that she restart peritoneal dialysis. Briefly describe this medical treatment, including its mechanism, and how it differs from hemodialysis.

II.   Understanding the Nutrition Therapy

7.   This patient was prescribed the following diet in the hospital:

1500 kcal, 75 g pro, 3000 mg Na, 3500 mg K, 1000 mg P, 2000 cc fluid

Explain the rationale for each component of her nutrition therapy Rx. How might this change once she has started peritoneal dialysis?

III.   Nutrition Assessment

8.   Assess Mrs. Caldwell's height and weight. Calculate her BMI and her % usual body weight. How would edema affect your interpretation of this information? Using the KDOQI guidelines, what is Mrs. Caldwell's adjusted body weight?

9.   Determine Mrs. Caldwell's energy and protein requirements. Explain the rationale for the method you used to calculate these requirements.

10. List all medications that Mrs. Caldwell is receiving. Determine the action of each medication and identify any drug–nutrient interactions that you should monitor for.

11. Mrs. Caldwell's laboratory values that you discussed previously in this case indicate she has anemia. Why do renal patients suffer from anemia? How is this typically treated in dialysis patients?

12. What factors in Mrs. Caldwell's history may affect her ability to eat? What are the most likely causes of these symptoms? Is it realistic to expect that they will change?

13. Evaluate Mrs. Caldwell's diet history and 24-hour recall. Is her usual diet consistent with her inpatient diet order?

IV.   Nutrition Diagnosis

14. Identify the pertinent nutrition problems and the corresponding nutrition diagnoses.

15. Write a PES statement for each high-priority nutrition problem.

V.   Nutrition Intervention

Mrs. Caldwell was discharged from the hospital and was prescribed the following regimen of peritoneal dialysis to begin at home:

CCPD daily. Ca 2.50; Mg 0.5, Dextrose 2.5%. Total fills (or exchanges) = 3 (3 fills/cycle @ 2500 mL). Total fill volume/24 hours: 7500 mL.

16. Determine the amount of energy that Mrs. Caldwell's PD prescription will provide each day. How will this affect your nutrition recommendations?

17. Using the KDOQI adult guidelines for peritoneal dialysis patients, determine Mrs. Caldwell's nutrition prescription for outpatient use. (Include energy, protein, phosphorus, calcium, potassium, sodium, and fluid.)

18. Using the identified nutrition problems (and with the understanding that Mrs. Caldwell has received a significant amount of nutrition education in the past), what would you determine to be the most important topics for nutrition education when she returns to the PD clinic?

VI.   Nutrition Monitoring and Evaluation

19. List factors that you would monitor to assess Mrs. Caldwell's nutritional status when she returns to the PD clinic.

Bibliography

Academy of Nutrition and Dietetics Nutrition Care Manual. Chronic Kidney Disease (CKD) Stage 5 Dialysis. https://www.nutritioncaremanual.org/topic.cfm?ncm _category_id=1&lv1=5537&lv2=255347&ncm_toc _id=255666&ncm_heading=Nutrition%20Care. Accessed 03/30/15.

Academy of Nutrition and Dietetics Nutrition Care Manual. Kidney Transplant. https://www .nutritioncaremanual.org/content.cfm?ncm_content _id=92237&ncm_category_id=1. Accessed 3/30/15.

Ash S, Campbell KL, Bogard J, Millichamp A. Nutrition prescription to achieve positive outcomes in chronic kidney disease: A systematic review. *Nutrients*. 2014;6:416–451.

Beto JA, Ramirez WE, Bansal VK. Medical nutrition therapy in adults with chronic kidney disease: Integrating evidence and consensus into practice for the generalist registered dietitian nutritionist. *J Acad Nutr Diet*. 2014;114:1077–1087.

Inker LA, Astor BC, Fox CH, et al. KDOQI US commentary on the 2012 KDIGO clinical practice guideline for the evaluation and management of CKD. *Am J Kidney Dis*. 2014;63:713–735.

Kopple JD, Massry SG, eds. *Nutrition Management of Renal Disease*. 2nd ed. Philadelphia, PA: Lippincott Williams & Wilkins; 2004.

Lacey K, Nahikian-Nelms ML. Diseases of the renal system. In: Nelms M, Sucher K, Lacey K. *Nutrition Therapy and Pathophysiology*. 3rd ed. Belmont, CA: Cengage Learning; 2016:521–561.

Lee R, Nieman D. *Nutritional Assessment*. 6th ed. New York, NY: McGraw-Hill; 2013.

Luttrell KJ, Beto JA, Tangney CC. Selected nutrition practices of women on hemodialysis and peritoneal dialysis: Observations from the NKF-CRN Second National Research Question Collaborative Study. *J Ren Nutr*. 2014;24:81–91.

McCann L, ed. *Pocket Guide to Nutrition Assessment of the Patient with Chronic Kidney Disease*. 3rd ed. New York, NY: National Kidney Foundation Council on Renal Nutrition; 2002.

Moore L. Implications for nutrition practice in the mineral-bone disorder of chronic kidney disease. *Nutr Clin Pract*. 2011;26:391–400.

National Kidney Foundation. KDOQI Clinical Practice Guidelines. Available at: http://www.kidney.org /professionals/kdoqi/guidelines. Accessed 5/12/15.

Skelton SL, Waterman AD, Davis LA, Peipert JD, Fish AF. Applying best practices to designing patient education for patients with end-stage renal disease pursuing kidney transplant. *Prog Transplant*. 2015;25:77–84.

Yilmaz R, Aricic M. How to prepare a chronic kidney disease patient for transplant. In: Arici M. *Management of Chronic Kidney Disease, A Clinician's Guide*. Springer; 2014:463–474.

Internet Resources

AND Evidence Analysis Library: http://www.andeal.org

American Association of Kidney Patients: http://www .aakp.org

International Society for Peritoneal Dialysis: http://www .ispd.org

National Institute of Diabetes and Digestive and Kidney Diseases of the National Institute of Health: http:// www.niddk.nih.gov

National Kidney Foundation: http://www.kidney.org

Nutrition Care Manual: http://www.nutritioncaremanual.org\

Drug Bank – Open Data Drug and Drug Target database: http://www.drugbank.ca

Case 21

Acute Kidney Injury (AKI)

Objectives

After completing this case, the student will be able to:

1. Define and describe the classifications of acute kidney injury (AKI) and its potential etiologies.
2. Describe the pathophysiology of AKI.
3. Identify and explain common nutritional problems associated with AKI.
4. Interpret laboratory parameters for nutritional implications and significance.
5. Analyze nutrition assessment data to evaluate nutritional status, identify specific nutrition problems, and document corresponding PES statements.

6. Develop a nutrition care plan—with appropriate measurable goals, interventions, and strategies for monitoring and evaluation—that addresses the nutrition diagnoses of this case.

Mr. Randall Maddox is a 67-year-old male admitted for a planned coronary bypass surgery 7 days ago. Postoperatively he experienced respiratory distress and infection, and now his urine output has suddenly decreased. It is now day 7 and a new nutrition consult has been ordered for Mr. Maddox.

Maddox, Randall, Male, 67 y.o.
Allergies: Penicillin, sulfa   **Code:** FULL   **Isolation:** Contact
Pt. Location: CICU   **Physician:** C. Taylor   **Admit Date:** 10/8

Patient Summary: Patient is a 67-year-old male who is s/p CABG on 10/9. Surgery was successful with 3-vessel bypass. He experienced a hypotensive event in recovery but responded to IV fluids. Further postoperative recovery has been complicated by respiratory distress, subsequent intubation, and infection.

History:
Onset of disease: Diagnosed with acute kidney injury postoperative day 7 (10/16)
Medical history: CAD, s/p MI 15 years ago, hyperlipidemia, and type 2 DM
Surgical history: s/p 3-vessel CABG 6 days ago
Medications at home: Lovostatin, Lasix, Lopressor
Tobacco use: 2 packs per day, 20 years of use; stopped tobacco use 1 year ago
Alcohol use: Socially
Family history: Mother—diabetes, breast cancer; father—heart disease, lung cancer

Demographics:
Marital status: Divorced; father of 4
Years education: 14+
Language: English only
Occupation: Retired from computer sales
Hours of work: N/A
Household members: Lives by himself
Ethnicity: Caucasian
Religious affiliation: Methodist

MD Progress Note 10/16:
Patient is now POD#7. Experienced continued decrease in urine output—+5295 mL since admission. Urine output last 24 hours—125 mL.

Vital Signs: Temp: 98.4   Pulse: 77   Resp rate: 18
                   BP: 116/88   Height: 6'2"   Weight: 225 lbs (admission wt: 208 lbs)

Cardiovascular: s/p CABG × 3
Pulmonary: Postoperative atelectasis: Encourage aggressive respiratory therapy
Neurologic: Alert and oriented × 3; chronic pain control—scheduled oxycodone
Extremities: Warm with normal pulses
Skin: Cool, pale
Chest/lungs: Respirations are rapid but clear to auscultation and percussion. CXR viewed.
Peripheral vascular: Peripheral edema noted +3
Abdomen: Soft—nt, nd. Tolerated sips of oral intake.
Consult: Nephrology for acute kidney injury—will begin on CRRT today
Consult: Nutrition for enteral feeding—7 days post-op with negligible nutritional intake.

C. Taylor. MD

Maddox, Randall, Male, 67 y.o.
Allergies: Penicillin, sulfa
Pt. Location: CICU

Code: FULL
Physician: C. Taylor

Isolation: Contact
Admit Date: 10/8

Nursing Assessment	10/16
Abdominal appearance (concave, flat, rounded, obese, distended)	obese
Palpation of abdomen (soft, rigid, firm, masses, tense)	soft
Bowel function (continent, incontinent, flatulence, no stool)	continent
Bowel sounds (P=present, AB=absent, hypo, hyper)	
RUQ	P
LUQ	P
RLQ	P
LLQ	P
Stool color	dark brown
Stool consistency	soft
Tubes/ostomies	NA
Genitourinary	
Urinary continence	catheter
Urine source	catheter
Appearance (clear, cloudy, yellow, amber, fluorescent, hematuria, orange, blue, tea)	cloudy, amber
Integumentary	
Skin color	pale
Skin temperature (DI=diaphoretic, W=warm, dry, CL=cool, CLM=clammy, CD+=cold, M=moist, H=hot)	CL
Skin turgor (good, fair, poor, TENT=tenting)	good
Skin condition (intact, EC=ecchymosis, A=abrasions, P=petechiae, R=rash, W=weeping, S=sloughing, D=dryness, EX=excoriated, T=tears, SE=subcutaneous emphysema, B=blisters, V=vesicles, N=necrosis)	EC, P
Mucous membranes (intact, EC=ecchymosis, A=abrasions, P=petechiae, R=rash, W=weeping, S=sloughing, D=dryness, EX=excoriated, T=tears, SE=subcutaneous emphysema, B=blisters, V=vesicles, N=necrosis)	intact
Other components of Braden score: special bed, sensory pressure, moisture, activity, friction/shear (>18=no risk, 15–16=low risk, 13–14=moderate risk, ≤12=high risk)	13

Maddox, Randall, Male, 67 y.o.
Allergies: Penicillin, sulfa
Pt. Location: CICU

Code: FULL
Physician: C. Taylor

Isolation: Contact
Admit Date: 10/8

Intake/Output

Date		10/15 0701–10/16 0700			
Time		0701–1500	1501–2300	2301–0700	Daily total
IN	P.O.	**490**	**240**	**0**	**730**
	I.V. (mL/kg/hr)				
	I.V. piggyback				
	TPN				
	Total intake (mL/kg)	**490** (5.2)	**240** (2.5)	**0** (0)	**730** (7.7)
OUT	Urine (mL/kg/hr)	**0** (0)	**75** (0.10)	**50** (0.07)	**125** (0.05)
	Emesis output				
	Other				
	Stool	**170**	**0**	**0**	**170**
	Total output (mL/kg)	**170** (1.8)	**75** (0.8)	**50** (0.5)	**295** (3.1)
Net I/O		**+320**	**+165**	**−50**	**+435**
Net since admission (10/8)		**+5,180.4**	**+5,345.4**	**+5,295.4**	**+5,295.4**

Laboratory Results

	Ref. Range	10/21 0600
Chemistry		
Sodium (mEq/L)	136–145	138
Potassium (mEq/L)	3.5–5.1	5.7 !↑
Chloride (mEq/L)	98–107	102
Carbon dioxide (CO_2, mEq/L)	23–29	24
Bicarbonate (mEq/L)	23–28	16 !↓
BUN (mg/dL)	6–20	38 !↑
Creatinine serum (mg/dL)	0.6–1.1 F 0.9–1.3 M	6.6 !↑
BUN/Crea ratio	10.0–20.0	5.7 !↓
Uric acid (mg/dL)	2.8–8.8 F 4.0–9.0 M	4.1
Est GFR, non-Afr Amer (mL/min/1.73 m²)	>60	8 !↓
Glucose (mg/dL)	70–99	123 !↑

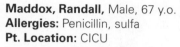

Maddox, Randall, Male, 67 y.o.
Allergies: Penicillin, sulfa
Pt. Location: CICU

Code: FULL
Physician: C. Taylor

Isolation: Contact
Admit Date: 10/8

Laboratory Results *(Continued)*

	Ref. Range	10/21 0600
Phosphate, inorganic (mg/dL)	2.2–4.6	5.3 !↑
Magnesium (mg/dL)	1.5–2.4	2.3
Calcium (mg/dL)	8.6–10.2	8.6
Anion gap (mmol/L)	10–20	20
Osmolality (mmol/kg/H_2O)	275–295	296 !↑
Bilirubin total (mg/dL)	≤1.2	0.7
Bilirubin, direct (mg/dL)	<0.3	0.29
Protein, total (g/dL)	6–7.8	5.0 !↓
Albumin (g/dL)	3.5–5.5	2.5 !↓
Prealbumin (mg/dL)	18–35	12 !↓
Ammonia (NH_3, µg/L)	6–47	11
Alkaline phosphatase (U/L)	30–120	141 !↑
ALT (U/L)	4–36	43 !↑
AST (U/L)	0–35	48 !↑
CPK (U/L)	30–135 F 55–170 M	190 !↑
Lactate dehydrogenase (U/L)	208–378	382 !↑
CRP (mg/L)	<1.0	125 !↑
Coagulation (Coag)		
PT (sec)	11–13	14.7 !↑
INR	0.9–1.1	1.3 !↑
Hematology		
WBC ($\times 10^3$/mm^3)	3.9–10.7	12.9 !↑
RBC ($\times 10^6$/mm^3)	4.2–5.4 F 4.5–6.2 M	2.95 !↓
Hemoglobin (Hgb, g/dL)	12–16 F 14–17 M	9.1 !↓
Hematocrit (Hct, %)	37–47 F 41–51 M	28.6 !↓
Mean cell volume (µm^3)	80–96	94.5
Mean cell Hgb (pg)	28–32	25.9 !↓
Mean cell Hgb content (g/dL)	32–36	19.5 !↓
RBC distribution (%)	11.6–16.5	16.8 !↑

Note: Values and units of measurement listed in these tables are derived from several resources. Substantial variation exists in the ranges quoted as "normal" and these may vary depending on the assay used by different laboratories.

Case Questions

I.   Understanding the Diagnosis and Pathophysiology

1. Define Mr. Maddox's diagnosis of acute kidney injury.

2. What are the risk factors associated with the development of AKI in critically ill adults?

3. Explain the major causes of prerenal, postrenal, and intrarenal/intrinsic AKI. Identify the staging for AKI. What do you suspect is the major etiology of Mr. Maddox's AKI?

4. Explain the major nutrient/metabolic changes (glucose, lipid, protein, and energy expenditure) that may occur during AKI and that would potentially affect your nutrition recommendations.

5. What laboratory values or other tests support Mr. Maddox's diagnosis of AKI? List all abnormal values and explain the likely cause for each abnormal value.

6. Mr. Maddox will be started on continuous renal replacement therapy (CRRT). Describe the basic mechanisms of this therapy.

7. Explain how nutrition therapy recommendations for an AKI patient may differ if he is receiving CRRT versus not receiving any dialysis treatment.

II. Understanding the Nutrition Therapy

8. Mr. Maddox has not eaten since his surgery. He was started on clear liquids several days ago but has taken in very little. Using the ASPEN guidelines, justify his requirement for nutrition support.

III. Nutrition Assessment

9. Assess Mr. Maddox's height, weight, and BMI. What factors from his medical record will affect your interpretation of his weight?

10. While conducting a nutrition-focused physical examination, the RD discovers that Mr. Maddox exhibits evidence of temporal wasting and loss of preorbital fat pads, as well as some evidence of triceps fat loss. How might this impact the nutrition recommendations the RD will make? Describe the etiology of the protein-energy wasting that may occur with AKI.

11. Determine Mr. Maddox's energy and protein requirements. Explain the rationale for the method you used to calculate these requirements.

IV.   Nutrition Diagnosis

12. Identify the pertinent nutrition problems and the corresponding nutrition diagnoses.

13. Write two PES statements for two high-priority nutrition problems.

V.   Nutrition Intervention

14. Outline the appropriate nutrition support plan for Mr. Maddox.

15. Should any micronutrients be supplemented for the AKI patient treated with CRRT? Are there other micronutrients that should be avoided during an episode of AKI treated with CRRT?

VI.   Nutrition Monitoring and Evaluation

16. Write your ADIME note for the nutrition support recommendations.

Bibliography

Academy of Nutrition and Dietetics Nutrition Care Manual. Renal Replacement Therapy. https://www.nutritioncaremanual.org/topic.cfm?ncm_category_id=1&lv1=5537&lv2=255347&ncm_toc_id=22459&ncm_heading=Nutrition%20Care. Accessed 03/30/15.

Bellomo R, Kellum JA, Ronco C. Acute kidney injury. *Lancet.* 2012;380:756–766.

Brown RO, Compher C, ASPEN Board of Directors. ASPEN Clincal Guidelines: Nutrition support in adult acute and chronic renal failure. *JPEN.* 2010;34:366–377.

Dirkes S. Acute kidney injury: Not just acute renal failure anymore. *Crit Care Nurs.* 2011;31:37–50.

Fiaccadori E, Regolisti G, Cabassi A. Specific nutritional problems in acute kidney injury, treated with non-dialysis and dialytic modalities. *NDTPlus.* 2010;3:1–7.

Gervasio JM, Garmon WP, Holowatyj M. Nutrition support in acute kidney injury. *Nutrition in Clinical Practice.* 2011;26:374–381.

Kalista-Richards M. Acute kidney injury. In: Byham-Gray LD, Burrowes JD, Chertow GM. *Nutrition in Kidney Disease.* New York: Humane Press, Springer Science & Business Media; 2014:231–246.

Kariyawasam D. Nutritional requirements in acute kidney injury. *J Ren Nurs.* 2012;4:231–235.

Kopple JD, Massry SG, eds. *Nutrition Management of Renal Disease.* 2nd ed. Philadelphia, PA: Lippincott Williams & Wilkins; 2004.

Lacey K, Nahikian-Nelms ML. Diseases of the renal system. In: Nelms M, Sucher K, Lacey K. *Nutrition Therapy and Pathophysiology.* 3rd ed. Belmont, CA: Cengage Learning; 2016:521–561.

Lewicki M, Ng I, Schneider AG. HMG CoA reductase inhibitors (statins) for preventing acute kidney injury after surgical procedures requiring cardiac bypass. *Cochrane Database Syst Rev.* 2015;3:CD010480.

Li Y, Tang X, Zhang J, Wu T. Nutritional support for acute kidney injury. *Cochrane Database Syst Rev.* 2010;1:CD005426.

Maursetter L, Kight CE, Mennig J, Hofmann RM. Review of the mechanism and nutrition recommendations for patients undergoing continuous renal replacement therapy. *Nutr Clin Prac.* 2011;26:382–390.

McCarthy MS, Phipps SC. Special nutrition challenges: Current approach to acute kidney injury. *Nutr Clin Pract.* 2014;29:56–62.

McClave S, Martindale RG, Vanek VW, et al. Guidelines for the provision and assessment of nutrition support therapy in the adult critically ill patient: SCCM and ASPEN. *JPEN.* 2009;33:277–316.

Obermüller N, Geiger H, Weipert C, Urbschat A. Current developments in early diagnosis of acute kidney injury. *Int Urol Nephrol.* 2014;46(1):1–7.

Patel N, Rogers CA, Angelini GD, Murphy GJ. Pharmacological therapies for the prevention of acute kidney injury following cardiac surgery: A systematic review. *Heart Failure Review.* 2011;16:553–567.

Tranter S. Cochrane Nursing Care Corner: Nutritional support for acute kidney injury. *Ren Soc Aust J.* 2011;7:36–37.

Valencia E, Marin A, Hardy G. Nutrition therapy for acute renal failure: A new approach based on "risk, injury, failure, loss and end-stage kidney" classification (RIFLE). *Curr Opin Clin Nutr Metabolic Care.* 2009;12:241–244.

Ukleja A, Freeman KL, Gilbert K, et al. Standards for nutrition support: Adult hospitalized patients. *Nutr Clin Pract.* 2010; 25: 403–414.

Wiesen P, Preiser JC. Nutrition support of critically ill patients with renal failure. In: Faber P, Siervo M. *Nutrition in Critical Care.* 1st ed. New York: Cambridge University Press; 2014:163–174.

Wiesen P, Van Overmeire L, Delanaye P, Dubois B, Preiser JC. Nutrition disorders during acute renal failure and renal replacement therapy. *JPEN J Parenter Enteral Nutr.* 2011;35:217–222.

Yang F, Zhang L, Wu H, Zou H, Du Y. Clinical analysis of cause, treatment and prognosis in acute kidney injury patients. *PLoS ONE.* 2014;9:e85214.

🌐 Internet Resources

AND Evidence Analysis Library: http://www.andeal.org

American Association of Kidney Patients: http://www.aakp.org

Cleveland Clinic Center for Continuing Education: http://www.clevelandclinicmeded.com/medicalpubs/diseasemanagement/nephrology/acute-kidney-injury/

National Institute of Diabetes and Digestive and Kidney Diseases of the National Institutes of Health: http://www2.niddk.nih.gov/

National Kidney Foundation: http://www.kidney.org

Nutrition Care Manual: http://www.nutritioncaremanual.org

Unit Eight

NUTRITION THERAPY FOR NEUROLOGICAL DISORDERS

Case 22 addresses neurological conditions through one of the most common diagnoses: stroke. According to the Centers for Disease Control and Prevention, stroke is the fifth leading cause of death in the United States (http://www.cdc.gov/nchs/fastats/stroke.htm, accessed March 31, 2015). The health consequences resulting from stroke are significant and, as in many neurological conditions, may involve impairment in the ability to maintain nutritional status. Symptoms such as impaired vision or ambulation may result in the inability to shop or prepare adequate meals. Depending on the severity of the stroke, symptoms may interfere with chewing, swallowing, or feeding oneself. These problems are often not easily identified or easily solved. Each situation is highly individualized and requires a comprehensive nutrition assessment. Throughout the course of the disease and rehabilitation, nutrition therapy plays a crucial role in the maintenance of nutritional status and quality of life.

Parkinson's disease and traumatic brain injury are additional diagnoses for which you will plan nutrition interventions for neurological disease. Consequences of these devastating diseases can interfere with all phases of obtaining, eating, and enjoying food. Cases 23 and 24 examine these consequences and allow for discussion about the role of the registered dietitian during terminal illness. Case 25 is a new case that will allow you to explore a pediatric chronic condition—cerebral palsy—and its subsequent nutritional concerns.

Case 22

Ischemic Stroke

Objectives

After completing this case, the student will be able to:

1. Apply a working knowledge of stroke pathophysiology to the nutrition care process.
2. Analyze nutrition assessment data to establish baseline nutritional status.
3. Identify and explain the role of nutrition support in recovery and rehabilitation from stroke.
4. Assess and identify nutritional risks in dysphagia.
5. Establish the nutrition diagnosis and compose a PES statement.
6. Create strategies to maximize calorie and protein intake.
7. Apply current recommendations for nutritional supplementation and determine appropriate nutrition interventions.

Mrs. Yvette Washington, a 63-year-old woman, is transported to the ED of University Hospital with the following symptoms: slurred speech, numbness on the right side of her face, and weakness of her right arm and leg.

Washington, Yvette, Female, 63 y.o.
Allergies: NKA
Pt. Location: RM 926

Code: FULL
Physician: S. Young

Isolation: None
Admit Date: 8/12

Patient Summary: Patient is brought to the hospital with right-sided hemiparesis and slurred speech.

History:
Onset of disease: N/A
Medical history: HTN × 10 years, hyperlipidemia × 2 years
Surgical history: Hysterectomy 10 years ago
Medications at home: Captopril 25 mg twice daily; lovastatin 20 mg once daily
Tobacco use: No
Alcohol use: No
Family history: Noncontributory

Demographics:
Marital status: Married—lives with husband; *Spouse name:* Robert
Number of children: Children are grown and do not live at home.
Years education: High school diploma
Language: English only
Occupation: Retired hairdresser
Hours of work: N/A
Ethnicity: African American
Religious affiliation: Protestant—AME

Admitting History/Physical:
Chief complaint: Mr. Washington states that his wife woke up this morning with everything pretty normal, but midmorning she became dizzy and then she couldn't talk or move one side of her body.
General appearance: African-American female who is unable to speak; unable to move right side

Vital Signs: Temp: 98.8   Pulse: 91   Resp rate: 19
                    BP: 138/88   Height: 5'2"   Weight: 185 lbs

Heart: Regular rate and rhythm, no gallops or rubs, point of maximal impulse at the fifth intercostal space in the midclavicular line
HEENT: Head: Normocephalic
          Eyes: Wears glasses for myopia
          Ears: Tympanic membranes normal
          Nose: WNL
          Throat: Slightly dry mucous membranes w/out exudates or lesions
Genitalia: Normal w/out lesions
Neurologic: New-onset weakness of the right side involving right arm and leg. Face and arm weakness is disproportionate to leg weakness and sensation is impaired on the contralateral side. Dysarthria with tongue deviation. Cranial nerves III, V, VII, XII impaired. Motor function tone and strength diminished. Plantar reflex decreased on right side. Blink reflex intact.

Washington, Yvette, Female, 63 y.o.
Allergies: NKA
Pt. Location: RM 926

Code: FULL
Physician: S. Young

Isolation: None
Admit Date: 8/12

Extremities: Reduced strength, bilaterally
Skin: Normal without lesions
Chest/lungs: Respirations normal; no crackles, rhonchi, wheezes, or rubs noted
Peripheral vascular: Bilateral, 3+ pedal pulses
Abdomen: Normal bowel sounds. No hepatomegaly, splenomegaly, masses, inguinal lymph nodes, or abdominal bruits.

Nursing Assessment	8/12
Abdominal appearance (concave, flat, rounded, obese, distended)	rounded, obese
Palpation of abdomen (soft, rigid, firm, masses, tense)	soft
Bowel function (continent, incontinent, flatulence, no stool)	incontinent
Bowel sounds (P=present, AB=absent, hypo, hyper)	
RUQ	P
LUQ	P
RLQ	P
LLQ	P
Stool color	brown
Stool consistency	formed
Tubes/ostomies	N/A
Genitourinary	
Urinary continence	catheter
Urine source	catheter
Appearance (clear, cloudy, yellow, amber, fluorescent, hematuria, orange, blue, tea)	yellow
Integumentary	
Skin color	pale
Skin temperature (DI=diaphoretic, W=warm, dry, CL=cool, CLM=clammy, CD+=cold, M=moist, H=hot)	CL
Skin turgor (good, fair, poor, TENT=tenting)	fair
Skin condition (intact, EC=ecchymosis, A=abrasions, P=petechiae, R=rash, W=weeping, S=sloughing, D=dryness, EX=excoriated, T=tears, SE=subcutaneous emphysema, B=blisters, V=vesicles, N=necrosis)	intact
Mucous membranes (intact, EC=ecchymosis, A=abrasions, P=petechiae, R=rash, W=weeping, S=sloughing, D=dryness, EX=excoriated, T=tears, SE=subcutaneous emphysema, B=blisters, V=vesicles, N=necrosis)	intact
Other components of Braden score: special bed, sensory pressure, moisture, activity, friction/shear (>18=no risk, 15–16=low risk, 13–14=moderate risk, ≤12=high risk)	sensory pressure, 12

Washington, Yvette, Female, 63 y.o.

Allergies: NKA	**Code:** FULL	**Isolation:** None
Pt. Location: RM 926	**Physician:** S. Young	**Admit Date:** 8/12

Orders:

Administer 0.6 mg/kg intravenous rtPA over 1 hour with 10% of total dose given as an initial intravenous bolus over one minute. Total dose of 67.5 mg.

Vital signs: q 15 minutes × 2 hours; then q 30 minutes × 6 hours; then q 1 hour × 16 hours.

Neuro checks: Level of consciousness and extremity weakness (use NIHSS scoring): q 30 minutes × 6 hours, then q 1 hour × 16 hours

IV: 0.9 NS at 75 cc/hr

O_2 at 2 liters/minute via nasal cannula (if needed to keep O_2 sats ≥95%)

Continuous cardiac monitoring

Strict Intake/Output records

Diet: NPO except medications for 24 hours

Noncontrast CT scan

Labs: Chem 16, coagulation times, CBC

Medications: Acetaminophen 650 mg po PRN for pain q 4 to 6 hours

No heparin, warfarin, or aspirin for 24 hours. After 24 hrs: CT to exclude intracranial hemorrhage before any anticoagulants.

Bedside swallowing assessment. Endoscopy with modified barium swallow.

Speech-language pathologist and dietitian to determine staged dysphagia diet.

Nutrition:

History: Mr. Washington states that his wife has a good appetite. She has not followed any special diet except for trying to avoid fried foods, and she has stopped adding salt at the table. She made these changes several years ago.

24-hour recall: According to Mr. Washington, his wife ate the following:

Breakfast:	Orange juice—1 c
	Raisin bran—1 c with 6 oz 2% milk
	1 banana
	8 oz coffee with 2 tbsp 2% milk and sweetener
Lunch:	Chicken tortellini soup (cheese tortellini cooked in chicken broth)—2 c
	Saltine crackers—about 8
	Canned pears—2 halves
	6 oz iced tea with sweetener
Dinner:	Fried pork chop—4–6 oz
	Baked sweet potato—1 medium—with 2 tbsp margarine
	Steamed broccoli—approx. 1 c with 1 tsp margarine
	Canned peaches in juice—6–8 slices
	6 oz iced tea with sweetener

Food allergies/intolerances/aversions: None

Previous nutrition therapy? No

Current diet: NPO

Food purchase/preparation: Mrs. Washington and spouse

Vit/min intake: Multivitamin/mineral supplement daily, 500 mg calcium 3 × daily

Washington, Yvette, Female, 63 y.o.
Allergies: NKA
Pt. Location: RM 926

Code: FULL
Physician: S. Young

Isolation: None
Admit Date: 8/12

Laboratory Results

	Ref. Range	8/12 1215
Chemistry		
Sodium (mEq/L)	136–145	141
Potassium (mEq/L)	3.5–5.1	3.8
Chloride (mEq/L)	98–107	101
Carbon dioxide (CO_2, mEq/L)	23–29	27
Bicarbonate (mEq/L)	23–28	25
BUN (mg/dL)	6–20	19
Creatinine serum (mg/dL)	0.6–1.1 F 0.9–1.3 M	1.2 !↑
BUN/Crea ratio	10.0–20.0	15.8
Uric acid (mg/dL)	2.8–8.8 F 4.0–9.0 M	5.9
Est GFR, Afr-Amer (mL/min/1.73 m²)	>60	56 !↓
Glucose (mg/dL)	70–99	99
Phosphate, inorganic (mg/dL)	2.2–4.6	4.2
Magnesium (mg/dL)	1.5–2.4	2.1
Calcium (mg/dL)	8.6–10.2	9.2
Osmolality (mmol/kg/H_2O)	275–295	294
Bilirubin total (mg/dL)	≤1.2	0.9
Bilirubin, direct (mg/dL)	<0.3	0.2
Protein, total (g/dL)	6–7.8	6.3
Albumin (g/dL)	3.5–5.5	4.6
Prealbumin (mg/dL)	18–35	31
Ammonia (NH_3, µg/L)	6–47	15
Alkaline phosphatase (U/L)	30–120	119
ALT (U/L)	4–36	21
AST (U/L)	0–35	33
CPK (U/L)	30–135 F 55–170 M	131
Lactate dehydrogenase (U/L)	208–378	371
Cholesterol (mg/dL)	<200	210 !↑
HDL-C (mg/dL)	>59 F, >50 M	40 !↓

(Continued)

Washington, Yvette, Female, 63 y.o.
Allergies: NKA
Pt. Location: RM 926

Code: FULL
Physician: S. Young

Isolation: None
Admit Date: 8/12

Laboratory Results *(Continued)*

	Ref. Range	8/12 1215
VLDL (mg/dL)	7–32	39 !↑
LDL (mg/dL)	<130	155 !↑
LDL/HDL ratio	<3.22 F <3.55 M	3.8 !↑
Triglycerides (mg/dL)	35–135 F 40–160 M	198 !↑
HbA$_{1c}$ (%)	<5.7	4.9
Coagulation (Coag)		
PT (sec)	11–13	11.5
INR	0.9–1.1	0.98
Hematology		
WBC ($\times 10^3$/mm^3)	3.9–10.7	10.1
RBC ($\times 10^6$/mm^3)	4.2–5.4 F 4.5–6.2 M	4.5
Hemoglobin (Hgb, g/dL)	12–16 F 14–17 M	13.7
Hematocrit (Hct, %)	37–47 F 41–51 M	38.1
Platelet count ($\times 10^3$/mm^3)	150–350	243

Note: Values and units of measurement listed in these tables are derived from several resources. Substantial variation exists in the ranges quoted as "normal" and these may vary depending on the assay used by different laboratories.

Case Questions

I. Understanding the Disease and Pathophysiology

1. Define *stroke*. Describe the differences between ischemic and hemorrhagic strokes.

2. The noncontrast CT confirmed that Mrs. Washington had suffered a lacunar ischemic stroke—NIH Stroke Scale Score of 14. What does Mrs. Washington's score for the NIH stroke scale indicate?

3. What factors place an individual at risk for stroke?

4. What specific signs and symptoms noted with Mrs. Washington's exam and history are consistent with her diagnosis? Which symptoms place Mrs. Washington at nutritional risk? Explain your rationale.

5. What is rtPA? Why was it administered?

II. Understanding the Nutrition Therapy

6. Define *dysphagia*. What is the primary nutrition implication of dysphagia?

7. Describe the four phases of swallowing:

   a. Oral preparation

   b. Oral transit

   c. Pharyngeal

   d. Esophageal

8. The National Dysphagia Diet defines three levels of solid foods and four levels of fluid consistency to be used when planning a diet for someone with dysphagia. Describe each of these levels of diet modifications.

9. It is determined that Mrs. Washington's dysphagia is centered in the esophageal transit phase and she has reduced esophageal peristalsis. Which dysphagia diet level is appropriate to try with Mrs. Washington?

10. Describe a bedside swallowing assessment. What are the background and training requirements of a speech-language pathologist?

11. Describe a modified barium swallow or fiberoptic endoscopic evaluation of swallowing.

12. Thickening agents and specialty food products are often used to provide texture changes needed for the dysphagia diet. Describe one of these products and how it may be incorporated into the diet.

III. Nutrition Assessment

13. Mrs. Washington's usual body weight is approximately 165 lbs. Calculate and interpret her BMI and her %UBW.

14. Estimate Mrs. Washington's energy and protein requirements. Should weight loss or weight gain be included in this estimation? What is your rationale?

15. Using Mrs. Washington's usual dietary intake, calculate the total number of kilocalories she consumed as well as the energy distribution of kilocalories for protein, carbohydrate, and fat.

16. Compare this to the nutrient recommendations for an individual with hyperlipidemia and hypertension. Should these recommendations apply for Mrs. Washington during this acute period after her stroke?

17. Estimate Mrs. Washington's fluid needs.

18. Review Mrs. Washington's labs upon admission. Identify any that are abnormal. For each abnormal value, explain the reason for the abnormality and describe the clinical significance and nutritional implications for Mrs. Washington.

IV.   Nutrition Diagnosis

19. Select two nutrition problems and complete the PES statement for each.

V.   Nutrition Intervention

20. For each of the PES statements that you have written, establish an ideal goal (based on the signs and symptoms) and an appropriate intervention (based on the etiology).

VI.   Nutrition Monitoring and Evaluation

21. To maintain or attain normal nutritional status while reducing danger of aspiration and choking, the texture of foods and/or viscosity of fluids are personalized for a patient with dysphagia. Define and give an example of each of the following terms used to describe characteristics of foods/fluids.

Consistency:

Texture:

Viscosity:

22. Using Mrs. Washington's 24-hour recall, make suggestions for consistency changes or food substitutions (if needed) to Mrs. Washington and her family.

Orange juice:

Raisin bran:

2% milk:

Banana:

Coffee:

Sweetener:

Chicken tortellini soup:

Saltine crackers:

Canned pears:

Iced tea:

Fried pork chop:

Baked sweet potato:

Steamed broccoli:

Margarine:

Canned peaches:

23. Describe Mrs. Washington's potential nutritional problems upon discharge. What recommendations could you make to her husband to prevent each problem you identified? How would you monitor her progress?

24. Would Mrs. Washington be an appropriate candidate for a stroke rehabilitation program? Why or why not?

Bibliography

Academy of Nutrition and Dietetics Nutrition Care Manual. Cerebrovascular Disease. Available from https://www.nutritioncaremanual.org/topic.cfm?ncm_category_id=1&lv1=5803&lv2=8233&ncm_toc_id=8233&ncm_heading=Nutrition%20Care. Accessed 03/30/15.

Asin Prieto G, Cano-de-la-Cuerda R, Lopez-Larraz J, et al. Emerging perspectives in stroke rehabilitation. In: Pons JL, Torricelli D. *Emerging Therapies in Neuro-rehabilitation.* Berlin; Springer Science & Business Media; 2014:3–21.

Belafsky P, Kuhn M. The videofluoroscopic swallow study technique and protocol. In: Belafsky PC, Kuhn M. *The Clinician's Guide to Swallowing Fluoroscopy.* New York; Springer; 2014:7–13.

Brody RA, Tougher-Decker R, VonHagen S, et al. Role of registered dietitians in dysphagia screening. *J Am Diet Assoc.* 2000;100(9):1029–1037.

Crary MA, Humphrey JL, Carnaby-Mann G, et al. Dysphagia, nutrition and hydration in ischemic stroke patients at admission and discharge from acute care. *Dysphagia.* 2013;28:69–76.

Dennis M, Lewis S, Cranswick G, Forbes J, FOOD Trial Collaboration. FOOD: A multicentre randomised trial evaluating feeding policies in patients admitted to hospital with a recent stroke. *Health Technol Assess.* 2006;10(2):iii–iv, ix–x, 1–120.

Go AS, Mozaffarian D, Roger VL, et al. Executive summary: Heart disease and stroke statistics—2014 update: A report from the American Heart Association. *Circulation.* 2014;129:399–410.

Grise EM, Adeoye O, Lindsell C, et al. Emergency department adherence to American Heart Association Guidelines for blood pressure management in acute ischemic stroke. *Stroke.* 2012;43:557–559.

Hinkle JL. Reliability and validity of the National Institutes of Health Stroke Scale for neuroscience nurses. *Stroke.* 2014;45: e32–34.

Jauch EC, Saver JL, Adams HP, et al. Guidelines for the early management of patient with acute ischemic stroke: A guideline for healthcare professionals from the American Heart Association/American Stroke Association. *Stroke.* 2013;44:870–947.

Johnson S, Brody R, Touger-Decker R, Fleish Marcus A. Knowledge and performance of dysphagia risk screening among registered dietitians in clinical practice. *JAND.* 2014;114 (9supp):A26.

Maasland L, Koudstaal PJ, Habbema JD, Dippel DW. Knowledge and understanding of disease process, risk factors and treatment modalities in patients with a recent TIA or minor ischemic stroke. *Cerebrovasc Dis.* 2007;23(5–6):435–440.

Morgenstern LB, Hemphill JC, Anderson C, et al. AHA/ASA Guideline: Guidelines for the management of spontaneous intracerebral hemorrhage. *Stroke.* 2010;41:2108–2129.

Paquereau J, Allart E, Romon M, Rousseaux M. The long-term nutritional status in stroke patients and its predictive factors. *Journal of Stroke and Cerebrovascular Diseases.* 2014;23:1628–1633.

Smith EE, Saver JL, Alexander DN, et al. Clinical performance measures for adults hospitalized with acute ischemic stroke: Performance measures for healthcare professionals from the American Heart Association/American Stroke Association. *Stroke.* 2014;45:3472–3498.

Torbey MT, Bosel J, Thoney DH, et al. Evidence-based guidelines for the management of large hemispheric infarction. *Neurocrit Care.* 2015;22:146–164.

Internet Resources

American Speech-Language-Hearing Association: http://www.asha.org

American Stroke Association: A Division of the American Heart Association: http://www.strokeassociation.org

National Institute of Neurological Disorders and Stroke: http://www.ninds.nih.gov/disorders/stroke/stroke.htm

NIH Stroke Scale and Scoring: http://www.strokecenter.org/trials/scales/nihss.html

USDA Choose My Plate – Supertracker: http://www.choosemyplate.gov/supertracker-tools/supertracker.html

Video Link for Evaluation of Stages of Swallowing: http://www.linkstudio.info/images/portfolio/medani/Swallow.swf

Case 23

Progressive Neurological Disease: Parkinson's Disease

Objectives

After completing this case, the student will be able to:

1. Demonstrate a working knowledge of the pathophysiology of Parkinson's disease and its current medical care.
2. Describe the potential drug–nutrient interactions for Parkinson's disease.
3. Discuss the current understanding of nutrient supplementation in treatment of Parkinson's disease.
4. Assess for and identify nutritional health risks in dysphagia.
5. Analyze nutrition assessment data to evaluate nutritional status, identify specific nutrition problems, and document corresponding PES statements.
6. Use current assessment data to assess for and diagnose malnutrition.
7. Interpret laboratory parameters for nutritional implications and significance.
8. Develop a nutrition care plan—with appropriate measurable goals, interventions, and strategies for monitoring and evaluation—that addresses the nutrition diagnoses of this case.

Rita McCormick is admitted to University Hospital with fever, cough, and respiratory symptoms for an assessment to R/O pneumonia. Her family states that she is experiencing coughing, choking, and difficulty eating. She was diagnosed with Parkinson's disease 10 years ago and has experienced continued progression of her disease.

McCormick, Rita, Female, 69 y.o.
Allergies: NKA
Pt. Location: 1101

Code: FULL
Physician: S. Goldman

Isolation: None
Admit Date: 2/13

Patient Summary: The patient is a 69-year-old female with Parkinson's disease. At her physician's office, she presented with fever and increased white blood cell count. Her family relates that she has had increasing difficulty eating. She often coughs and appears to choke during meals.

History:

Onset of disease: Diagnosed initially 10 years ago
Medical history: Parkinson's disease
Surgical history: Bilateral salpingo-oophorectomy
Medications at home: Sinemet: carbidopa/levodopa, 50/200 mg controlled-release tablet twice daily; citalopram 20 mg daily; esomeprazole 20 mg daily; omega-3-fatty acids 1000 mg daily
Tobacco use: Quit over 30 years ago
Alcohol use: Socially
Family history: Mother—Alzheimer's disease; father—CAD

Demographics:

Marital status: Widowed
Years education: 2 year college
Language: English
Occupation: Retired dental assistant
Household members: Lives with son (45) and his wife (42)
Ethnicity: Caucasian
Religious affiliation: Methodist

Admitting History/Physical:

Chief complaint: "Every time I eat, something gets stuck in my throat. I cough and feel like I'm choking. It just scares me to eat."

Vital Signs:
Temp: 101.5   Pulse: 80   Resp rate: 22
BP: 135/85   Height: 60"   Weight: 90 lbs
UBW: 110 lbs (six months previous)

Heart: RRR. No gallops or rubs, point of maximal impulse at the fifth intercostal space in the midclavicular line.
HEENT: Head: Normocephalic; dry, dull hair; sunken cheeks; evidence of temporal wasting
       Eyes: Glasses for myopia; bilateral redness, fissured eyelid corners; reduced subcutaneous fat within orbital area
       Ears: Tympanic membranes normal
       Nose: Dry mucous membranes without lesions
       Throat: Slightly dry mucous membranes without exudates or lesions
Genitalia: WNL
Neurologic: Alert and oriented × 3; decreased blink reflex; positive palmomental; diminished postural reflexes. Family reports 3 falls in past 6 months. UPDRS: Stage 3.

McCormick, Rita, Female, 69 y.o.
Allergies: NKA   **Code:** FULL   **Isolation:** None
Pt. Location: 1101   **Physician:** S. Goldman   **Admit Date:** 2/13

Extremities: Reduced strength, evidence of muscle loss in quadriceps and gastrocnemius; koilonychias, bilateral tremor
Skin: Warm, dry, poor turgor, angular stomatitis and cheilosis noted on lips
Chest/lungs: Respirations rapid; crackles, rhonchi noted
Peripheral vascular: Bilateral, 3+pedal pulses
Abdomen: Normal bowel sounds—in all regions, without masses or splenomegaly

Nursing Assessment	2/13
Abdominal appearance (concave, flat, rounded, obese, distended)	flat
Palpation of abdomen (soft, rigid, firm, masses, tense)	soft
Bowel function (continent, incontinent, flatulence, no stool)	continent
Bowel sounds (P=present, AB=absent, hypo, hyper)	
RUQ	P
LUQ	P
RLQ	P
LLQ	P
Stool color	dark brown
Stool consistency	hard
Tubes/ostomies	none
Genitourinary	
Urinary continence	yes
Urine source	clean catch
Appearance (clear, cloudy, yellow, amber, fluorescent, hematuria, orange, blue, tea)	cloudy, amber
Integumentary	
Skin color	pale
Skin temperature (DI=diaphoretic, W=warm, dry, CL=cool, CLM=clammy, CD+=cold, M=moist, H=hot)	W
Skin turgor (good, fair, poor, TENT=tenting)	poor
Skin condition (intact, EC=ecchymosis, A=abrasions, P=petechiae, R=rash, W=weeping, S=sloughing, D=dryness, EX=excoriated, T=tears, SE=subcutaneous emphysema, B=blisters, V=vesicles, N=necrosis)	EC
Mucous membranes (intact, EC=ecchymosis, A=abrasions, P=petechiae, R=rash, W=weeping, S=sloughing, D=dryness, EX=excoriated, T=tears, SE=subcutaneous emphysema, B=blisters, V=vesicles, N=necrosis)	intact, D
Other components of Braden score: special bed, sensory pressure, moisture, activity, friction/shear (>18=no risk, 15–16=low risk, 13–14=moderate risk, ≤12=high risk)	15

McCormick, Rita, Female, 69 y.o.
Allergies: NKA
Pt. Location: 1101

Code: FULL
Physician: S. Goldman

Isolation: None
Admit Date: 2/13

Admission Orders:

Laboratory: CBC, Chem 27, CXR
Initiate azithromycin 500 mg IV once daily
Vital Signs: Per protocol
Diet: NPO—Nutrition consult
Gastroenterology consult for MBS (Modified Barium Swallow)
SLP Consult: Flexible endoscopic evaluation of swallowing

Nutrition:

Meal type: Previously regular at home—now NPO
History: Mostly liquids, because solids are difficult to swallow
Usual dietary intake: Before developing current difficulty with swallowing, Mrs. McCormick usually ate the following:
Breakfast: ½ scrambled egg, ½ slice toast or English muffin, 1 tsp jelly, coffee with 2% milk and artificial sweetener
Lunch: ½ ham or turkey sandwich, 6–7 chips, iced tea with artificial sweetener
Dinner: ¾ c spaghetti with ½ c meat sauce, 2–3 tbsp green peas or other vegetable, ½ c canned fruit cocktail, ½ slice bread with 1 tsp butter, iced tea with artificial sweetener

Intake/Output

Date		2/13 0701–2/14 0700			
Time		0701–1500	1501–2300	2301–0700	Daily total
IN	P.O.	0	0	0	0
	I.V.	400	400	400	1200
	(mL/kg/hr)	(1.22)	(1.22)	(1.22)	(1.22)
	I.V. piggyback	250	0	0	250
	TPN				
	Total intake	650	400	400	1450
	(mL/kg)	(15.89)	(9.78)	(9.78)	(35.45)
OUT	Urine	320	310	200	830
	(mL/kg/hr)	(0.98)	(0.95)	(0.61)	(0.84)
	Emesis output				
	Other				
	Stool	×1			
	Total output	320	310	200	830
	(mL/kg)	(7.82)	(7.58)	(4.89)	(20.29)
Net I/O		+330	+90	+200	+620
Net since admission (2/13)		+330	+420	+620	+620

McCormick, Rita, Female, 69 y.o.
Allergies: NKA
Pt. Location: 1101

Code: FULL
Physician: S. Goldman

Isolation: None
Admit Date: 2/13

Laboratory Results

	Ref. Range	2/13 0900
Chemistry		
Sodium (mEq/L)	136–145	145
Potassium (mEq/L)	3.5–5.1	4.1
Chloride (mEq/L)	98–107	101
Carbon dioxide (CO_2, mEq/L)	23–29	24
Bicarbonate (mEq/L)	23–28	23
BUN (mg/dL)	6–20	14
Creatinine serum (mg/dL)	0.6–1.1 F 0.9–1.3 M	1.1
BUN/Crea ratio	10.0–20.0	12.7
Uric acid (mg/dL)	2.8–8.8 F 4.0–9.0 M	3.1
Est GFR, non-Afr Amer (mL/min/1.73 m²)	>60	51 !↓
Glucose (mg/dL)	70–99	78
Phosphate, inorganic (mg/dL)	2.2–4.6	2.2
Magnesium (mg/dL)	1.5–2.4	1.5
Calcium (mg/dL)	8.6–10.2	8.9
Osmolality (mmol/kg/H_2O)	275–295	299 !↑
Bilirubin total (mg/dL)	≤1.2	1.0
Bilirubin, direct (mg/dL)	<0.3	0.2
Protein, total (g/dL)	6–7.8	5.8 !↓
Albumin (g/dL)	3.5–5.5	2.9 !↓
Prealbumin (mg/dL)	18–35	17 !↓
Ammonia (NH_3, μg/L)	6–47	8
Alkaline phosphatase (U/L)	30–120	45
ALT (U/L)	4–36	21
AST (U/L)	0–35	17
CPK (U/L)	30–135 F 55–170 M	88
Lactate dehydrogenase (U/L)	208–378	301
Cholesterol (mg/dL)	<200	145
HDL-C (mg/dL)	>59 F, >50 M	62
VLDL (mg/dL)	7–32	13

(Continued)

McCormick, Rita, Female, 69 y.o.
Allergies: NKA
Pt. Location: 1101

Code: FULL
Physician: S. Goldman

Isolation: None
Admit Date: 2/13

Laboratory Results *(Continued)*

	Ref. Range	2/13 0900
LDL (mg/dL)	<130	71
LDL/HDL ratio	<3.22 F <3.55 M	1.14
Triglycerides (mg/dL)	35–135 F 40–160 M	68
Hematology		
WBC (× 10³/mm³)	3.9–10.7	11.9 !↑
RBC (× 10⁶/mm³)	4.2–5.4 F 4.5–6.2 M	3.8 !↓
Hemoglobin (Hgb, g/dL)	12–16 F 14–17 M	10.5 !↓
Hematocrit (Hct, %)	37–47 F 41–51 M	32.4 !↓
Transferrin (mg/dL)	250–380 F 215–365 M	391 !↑
Ferritin (mg/mL)	20–120 F 20–300 M	11 !↓
Total iron binding capacity (mg/dL)	240–460	463 !↑

Note: Values and units of measurement listed in these tables are derived from several resources. Substantial variation exists in the ranges quoted as "normal" and these may vary depending on the assay used by different laboratories.

Case Questions

I.   Understanding the Diagnosis and Pathophysiology

1. Describe our current understanding of the pathophysiology of Parkinson's disease.

2. How does this pathophysiology translate into the cardinal signs and symptoms of Parkinson's? Which may contribute to nutritional risk? Which of these are noted in Mrs. McCormick's history and physical?

3. Currently the disease status is often described using the Unified Parkinson's Disease Rating Scale (UPDRS). What is this, and how would you interpret Mrs. McCormick's staging?

4. Identify and describe the primary medical interventions that are used for treatment of Parkinson's disease.

5. One of the major medications used to treat Parkinson's is levodopa. How does diet potentially play a role in this medication's efficacy? Identify all drug–nutrient interactions for Mrs. McCormick's prescribed medications.

II.   Understanding the Nutrition Therapy

6. Define *dysphagia*. What medical and nutritional complications may be associated with dysphagia?

7. Mrs. McCormick is having an SLP consult and a FEES test completed. What training does a speech-language therapist have? What is a FEES? What type of information will this provide for the MD and the RD?

8. What is an MBS? What information will this test provide?

9. Discuss the major nutrition concerns associated with Parkinson's. Provide evidence for any of these that Mrs. McCormick may be experiencing.

10. Mrs. McCormick's MD discusses the potential for the placement of a PEG tube for this patient. Provide any justification for nutrition support using the appropriate criteria and guidelines.

11. There are a number of supplements that have been studied as components of Parkinson's treatment. Discuss the use of coenzyme Q, omega-3-fatty acids, and creatine and their potential efficacy for patients with Parkinson's.

III.   Nutrition Assessment

12. Evaluate Mrs. McCormick's weight by calculating her BMI and %UBW.

13. After examining Mrs. McCormick's history and physical, identify any clinical signs and symptoms that may alert you to a nutrient deficiency. Describe the nutrition-focused physical examination and address the important components that may be used to fully assess Mrs. McCormick's nutritional status.

14. Evaluate Mrs. McCormick's laboratory values. List all abnormal values and explain the likely cause for each abnormal value.

15. Determine Mrs. McCormick's energy and protein requirements. Explain the rationale for the method you used to calculate these requirements.

16. Assess Mrs. McCormick's diet prior to having difficulty swallowing. Compare her energy and protein intakes to her estimated nutrient needs.

IV.   Nutrition Diagnosis

17. What criteria would you assess to determine if Mrs. McCormick meets the criteria for malnutrition using the proposed definitions of malnutrition associated with chronic disease?

18. Identify two pertinent nutrition problems and the corresponding nutrition diagnoses.

19. Write your PES statement for each nutrition problem.

V.   Nutrition Intervention

20. The National Dysphagia Diet defines three levels of solid foods and four levels of fluid consistency to be used when planning a diet for someone with dysphagia. Describe each of these levels of diet modifications.

21. The Dysphagia Outcome and Severity Scale (DOSS) is used to determine the nutrition prescription for a patient. Discuss this scale and how it corresponds to the level of dysphagia diet that is recommended.

22. The FEES and MBS indicate the following: "Patient demonstrates difficulty initiating the swallow and bolus was held in the mouth for an excessive amount of time. Spillage into the larynx is noted with some aspiration." Identify the diet you would recommend at this time.

23. Using the data collected during your nutrition assessment, what vitamin and mineral supplementation would you recommend?

VI.   Nutrition Monitoring and Evaluation

24. Identify factors that you will need to monitor to ensure adequacy of her nutrition intervention.

25. What criteria would you use to determine whether Mrs. McCormick requires enteral feeding?

Bibliography

Bachmann CG, Trenkwalder C. Body weight in patients with Parkinson's disease. *Mov Disord*. 2006;21(11):1824–1830.

Bariachella M, Cerada E, Pezzoli G. Major nutritional issues in the management of Parkinson's disease. *Mov Disord*. 2009;24:1881–1892.

Barichella M, Marczewska A, De Notaris R, et al. Special low-protein foods ameliorate postprandial off in patients with advanced Parkinson's disease. *Mov Disord*. 2006;21(10):1682–1687.

Bender A, Koch W, Elstner M, et al. Creatine supplementation in Parkinson disease: A placebo-controlled randomized pilot trial. *Neurology*. 2006;67(7):1262–1264.

Caviness JN. Pathophysiology of Parkinson's disease behavior—a view from the network. *Parkinsonism Relat Disord*. 2014;20 Suppl 1:S39–S43.

Chao J, Leung Y, Wang M, Chuen-Chung Chang R. Nutraceuticals and their preventive or potential value in Parkinson's disease. *Nutr Rev*. 2012;70:373–386.

Cintra MT, de Rezende NA, de Moraes EN, Cunha LC, da Gama Torres HO. A comparison of survival, pneumonia, and hospitalization in patients with advanced dementia and dysphagia receiving either oral or enteral nutrition. *J Nutr Health Aging*. 2014(10);18: 894–899.

Cushing ML, Traviss KA, Caine SM. Parkinson's disease: Implications for nutritional care. *Canadian J Diet Prac Res*. 2002;63:81–87.

Delikanaki-Skaribas E, Trail M, Wong WW, Lai EC. Daily energy expenditure, physical activity, and weight loss in Parkinson's disease patients. *Mov Disord*. 2009;24:667–671.

Evatt ML. Nutritional therapies in Parkinson's disease. *Curr Treat Options Neurol*. 2007;9:198–204.

Fu LM, Fu KA. Analysis of Parkinson's disease pathophysiology using an integrated genomics-bioinformatics approach. *Pathophysiology*. 2015;22(1):15–29.

Giladi N, Manor Y, Hilel A, Gurevich T. Interdisciplinary teamwork for the treatment of people with Parkinson's disease and their families. *Curr Neurol Neurosci Rep*. 2014;14:493.

Goetz CG, Pal G. Initial management of Parkinson's disease. *BMJ*. 2014;349:g6258.

Leckie RL, Manuck SB, Bhattacharjee N, Muldoon MF, Flory JM, Erickson KI. Omega-3 fatty acids moderate effects of physical activity on cognitive function. *Neuropsychologia*. 2014;59:103–111.

Lewitt PA. Levodopa therapy for Parkinson's disease: Pharmacokinetics and pharmacodynamics. *Mov Disord*. 2015;30:64–72.

Li Z, Wang P, Yu Z, et al. The effect of creatine and co-enzyme Q10 combination therapy on mild cognitive impairment in Parkinson's disease. *Eur Neurol*. 2015;73:205–211.

Marcason W. What are the primary nutritional issues for a patient with Parkinson's disease? *J Am Diet Assoc*. 2009;109:1316.

Nahikian-Nelms ML. Diseases and disorders of the neurological system. In: Nelms M, Sucher K, Lacey K. *Nutrition Therapy and Pathophysiology*. 3rd ed. Belmont, CA: Cengage Learning; 2016:596–634.

Nahikian-Nelms ML. Diseases of the upper gastrointestinal tract. In: Nelms M, Sucher K, Lacey K. *Nutrition Therapy and Pathophysiology*. 3rd ed. Belmont, CA: Cengage Learning; 2016:342–435.

NINDS NET-PD Investigators. A randomized clinical trial of coenzyme Q10 and GPI-1485 in early Parkinson disease. *Neurology*. 2007;68:20–28

Olanow CW. Levodopa: Effect on cell death and the natural history of Parkinson's disease. *Mov Disord*. 2015;30:37–44.

O'Neil, Purdy M, Falk J, Gallo L. The dysphagia outcome and severity scale. *Dysphagia*. 1999;14:139–145.

Seidl SE, Santiago JA, Bilyk H, Potashkin JA. The emerging role of nutrition in Parkinson's disease. *Front Aging Neurosci*. 2014;6:36.

Smith RN, Agharkar AS, Gonzales EB. A review of creatine supplementation in age-related diseases: More than a supplement for athletes. *F1000Res*. 2014;3:222.

Soo-Peary K, Hsu A. The pharmcokinetics and pharmocodynamics of levodopa in the treatment of Parkinson's disease. *Current Clinical Pharmacology*. 2007;2:234–243.

Storch A, Jost WH, Vieregge P, et al. Randomized, double-blind, placebo-controlled trial on symptomatic effects of coenzyme Q(10) in Parkinson disease. *Arch Neurol*. 2007;64:938–944.

Tappendan KA, Quatrara B, Parkhurst ML, Malone AM, Fanjang G, Zeigler TR. Critical role of nutrition in improving quality of care: An interdisciplinary call to action to address adult hospital malnutrition. *JPEN*. 2013;17:482–497.

White JV, Guenter P, Jensen G, Malone A, Schofield M, Academy of Nutrition and Dietetics Malnutrition Work Group, A.S.P.E.N. Malnutrition Task Force, A.S.P.E.N. Board of Directors. Consensus statement of the Academy of Nutrition and Dietetics/American Society of Parenteral and Enteral Nutrition: Characteristics recommended for the identification and documentation of adult malnutrition. *J Acad Nutr Diet*. 2012;112:730–738.

Internet Resources

American Speech Language Hearing Association: Dysphagia Diets: http://www.asha.org/SLP/clinical/dysphagia/Dysphagia-Diets/

MedScape: Overview of Aspiration Pneumonia: http://emedicine.medscape.com/article/296198-overview

GI Motility Online: http://www.nature.com/gimo/contents/pt1/full/gimo28.html

International Parkinson and Movement Disorder Society: MDS-UPDRS: http://www.movementdisorders.org/MDS-Files1/Resources/PDFs/MDS-UPDRS.pdf

National Institute of Neurological Disorders and Stroke: http://www.ninds.nih.gov/disorders/parkinsons_disease/parkinsons_disease.htm

Nutrition Care Manual: http://www.nutritioncaremanual.org

Parkinson's Disease Foundation: www.pdf.org

Adult Traumatic Brain Injury

Objectives

After completing this case, the student will be able to:

1. Describe the pathophysiology of traumatic brain injury.
2. Describe the metabolic response to stress and trauma.
3. Determine nutrient, fluid, and electrolyte requirements for a critically ill patient.
4. Evaluate nutrition assessment data to determine nutritional status and identify specific nutrition problems.

5. Determine nutrition diagnoses and write appropriate PES statements.
6. Use evidence-based guidelines to design an enteral nutrition support plan.
7. Determine steps to monitor and evaluate enteral nutrition support and the transition to an oral diet.

Mr. Ryan Walker is a 25-year-old admitted through the ED after an MVC collision with tree.

Walker, Ryan, Male, 25 y.o.
Allergies: NKA
Pt. Location: SICU Bed #1

Code: FULL
Physician: L. King

Isolation: None
Admit Date: 6/6

Patient Summary: Ryan Walker is a 25-year-old white male admitted through ED after motor vehicle collision with tree. Last pm, 911 call indicated that 25 yo white male swerved to miss deer crossing the highway, lost control of his vehicle, hit guardrail and then tree which stopped his projectory. Mr. Walker was unconscious at the scene with unstable vitals. He was transported via Lifeflight to University Hospital.

History:
Onset of disease: Mr. Walker, restrained single driver in MVC with deer at 8:00 pm tonight. Intubated in ED emergently. He is transferred to SICU from the ED after stabilization.
Medical history: no significant medical history
Surgical history: appendectomy age 20
Medications at home: none
Tobacco use: nonsmoker
Alcohol use: social drinker per family—2–3 drinks per week
Family history: mother—breast cancer; father—hypertension, hyperlipidemia; brother (age 14)—leukemia now in remission

Demographics:
Marital status: single
Years education: 16 years—BS in mechanical engineering
Language: English, Spanish
Occupation: Engineer—Bismarck Airline Corporation
Hours of work: 9–5
Household members: lives with roommate
Ethnicity: Caucasian
Religious affiliation: none

Admitting History/Physical:
Chief complaint: Patient is alternating between moaning and unconsciousness.
General appearance: Multiple lacerations on head, face and arms.

Vital Signs: Temp: 100.5   Pulse: 105   Resp rate: 26
                    BP: 90/70   Height: 5'11"   Weight: 172 lbs
Heart: Regular rate and rhythm
HEENT: Head: multiple lacerations head, face and neck.
      Eyes: Pupils 4 mm reactive—opens to painful stimuli
      Ears: Clear
      Nose: Clear
      Throat: WNL
Genitalia: +rectal tone, heme negative

Walker, Ryan, Male, 25 y.o.
Allergies: NKA   **Code:** FULL   **Isolation:** None
Pt. Location: SICU Bed #1   **Physician:** L. King   **Admit Date:** 6/6

Neurologic: GCS = 8 E2 V2 M4. Withdrawal and moaning when touched. Some incomprehensible words.
Extremities: Flexion withdrawal from painful stimuli. Lacerations on both knees.
Skin: Warm and dry
Chest/lungs: Intubated in ED
Peripheral vascular: Pulse 4 + bilaterally, warm, no edema
Abdomen: Active bowel sounds × 4; nondistended

Orders:

Neuro checks q hour; Position HOB 30 degrees or greater.
Vital signs every hour—Maintain systolic blood pressure greater than 180 or less than 90; diastolic blood pressure greater than 100 or less than 60; heart rate greater than 110 or less than 60; respiratory rate greater than 24 or less than 10; temperature greater than 101.5; SaO2 less than 92%.
Cardiac monitoring
Continuous pulse oximetry
Intake/output
Weigh daily
Oral care per ventilator protocol.
Arterial line care per protocol.
Sedation Dose titration—Follow unit ICU sedation protocol for mechanical ventilation. If sedation weaning/interruption is not performed, document contraindications in patient chart.
Blood glucose every 6 hours—If any blood glucose is greater than 300mg/dl, then repeat blood glucose (POC device) in 2 hours. If the initial blood glucose was greater than 300mg/dl and if second blood glucose is greater than 200mg/dl, then notify house officer.
Medications: Diprivan (Propofol) 30 mcg/kg/min
               Fentanyl 25 mcg/hr
               Cefazolin (ANCEF) in 0.9% sodium chloride—2 g.
               Hydromorphone 0.5–1 mg every four hours
               4 g calcium gluconate, 4 g magnesium sulfate in 0.9% sodium chloride 75 mL/hr
               Tetanus and diphtheria toxoids vaccine injection 0.5 mL

Department of Radiology—CT Report
Date: 6/6
Patient: Ryan Walker
Physician: L. King, MD
Two areas of increased density in L frontal lobe near vertex and possibly left central modality
Victoria Roundtree, MD, Dept. of Radiology

Walker, Ryan, Male, 25 y.o.
Allergies: NKA
Pt. Location: SICU Bed #1

Code: FULL
Physician: L. King

Isolation: None
Admit Date: 6/6

Department of Radiology—MRI Report

Date: 6/6
Patient: Ryan Walker
Physician: *L. King, MD*
MRI showed areas of hemorrhagic edema in deep white matter of L frontal lobe anteriorly.
Additionally, heme and edema found in the splenium of corpus callosum.
3.4 cm × 4.2 cm × 1.0 cm representing areas of shearing injury.
H. Loews, MD, Dept. of Radiology

Nursing Assessment	6/6
Abdominal appearance (concave, flat, rounded, obese, distended)	flat
Palpation of abdomen (soft, rigid, firm, masses, tense)	soft
Bowel function (continent, incontinent, flatulence, no stool)	incontinent
Bowel sounds (P=present, AB=absent, hypo, hyper)	
RUQ	P
LUQ	P
RLQ	P
LLQ	P
Stool color	light brown
Stool consistency	soft
Tubes/ostomies	Foley catheter in place
Genitourinary	
Urinary continence	catheter
Urine source	catheter
Appearance (clear, cloudy, yellow, amber, fluorescent, hematuria, orange, blue, tea)	cloudy, hematuria
Integumentary	
Skin color	pale
Skin temperature (DI=diaphoretic, W=warm, dry, CL=cool, CLM=clammy, CD+=cold, M=moist, H=hot)	W
Skin turgor (good, fair, poor, TENT=tenting)	good
Skin condition (intact, EC=ecchymosis, A=abrasions, P=petechiae, R=rash, W=weeping, S=sloughing, D=dryness, EX=excoriated, T=tears, SE=subcutaneous emphysema, B=blisters, V=vesicles, N=necrosis)	EC, A
Mucous membranes (intact, EC=ecchymosis, A=abrasions, P=petechiae, R=rash, W=weeping, S=sloughing, D=dryness, EX=excoriated, T=tears, SE=subcutaneous emphysema, B=blisters, V=vesicles, N=necrosis)	intact
Other components of Braden score: special bed, sensory pressure, moisture, activity, friction/shear (>18=no risk, 15–16=low risk, 13–14=moderate risk, ≤12=high risk)	13

Walker, Ryan, Male, 25 y.o.
Allergies: NKA
Pt. Location: SICU Bed #1

Code: FULL
Physician: L. King

Isolation: None
Admit Date: 6/6

Nutrition:

Meal type:	NPO
History:	Family indicates that patient is a lacto-ovo-vegetarian and has always been very health-conscious.
AM:	smoothie made with whey protein, Greek yogurt, 1–2 fruits and 1–2 vegetables
Lunch:	eats in work cafeteria—salad with some tofu, nuts, and cheese; bread or crackers
Dinner:	usually cooks—likes all vegetables, fruits, grains, nuts, eggs and dairy products. Does eat out some days—likes all kinds of ethnic foods—Greek, Indian, Chinese, Mexican, Thai.

MD Progress Note:

6/8 0750
Subjective: Previous 24 hours reviewed. Stable overnight.
Nasogastric tube placed for enteral feeding. ICP WNL.
Vitals: Temp: 99.6, Pulse: 83, Resp rate: 33, BP: 129/92 Wt. 79.2 kg
Urine output: 3720 mL (46.9 mL/kg)

Physical Exam
General: MRI showed areas of hemorrhagic edema in deep white matter of L frontal lobe anteriorly. Additionally, heme and edema found in the splenium of corpus callosum. 3.4 cm × 4.2 cm × 1.0 cm representing areas of shearing injury. Continues to arouse easily. One-level commands followed. Oriented to family but not place or time.
Neck: WNL
Heart: WNL
Lungs: Clear to auscultation
Abdomen: Active bowel sounds

Assessment/Plan:

Dx: Traumatic Brain Injury secondary to MVA collision—GCS = 8 E2 V2 M4.
Plan: PT, OT consult. Begin attempts to wean from ventilator — consult for spontaneous breathing trial. Nutrition consult for enteral feeding.

.... *L King, MD*

Walker, Ryan, Male, 25 y.o.
Allergies: NKA
Pt. Location: SICU Bed #1

Code: FULL
Physician: L. King

Isolation: None
Admit Date: 6/6

Intake/Output

Date		6/6 1900–6/7 0700 78.1 kg			
Time		0701–1500	1501–2300	2301–0700	Daily total
IN	P.O.	**0**	0	0	0
	I.V. (mL/kg/hr)			600 (0.96)	600 (0.96)
	I.V. piggyback			150	
	TPN			0	
	Total intake (mL/kg)			750 (9.6)	750 (9.6)
OUT	Urine (mL/kg/hr)			450 (0.72)	450
	Emesis output			**0**	
	Other			**0**	
	Stool			**0**	
	Total output (mL/kg)			**450 (5.76)**	**450 (5.76)**
Net I/O				+300	+300
Net since admission (6/6)				+300	+300

Walker, Ryan, Male, 25 y.o.
Allergies: NKA
Pt. Location: SICU Bed #1

Code: FULL
Physician: L. King

Isolation: None
Admit Date: 6/6

Intake/Output

Date		6/7 0700–6/8 0700 79.2 kg			
Time		0701–1500	1501–2300	2301–0700	Daily total
IN	P.O.	0	0	0	0
	I.V.	600	600	600	1800
	(mL/kg/hr)	(0.94)	(0.94)	(0.94)	(0.94)
	I.V. piggyback		300		
	Enteral feeding		150	400	650
	Total intake	600	1050	1000	2450
	(mL/kg)	(7.57)	(13.2)	(12.6)	(30.93)
OUT	Urine	710	1300	1500	3510
	(mL/kg/hr)	(1.12)	(2.05)	(2.36)	(1.84)
	Emesis output	**0**	**0**	**0**	**0**
	NG to suction	**50**	**120**	**40**	**210**
	Stool	**0**	**0**	**0**	**0**
	Total output	**760**	**1420**	**1540**	**3720**
	(mL/kg)	**(9.5)**	**(17.9)**	**(19.4)**	**(46.9)**
Net I/O		−160	−370	−540	−1270
Net since admission (6/6)					−770

Walker, Ryan, Male, 25 y.o.
Allergies: NKA
Pt. Location: SICU Bed #1

Code: FULL
Physician: L. King

Isolation: None
Admit Date: 6/6

Laboratory Results

	Ref. Range	6/6 1615	6/7 0600
Chemistry			
Sodium (mEq/L)	136–145	137	135
Potassium (mEq/L)	3.5–5.1	3.8	3.7
Chloride (mEq/L)	98–107	101	99
Carbon dioxide (CO_2, mEq/L)	23–29	29	27
Bicarbonate (mEq/L)	23–28	28	27.5
BUN (mg/dL)	6–20	19	18
Creatinine serum (mg/dL)	0.6–1.1 F 0.9–1.3 M	0.96	1.0
BUN/Crea ratio	10.0–20.0	20	18
Uric acid (mg/dL)	2.8–8.8 F 4.0–9.0 M	6.1	
Est GFR, non-Afr Amer (mL/min/1.73 m^2)	>60	109	104
Glucose (mg/dL)	70–99	97	125 !↑
Lactate (mmol/L)	0.50–1.60	2.77 !↑	2.8 !↑
Phosphate, inorganic (mg/dL)	2.2–4.6	2.5	2.1 !↓
Magnesium (mg/dL)	1.5–2.4	1.6	1.4 !↓
Calcium (mg/dL)	8.6–10.2	8.6	8.4
Anion gap (mmol/L)	10–20	8.0 !↓	
Osmolality (mmol/kg/H_2O)	275–295	286	283
Bilirubin total (mg/dL)	≤1.2	0.9	1.1
Bilirubin, direct (mg/dL)	<0.3	0.1	0.2
Protein, total (g/dL)	6–7.8	6.5	6.1
Albumin (g/dL)	3.5–5.5	4.6	3.7
Prealbumin (mg/dL)	18–35	33	21
Ammonia (NH_3, µg/L)	6–47	21	19
Alkaline phosphatase (U/L)	30–120	141 !↑	145 !↑
ALT (U/L)	4–36	18	22
AST (U/L)	0–35	23	24
CPK (U/L)	30–135 F 55–170 M	220 !↑	235 !↑
Lactate dehydrogenase (U/L)	208–378	210	175
C-reactive protein (mg/dL)	<1.0	145 !↑	155 !↑

Walker, Ryan, Male, 25 y.o.
Allergies: NKA
Pt. Location: SICU Bed #1

Code: FULL
Physician: L. King

Isolation: None
Admit Date: 6/6

Laboratory Results *(Continued)*

	Ref. Range	6/6 1615	6/7 0600
Coagulation (Coag)			
PT (sec)	11–13	12.1	12.7
INR	0.9–1.1	1.0	0.9
PTT (sec)	24–34	25	26
Hematology			
WBC (×10³/mm³)	3.9–10.7	7.9	12.1 !↑
RBC (×10⁶/mm³)	4.2–5.4 F / 4.5–6.2 M	4.55	3.9 !↓
Hemoglobin (Hgb, g/dL)	12–16 F / 14–17 M	14.0	13.1 !↓
Hematocrit (Hct, %)	37–47 F / 41–51 M	41.2	39 !↓
Mean cell volume (μm³)	80–96	90.4	91
Mean cell Hgb (pg)	28–32	31.1	30
Mean cell Hgb content (g/dL)	32–36	34.1	33
RBC distribution (%)	11.6–16.5	12.7	11.7
Platelet count (×10³/mm³)	150–350	175	184
Transferrin (mg/dL)	250–380 F / 215–365 M	304	310
Hematology, Manual Diff			
Neutrophil (%)	40–70	57	73 !↑
Lymphocyte (%)	22–44	33.8	37
Monocyte (%)	0–7	7.8 !↑	8.1 !↑
Eosinophil (%)	0–5	0.8	1.0
Basophil (%)	0–2	0.6	0.7
Blasts (%)	3–10	3.7	3.1
Segs (%)	0–60	21	19
Bands (%)	0–10	3	12 !↑
Urinalysis			
Collection method	—	cath	
Color	—	yellow	
Appearance	—	cloudy	
Specific gravity	1.001–1.035	1.007	
pH	5–7	5.67	

(Continued)

Walker, Ryan, Male, 25 y.o.
Allergies: NKA
Pt. Location: SICU Bed #1

Code: FULL
Physician: L. King

Isolation: None
Admit Date: 6/6

Laboratory Results *(Continued)*

	Ref. Range	6/6 1615	6/7 0600
Protein (mg/dL)	Neg	Neg	
Glucose (mg/dL)	Neg	Neg	
Ketones	Neg	Neg	
Blood	Neg	+ !↑	
Bilirubin	Neg	Neg	
Nitrites	Neg	Neg	
Urobilinogen (EU/dL)	<1.0	0.12	
Leukocyte esterase	Neg	Neg	
Prot chk	Neg	Neg	
WBCs (/HPF)	0–5	3	
RBCs (/HPF)	0–2	4 !↑	
Bact	0	0	
Mucus	0	0	
Crys	0	0	
Casts (/LPF)	0	0	
Yeast	0	0	
Arterial Blood Gases (ABGs)			
pH	7.35–7.45	7.37	7.39
pCO$_2$ (mm Hg)	35–45	41.8	42
SO$_2$ (%)	≥95	98	97
CO$_2$ content (mmol/L)	25–30	29.4	28.1
O$_2$ content (%)	15–22	18	19
pO$_2$ (mm Hg)	≥80	452.9 !↑	310 !↑
HCO$_3$- (mEq/L)	21–28	23.7	24

Note: Values and units of measurement listed in these tables are derived from several resources. Substantial variation exists in the ranges quoted as "normal" and these may vary depending on the assay used by different laboratories.

Case Questions

I. Understanding the Diagnosis and Pathophysiology

1. Define traumatic brain injury (TBI). What is the Glasgow coma scale? What was Mr. Walker's GCS score? What findings from the physical exam are consistent with this score?

2. Read the radiology reports and the MD progress note dated 6/7. What causes edema and bleeding after a TBI? What general functions occur in the frontal lobe? How might Mr. Walker's injury affect him in the long term?

3. Secondary effects for this type of injury result from the complications initiated by the injury and may occur over days following the insult. These may include the following: inflammatory response, oxidative stress, ischemia, hypoxia, and increased intracranial pressure. Discuss three of these complications and how they may impact Mr. Walker's hospitalization and recovery.

II. Understanding the Nutrition Therapy

4. Head trauma patients are significantly catabolic. Describe this acute metabolic response to injury.

5. Using the ASPEN and/or AND evidence-based guidelines, describe the role of nutrition support in the care of the TBI patient.

6. Are there specific nutrients that are recommended to support the care of the patient with a TBI?

III. Nutrition Assessment

7. Assess Mr. Walker's admitting height and weight. Calculate and evaluate his BMI.

8. Determine Mr. Walker's energy, protein, and fluid requirements. Provide a rationale for the method you have used to estimate his needs.

9. Mr. Walker was started on Pivot 1.5 @ 50 mL/hr. How much energy and protein will this provide? Does it meet his estimated protein and energy needs that you determined in question #8?

10. Using the intake/output information for 6/7-6/8, answer the following:

    a. What was the total volume of feeding for 6/7–6/8?

    b. What was the nutritional value of his feeding? Calculate the total energy and protein that he received.

    c. What percentage of his needs was met? What factors may interfere with the patient receiving his prescribed nutrition support? What steps can be made to assure adequate delivery of nutrition support to the critically ill patient?

11. Assess Mr. Walker's laboratory values at admission and on 6/7. Explain any abnormal laboratory values.

IV.   Nutrition Diagnosis

12. Select two high-priority nutrition problems and complete the PES statement for each.

V.   Nutrition Intervention

13. Mr. Walker's MD started enteral feeding on day 2 of the admission. As the RD in the neurointensive care unit, outline the nutrition support recommendations you would make for Mr. Walker.

14. Mr. Walker has received propofol (diprivan) 25 mcg/kg/min or 8.2 ml/h. What is propofol? How many kcal would he receive from this prescription?

VI.   Nutrition Monitoring and Evaluation

15. Mr. Walker was extubated on day 4 of his admission. He received a swallowing evaluation that is described in the following report:

Department of Speech Pathology:

RE: Interpretation of FEES/Swallowing Evaluation—Ryan Walker

Date: 6/10

Patient, Ryan Walker, accepted applesauce with appropriate tongue lateralization and chewing skills but choked when offered 2–3 sips of water. Oral skills appropriate. Showed significant signs of fatigue and decreased cooperation after a few swallows, which inhibited PO feeding. No evidence of penetration or aspiration. Recommend to retry evaluation in 2–3 days.

C. Davie, MS, SLP

What is a FEES? What factors in the speech pathologist's report indicate the continued need for enteral feeding?

16. When Mr. Walker is cleared for an oral diet by the SLP and physician, what information would you use to determine the appropriate oral diet order? What guidelines would you use to determine when Mr. Walker can be weaned from his enteral feeding?

17. Mr. Walker will be transferred to the rehabilitation unit in the hospital for therapies with physical therapy, occupational therapy, and speech therapy. Summarize the training for each of these professionals and describe their potential role in Mr. Walker's recovery.

Bibliography

Academy of Nutrition and Dietetics Nutrition Care Manual. Critical Illness. https://www .nutritioncaremanual.org/topic.cfm?ncm_category _id=1&lv1=37030&ncm_toc_id=37030&ncm _heading=Nutrition%20Care. Accessed 07/06/15.

Bistrian BR, Askew W, Erdman JW, Oria MP. Nutrition and traumatic brain injury: A perspective from the Institute of Medicine report. *JPEN*. 2011;35:556–559.

Chourdakis M, Kraus MM, Tzellos T, et al. Effect of early compared with delayed enteral nutrition on endocrine function in patients with traumatic brain injury: An open-labeled randomized trial. *JPEN*. 2011;36:108–116.

Chowdhury T, Kowalksi S, Arabi Y, Dash HH. Prehospital and initial management of head injury patients: An update. *Saudi J Anesthesia*. 2014;8:115–119.

Collier BR, Cherry-Nukowiec JR, Mills MB. Trauma Surgery and Burns. In: *ASPEN Nutrition Support Curriculum*. 2nd ed. 2012. Silver Springs, MD. 392–411.

Costello LS, Lithander FE, Gruen RL, Williams LT. Nutrition therapy in the optimization of health outcomes in adult patients with moderate to severe traumatic brain injury: Findings from a scoping review. *Injury, Int'l J Care Injured*. 2014;45:1834–1841.

Frankenfield CD, Ashcraft CM. Description and prediction of resting metabolic rate after stroke and traumatic brain injury. *Nutrition*. 2012;28:906–911.

Ghajar J. Traumatic brain injury. *Lancet*. 2000;356:923–929.

Haddad SH, Arabi YM. Critical care management of severe traumatic brain injury in adults. *Scand J Traum Resc Emerg Med*. 2012;20:12–27.

Jones Irwin K, Hansen-Petrik M. Diseases and disorders of the neurological system. In: Nelms MN, Sucher K, Lacey K. *Nutrition Therapy and Pathophysiology*. 3rd ed. Belmont, CA: Cengage; 2016:596–634.

Koskinen LOD, Olivecrona M, Grande PO. Severe traumatic brain injury management and clinical outcome using the LUND concept. *Neuroscience*. 2014;283:245–255.

Lichtenberg K, Guay-Berry P, Pipitone A, Bondy A, Rotello L. Compensatory increased enteral feeding goal rates: A way to achieve optimal nutrition. *Nutr Clin Pract*. 2010;25(6):653–657.

Mandaville A, Ray A, Robertson H, Foster C, Jesser C. A retrospective review of swallow dysfunction in patients with severe traumatic brain injury. *Dysphagia*. 2014;29:310–318.

McClave SA, Martindale RG, Vanek VW, et al. Guidelines for the provision and assessment of nutrition support therapy in the adult critically ill patient. *JPEN*. 2009; 33: 277–316.

Nahikian-Nelms M. Metabolic stress and the critically ill. In: Nelms MN, Sucher K, Lacey K. *Nutrition Therapy and Pathophysiology*. 3rd ed. Belmont, CA: Cengage; 2016:665–685.

National Institute for Health and Care Excellence. Head Injury. NICE Clinical Guideline 176. 2014. Available from: guidance.nice.org.uk/cg176. Accessed 06/07/15.

Osuka A, Uno T, Nakanishi J, et al. Energy expenditure in patients with severe head injury: Controlled normothermia with sedation and neuromuscular blockade. *J Crit Care*. 2013;28:218.e9–218.e13.

Pinto TF, Rocha R, Pauala CA, DeJesus RP. Tolerance to enteral nutrition therapy in traumatic brain injury patients. *Brain Injury*. 2012;26:1113–1117.

Ruf L, Magnuson B, Hatton J, Cook A. Nutrition in Neurologic Impairment. In: *ASPEN Nutrition Support Curriculum*. 2nd ed. 2012. Silver Springs, MD. 363–376.

Taylor B, Brody R, Denmark R, Southard R, Byham-Gray L. Improving enteral delivery through the adoption of the "Feed Early Enteral Diet Adequately for Maximum Effect (FEED ME)" protocol in a surgical trauma ICU. *Nutr Clin* Pract. 2014;29:639–648.

Vinzzini A, Aranda-Michel J. Nutritional support in head injury. *Nutrition*. 2011;27:129–132.

Wang X, Dong Y, Han Xi, et al. Nutritional support for patients sustaining traumatic brain injury: A systematic review and meta-analysis of prospective studies. *PLOS One*. 2013;8:114.

Woodcock T, Morganti-Kossmann M. The role of markers of inflammation in traumatic brain injury. *Front. Neurol*. 2013;4:18. doi: 10.3389/fneur.2013.00018.

Internet Resources

AND Evidence Analysis Library: http://www.andeal.org

Centers for Disease Control: http://www.cdc.gov /TraumaticBrainInjury/

American Physical Therapy Association: http://www.apta .org/AboutPTs/

American Occupational Therapy Association: http://www .aota.org/About-Occupational-Therapy.aspx

American Speech Language Hearing Association: http://www.asha.org/.

Case 25

Pediatric Cerebral Palsy

Holly Estes Doetsch, MS, RDN,LD,CNSC
The Ohio State University

Objectives

After completing this case, the student will be able to:

1. Define cerebral palsy (CP) and describe its impact on functional capacity.
2. Identify common nutritional problems associated with CP.
3. Assess and interpret anthropometric measures in conjunction with overall growth patterns.
4. Estimate the nutritional needs for a pediatric patient with CP.
5. Determine nutrition diagnoses, measurable goals, relevant interventions, and appropriate plan for monitoring and evaluating the patient's progress.

Olivia Foster presents to the Neuromuscular Disorders Clinic at the local pediatric hospital for a routine assessment and baclofen pump refill. She was born prematurely and diagnosed with spastic quadriplegic cerebral palsy at 10 months of age when parents and pediatrician noticed Olivia was having difficulty achieving normal developmental milestones, particularly functional motor skills. During infancy she also experienced several seizures, which arc now well controlled with anti-epileptic therapy. In early childhood, Olivia failed to respond sufficiently to many common therapies for spasticity, including oral baclofen, botulinum toxin, and surgeries. She has responded positively to intrathecal baclofen, increasing her mobility and spending less time in her wheelchair. Olivia struggles with some oral-motor dysfunction, but has few cognitive limitations. At the current clinic visit, her mom expresses concerns regarding Olivia's weight as well as a recent fall that Olivia experienced a couple days earlier.

Foster, Olivia, Female, 10 y.o.
Allergies: NKA   **Code:** FULL   **Isolation:** None
Pt. Location: RM   **Physician:** K. Garrison   **Admit Date:** 4/13

Patient Summary: Olivia Foster is a10-year-old female with cerebral palsy, GMFCS level 3. Here for a baclofen pump refill and biannual assessment.

History:

Onset of disease: Patient was born premature at 32 weeks GA, birth weight of 1200 g. Diagnosed with cerebral palsy at 10 months.
Medical history: Spastic quadriplegic cerebral palsy, prematurity, developmental delay, seizure d/o, speech difficulties, GERD, constipation
Surgical history: ITB pump insertion (August 2013), multiple lower limb surgeries (2009–2012)
Medications: Polyethylene glycol 3350 8 g PO BID, Lansoprazole 20 mg PO daily, Baclofen (2000 mcg/mL) 274 mcg ITB infusion daily, Phenytoin 50 mg PO BID, pediatric gummy complete multivitamin 1 PO BID
Social history: Lives at home with her parents and younger brother. Attends school regularly and has several friends. Struggles with math (attends Resource Room for help) otherwise performing well in school. Communication frustrating for pt 2' to dysarthria. School provides SLP, OT, and PT services.
Family history: Mother—hypertension, irritable bowel syndrome, Father—kidney stones

Demographics:

Years education: Fifth grade
Language: English
Occupation: Student
Household members: Father age 42, mother age 39, brother age 4
Ethnicity: Caucasian
Religious affiliation: Seventh Day Adventist

Admitting History/Physical:

Chief complaint (per mom): "We're here for Olivia's baclofen refill. I think overall she's doing quite well and using her crutches often. She did fall on her hip the other day while playing with the dog, but she keeps telling me she's fine. I'm also a little concerned about her weight. I've noticed she looks a little thinner than usual. Maybe she's having a growth spurt? She still takes her multivitamin twice a day and her meals are pretty balanced."

Vital Signs: Temp: 98.6   Pulse: 72   Respiratory rate: 15   BP:110/76
                    Ht: 130.5 cm   Wt: 23.1 kg   BMI: 13.6

Physical Exam:

General Appearance: Thin, 10 y.o. female in no acute distress, smiles easily. Sitting in her wheelchair today.
HEENT: Dry mucous membranes

Foster, Olivia, Female, 10 y.o.
Allergies: NKA
Pt. Location: RM

Code: FULL
Physician: K. Garrison

Isolation: None
Admit Date: 4/13

Heart: Regular rate and rhythm
Extremities: Bruising at L hip, no swelling. Pt rates pain at a 4–5 with palpation.
Neuromuscular: Hypertonia, mild to moderate contractures in in upper and lower limbs. Altered gait (most recent PT assessment last fall).
Skin: Pale, dry, normal turgor
Chest/lungs: Respirations normal, no crackles or wheezing
Abdomen: Soft, nontender, nondistended, +BS. ITB pump lower L abdomen, no swelling or erythema.

Nutrition:

(See Appendix D for Olivia's growth charts.)
General: Olivia sits for most of the day in her classes, but walks the short distances between classes using crutches. She meets with the school physical therapist twice a week. She uses a wheelchair for longer distances, such as during school field trips and outings to the mall. Olivia self-feeds and declines assistance with eating from others, but her aide helps her carry school supplies and take notes during class. She has been following an advanced mechanical soft diet for most of her life due to some chewing difficulties. The entire family refrains from consuming meat, poultry, and fish. During the school day, Olivia consumes "whatever is being served at the cafeteria" that fits within the realm of a vegetarian and advanced mechanical soft diet. She dislikes most sweets. Her mom reports that although her daughter can be a picky eater, she eats fairly consistent portion sizes and at regular times from day to day. On average, Olivia takes around an hour to consume each meal and 20–30 minutes to eat snacks. When asked whether she could eat more if she had more time to do so, Olivia replies, "Probably." GERD is controlled with medication. No coughing or choking with eating and drinking. Bowel movements are fairly consistent; 1–2 soft stools every other day.

24 hour recall:
Breakfast—1 scrambled egg (w/ a couple tbsp 1% milk added), 6–8 oz water, 1/2 banana
Lunch—1/2 c cooked carrots, 4–6 oz chocolate milk, 1/2 cup macaroni and cheese (from school cafeteria)
After school snack—6 oz yogurt with diced strawberries, 6–8 oz water
Dinner—1/2 c rice and black bean casserole, 1/2 c diced peaches, 4–6 oz 1% milk
Bedtime snack—6–8 oz water, 1/2 c apple sauce + 1 tsp cinnamon sugar
Sips water periodically throughout the day
Food allergies/intolerances/aversions: NKFA
Previous nutrition therapy? Has seen RD in outpatient clinic and when hospitalized
Food purchase/preparation: Parents
Vit/min intake: pediatric gummy complete multivitamin 1 PO twice daily

Foster, Olivia, Female, 10 y.o.
Allergies: NKA
Pt. Location: RM

Code: FULL
Physician: K. Garrison

Isolation: None
Admit Date: 4/13

Laboratory Results

	Ref. Range	4/13 1634
Chemistry		
Sodium (mEq/L)	136–145	143
Potassium (mEq/L)	3.5–5.0	4.7
Chloride (mEq/L)	98–108	101
Carbon dioxide (CO_2, mEq/L)	22–30	25
BUN (mg/dL)	5–18	19 ↑!
Creatinine serum (mg/dL)	≤1.2	0.9
Glucose (mg/dL)	70–99	87
Phosphate, inorganic (mg/dL)	2.2–4.6	4
Magnesium (mg/dL)	1.6–2.6	2.4
Calcium (mg/dL)	8.6–10.5	10.5
Bilirubin total (mg/dL)	≤1.2	1.1
Protein, total (g/dL)	6–7.8	7.8
Albumin (g/dL)	3.5–5	4.9
Prealbumin (mg/dL)	17–39	21
Alkaline phosphatase (U/L)	<500	625 ↑!
ALT (U/L)	3–28	18
AST (U/L)	19–28	25
Hematology		
Hemoglobin (g/dL)	11–16	11.5
Hematocrit (%)	31–43	32
Vitamin D 25 hydroxy (ng/mL)	30–100	16 ↓!

Assessment and Plan: 10 y.o. female with spastic quadriplegic CP here for ITB pump refill and 6 month visit. Continuing to respond well to baclofen, spending less time in her wheelchair, though had a recent fall. Labs notable for low 25-OH vit D. Evaluate BMD (most recent DEXA 3 years ago). Pt's weight has deviated from curve over the past year, will discuss with Nutrition.

Medical Tx Plan: Refill ITB pump, 20 mL. Continue current dosing regimen.
Obtain GGT, B-ALP
L hip XR
DEXA scan
PT consult re: repeat gait analysis and fall prevention
Nutrition consult re: optimizing growth, vit D status.

Case Questions

I. **Understanding the Diagnosis and Pathophysiology**

1. What is cerebral palsy (CP)? Identify several risk factors for CP.

2. What functional abilities can be impacted by CP? What is the Gross Motor Function Classification System (GMFCS)? What does a GMFCS score of 3 indicate?

3. Describe the classifications of CP according to motor function and severity level. What is a baclofen pump and how is it used to manage CP?

4. Poor growth secondary to poor nutrition status is a common problem in pediatric patients with CP. Summarize at least three factors that may contribute to malnutrition and subsequent poor growth in CP.

II. **Understanding the Nutrition Therapy**

5. What are limitations to using standard height and weight measurement tools in CP patients? What are commonly used methods for assessing height and weight in children with CP? Are there other anthropometric measures that may be useful?

6. What are the limitations to using reference standards of growth in children with CP? What are factors to consider when interpreting growth data in this patient population?

7. What are factors that impact the caloric needs of CP patients? Which ones are relevant to the current patient?

8. Define "metabolic bone disease." What are factors that may increase the risk for metabolic bone disease in CP, and which factors apply to the current patient?

9. Briefly describe the process through which vitamin D deficiency impacts bone remodeling. Why is the serum calcium level often normal in patients with vitamin D deficiency?

III.   **Nutrition Assessment**

10. Review Olivia's growth chart and identify the percentiles that correspond with her current measurements (see Appendix D for Olivia's growth chart). Describe the patient's growth velocity over the past year. How would you interpret this information?

11. Determine Olivia's daily caloric, protein, and fluid intake based on her 24-hour recall. Calculate Olivia's caloric, protein, and fluid requirements. Support the methods you used to calculate these values.

12. Compare Olivia's reported intake with her estimated needs. Identify at least three key nutrients inadequate in her diet.

13. Identify the abnormal laboratory values, and for each one, describe potential causes for these abnormalities.

IV.   **Nutrition Diagnosis**

14. Identify two nutrition problems and develop a PES statement for each.

V.   **Nutrition Intervention**

15. For each PES statement, establish an appropriate goal (based on the signs and symptoms) and intervention (based on the etiology).

16. Power packing is a common nutrition intervention used for pediatric patients with poor growth. What is "power packing" and why might this be a useful nutrition intervention for this patient? Based on Olivia's 24-hour recall, what are specific power packing suggestions you could offer the patient?

17. Olivia takes a daily multivitamin supplement that includes 600 IUs of vitamin D. Would you recommend additional vitamin D supplementation? If so, outline your recommendation.

VI.   Nutrition Monitoring and Evaluation

18. Write an ADIME note for your initial nutrition assessment. When would be an appropriate time to follow up with Olivia and reassess her nutrition status?

19. Multidisciplinary treatment is essential to address the multiple co-morbidities associated with CP. List three other health professionals who commonly play a role in the care of CP patients. Describe the role of each one.

Bibliography

Andrew MJ, Sullivan PB. Growth in cerebral palsy. *Nutr Clin Pract.* 2010;25(4):357–361.

Arvedson JC. Feeding children with cerebral palsy and swallowing difficulties. *European J Clin Nutr.* 2013;67:S9–S12.

Behavioral Health Nutrition Dietetics Practice Group and Pediatric Nutrition Practice Group. Academy of Nutrition and Dietetics pocket guide to children with special health care and nutritional needs. Chicago, IL: Academy of Nutrition and Dietetics. 2012. https://publications.webauthor.com/pub/HCNPG/. Accessed 04/01/15.

Houlihan CM, Stevenson RD. Bone density in cerebral palsy. *Phys Med Rehabil Clin N Am.* 2009;20(3):493–508.

Kuperminc MN, Gottrand F, Samson-Fang L, et al. Nutritional management of children with cerebral palsy: A practical guide. *Eur J Clin Nutr.* 2013;67:S21–S23.

Kuperminc MN, Stevenson RD. Growth and nutrition disorders in children with cerebral palsy. *Dev Disabil Res Rev.* 2008;14(2):137–146.

Lark RK, Williams CL, Stadler D, et al. Serum prealbumin and albumin concentrations do not reflect nutritional state in children with cerebral palsy. *J Pediatr.* 2005;147:695–697.

Mughal MZ. Fractures in children with cerebral palsy. *Curr Osteoporos Rep.* 2014;12(3):313–318.

Samson-Fang L, Bell KL. Assessment of growth and nutrition in children with cerebral palsy. *Eur J Clin Nutr.* 2013;67:S5–S8.

Wittenbrook W. Nutritional assessment and intervention in cerebral palsy. *Pract Gastroenterol.* 2011;32(2):16, 21–32. http://www.medicine.virginia.edu/clinical/departments/medicine/divisions/digestive-health/clinical-care/nutrition-support-team/nutrition-articles/WittenbrookArticle.pdf. Accessed 04/01/15.

Internet Resources

Centers for Disease Control and Prevention. Cerebral Palsy: http://www.cdc.gov/ncbddd/cp/

Centers for Disease Control and Prevention. Growth Charts: http://www.cdc.gov/growthcharts/

National Institute of Neurological Disorders and Stroke: http://www.ninds.nih.gov/disorders/cerebral_palsy/cerebral_palsy.htm

Nutrition Care Manual: https://www.nutritioncaremanual.org/

Unit Nine

NUTRITION THERAPY FOR PULMONARY DISORDERS

The two cases in this section portray the interrelationship between nutrition and the respiratory system. In a healthy individual, the respiratory system receives oxygen for cellular metabolism and expires waste products—primarily carbon dioxide. Fuels—carbohydrate, protein, and lipid—are metabolized, using oxygen and producing carbon dioxide. The type of fuel an individual receives can affect physiological conditions and interfere with normal respiratory function. Malnutrition can impair the function of the respiratory system as well.

Nutritional status and pulmonary function are interdependent. Malnutrition can evolve from pulmonary disorders and can contribute to declining pulmonary status. The incidence of malnutrition is common for people with COPD, ranging anywhere from 25 percent to 50 percent. In respiratory disease, maintaining nutritional status improves muscle strength needed for breathing, decreases risk of infection, facilitates weaning from mechanical ventilation, and improves ability for physical activity.

The American Thoracic Society defines chronic obstructive pulmonary disease (COPD) as a disease process of chronic airway obstruction caused by chronic bronchitis, emphysema, or a combination of both. These conditions place a significant burden on the health care systems in the United States.

In Cases 26 and 27, nutritional assessment and evaluation demonstrate the effects of COPD on nutritional status. As the patient is started on nutrition support in Case 27, you will examine the impact of nutrition on declining respiratory status.

Case 26

Chronic Obstructive Pulmonary Disease

Objectives

After completing this case, the student will be able to:

1. Identify and explain common nutritional problems associated with this disease.
2. Identify effects of malnutrition on pulmonary status.
3. Identify effects of nutrient metabolism on pulmonary function.
4. Analyze nutrition assessment data to evaluate nutritional status and identify specific nutrition problems.
5. Determine nutrition diagnoses and write appropriate PES statements.
6. Plan interventions to increase an individual's intake of energy and protein.

Louise Hoffman was initially diagnosed with stage 1 COPD (emphysema) 5 years ago. She is now admitted with increasing shortness of breath and a possible upper respiratory infection.

Hoffman, Louise, Female, 62 y.o.
Allergies: NKA
Pt. Location: RM 704

Code: FULL
Physician: D. Bradshaw

Isolation: None
Admit Date: 1/25

Patient Summary: Acute exacerbation of COPD, increasing dyspnea, hypercapnia, r/o pneumonia

History:
Onset of disease: Initially diagnosed with stage 1 COPD (emphysema) five years ago. Medical records at last admission indicate pulmonary function tests: baseline FEV^1 = 0.7L, FVC = 1.5L, FEV/FVC 46%.
Medical history: No occupational exposures; history of bronchitis and upper respiratory infections during winter months for most of adult life. 4 live births; 2 miscarriages.
Surgical history: No surgeries
Medications at home: Combivent (metered-dose inhaler)—2 inhalations 4 times daily (each inhalation delivers 18 mcg ipratropium bromide; 130 mcg albuterol sulfate)
Tobacco use: Yes. 46 years, 1 PPD history—has not smoked for past year.
Alcohol use: No
Family history: What? CA. Who? Mother, 2 aunts died from lung cancer

Demographics:
Marital status: Married, lives with husband, aged 68, who has PMH of CAD
Years education: Completed two years of college
Language: English only
Occupation: Retired office manager for independent insurance agency
Hours of work: N/A
Ethnicity: Caucasian
Religious affiliation: Methodist

Admitting History/Physical:
Chief complaint: "I'm hardly able to do anything for myself right now. Even taking a bath or getting dressed makes me short of breath. My husband had to help me out of the shower this morning. I feel that I am gasping for air. I am coughing up a lot of phlegm that is a dark brownish-green. I am always short of breath, but I can tell when things change. I was at a church meeting with a lot of people—I might have caught something there. My husband says that I am confused in the morning. I do know it is hard for me to get going in the morning. Do you think my confusion is related to my COPD?"

Vital Signs: Temp: 98.8°F   Pulse: 92   Resp rate: 22
                    BP: 130/88   Height: 5'3"   Weight: 119 lbs

Heart: Regular rate and rhythm; mild jugular distension noted
HEENT: Eyes: PERRLA, no hemorrhages
          Ears: Slight redness
          Nose: Clear
          Throat: Clear
Genitalia: Deferred
Rectal: Not performed

Hoffman, Louise, Female, 62 y.o.
Allergies: NKA
Pt. Location: RM 704

Code: FULL
Physician: D. Bradshaw

Isolation: None
Admit Date: 1/25

Neurologic: Alert, oriented; cranial nerves intact
Extremities: 1+ bilateral pitting edema. No cyanosis or clubbing.
Skin: Warm, dry
Chest/lungs: Decreased breath sounds, percussion hyperresonant; prolonged expiration with wheezing; rhonchi throughout; using accessory muscles at rest
Abdomen: Liver, spleen palpable; nondistended, nontender, normal bowel sounds

Nursing Assessment	1/25
Abdominal appearance (concave, flat, rounded, obese, distended)	flat
Palpation of abdomen (soft, rigid, firm, masses, tense)	soft
Bowel function (continent, incontinent, flatulence, no stool)	continent
Bowel sounds (P=present, AB=absent, hypo, hyper)	
RUQ	P
LUQ	P
RLQ	P
LLQ	P
Stool color	brown
Stool consistency	soft
Tubes/ostomies	NA
Genitourinary	
Urinary continence	yes
Urine source	clean catch
Appearance (clear, cloudy, yellow, amber, fluorescent, hematuria, orange, blue, tea)	clear, yellow
Integumentary	
Skin color	pale
Skin temperature (DI=diaphoretic, W=warm, dry, CL=cool, CLM=clammy, CD+=cold, M=moist, H=hot)	W, D
Skin turgor (good, fair, poor, TENT=tenting)	fair
Skin condition (intact, EC=ecchymosis, A=abrasions, P=petechiae, R=rash, W=weeping, S=sloughing, D=dryness, EX=excoriated, T=tears, SE=subcutaneous emphysema, B=blisters, V=vesicles, N=necrosis)	intact
Mucous membranes (intact, EC=ecchymosis, A=abrasions, P=petechiae, R=rash, W=weeping, S=sloughing, D=dryness, EX=excoriated, T=tears, SE=subcutaneous emphysema, B=blisters, V=vesicles, N=necrosis)	intact
Other components of Braden score: special bed, sensory pressure, moisture, activity, friction/shear (>18 = no risk, 15–16 = low risk, 13–14 = moderate risk, ≤12 = high risk)	activity, 18

Hoffman, Louise, Female, 62 y.o.
Allergies: NKA   **Code:** FULL   **Isolation:** None
Pt. Location: RM 704   **Physician:** D. Bradshaw   **Admit Date:** 1/25

Orders:

O_2 1 L/minute via nasal cannula with humidity—keep O_2 saturation 90–91%
IVF D_5 / NS with 20 mEq KCL @ 75 cc/hr; Solumedrol 10 mg/kg q 6 hr; Ancef 500 mg q 6 hr;
Ipratropium bromide via nebulizer 2.5 mg q 30 minutes × 3 treatments then q 2 hr;
albuterol sulfate via nebulizer 4 mg q 30 minutes × 3 doses then 2.5 mg q 4 hr;
ABGs q 6 hours; CXR—EPA/LAT; Sputum cultures and Gram stain

Nutrition:

General: Patient states that her appetite is poor: "I fill up so quickly—after just a few bites." Relates that meal preparation is difficult: "By the time I fix a meal, I am too tired to eat it." In the previous two days, she states that she has eaten very little. Increased coughing has made it very hard to eat: "I don't think food tastes as good, either. Everything has a bitter taste." Highest adult weight was 145–150 lbs (5 years ago). States that her family constantly tells her how thin she has gotten: "I haven't weighed myself for a while but I know my clothes are bigger." Dentures are present but fit loosely.

Usual dietary intake:
AM: Coffee, juice or fruit, dry cereal with small amount of milk
Lunch: Large meal of the day—meat; vegetables; rice, potato, or pasta,but patient admits she eats only very small amounts.
Dinner/evening meal: Eats very light in evening—usually soup, scrambled eggs, or sandwich. Drinks Pepsi® throughout the day (usually 3 12-oz cans).

24-hr recall: ½ c coffee with nondairy creamer, few sips of orange juice, ½ c oatmeal with 1 tsp sugar, ¾ c chicken noodle soup, 2 saltine crackers, ½ c coffee with nondairy creamer; sips of Pepsi throughout the day and evening—estimated amount 32 oz.
Anthropometric data: Ht. 5'3", Wt. 119 lbs, UBW 145–150 lbs, last recorded weight: 139 lbs 1 year ago
Food allergies/intolerances/aversions: Avoids milk: "People say it will increase mucus production."
Previous nutrition therapy? No.
Food purchase/preparation: Self; "My daughters come and help sometimes."
Vit/min intake: None

Laboratory Results

	Ref. Range	1/25 0600	1/27 0600
Chemistry			
Sodium (mEq/L)	136–145	136	
Potassium (mEq/L)	3.5–5.1	3.7	
Chloride (mEq/L)	98–107	101	
Carbon dioxide (CO_2, mEq/L)	23–29	32 ↑	
Bicarbonate (mEq/L)	23–28	29 ↑	

Hoffman, Louise, Female, 62 y.o.

Allergies: NKA

Pt. Location: RM 704

Code: FULL

Physician: D. Bradshaw

Isolation: None

Admit Date: 1/25

Laboratory Results *(Continued)*

	Ref. Range	1/25 0600	1/27 0600
BUN (mg/dL)	6–20	9	
Creatinine serum (mg/dL)	0.6–1.1 F 0.9–1.3 M	0.9	
BUN/Crea ratio	10.0–20.0	10	
Uric acid (mg/dL)	2.8–8.8 F 4.0–9.0 M	4.1	
Est GFR, non-Afr Amer (mL/min/1.73 m^2)	>60	69	
Glucose (mg/dL)	70–99	92	
Phosphate, inorganic (mg/dL)	2.2–4.6	3.1	
Magnesium (mg/dL)	1.5–2.4	1.8	
Calcium (mg/dL)	8.6–10.2	9.1	
Anion gap (mmol/L)	10–20	6.0 !↓	
Osmolality (mmol/kg/H$_2$O)	275–295	280	
Bilirubin total (mg/dL)	≤1.2	0.9	
Bilirubin, direct (mg/dL)	<0.3	0.1	
Protein, total (g/dL)	6–7.8	5.8 !↓	
Albumin (g/dL)	3.5–5.5	3.3 !↓	
Prealbumin (mg/dL)	18–35	16 !↓	
Ammonia (NH$_3$, µg/L)	6–47	15	
Alkaline phosphatase (U/L)	30–120	99	
ALT (U/L)	4–36	8	
AST (U/L)	0–35	22	
CPK (U/L)	30–135 F 55–170 M	40	
Lactate dehydrogenase (U/L)	208–378	285	
Cholesterol (mg/dL)	<200	145	
HDL-C (mg/dL)	>59 F, >50 M	61	
VLDL (mg/dL)	7–32	19	
LDL (mg/dL)	<130	98	
LDL/HDL ratio	<3.22 F <3.55 M	1.61	
Triglycerides (mg/dL)	35–135 F 40–160 M	120	
HbA$_{1C}$ (%)	<5.7	4.6	

(Continued)

Hoffman, Louise, Female, 62 y.o.
Allergies: NKA
Pt. Location: RM 704

Code: FULL
Physician: D. Bradshaw

Isolation: None
Admit Date: 1/25

Laboratory Results *(Continued)*

	Ref. Range	1/25 0600	1/27 0600
Coagulation (Coag)			
PT (sec)	11–13	12.1	
INR	0.9–1.1	0.9	
Hematology			
WBC ($\times 10^3$/mm^3)	3.9–10.7	15.3 !↑	
RBC ($\times 10^6$/mm^3)	4.2–5.4 F 4.5–6.2 M	4.0 !↓	
Hemoglobin (Hgb, g/dL)	12–16 F 14–17 M	11.5 !↓	
Hematocrit (Hct, %)	37–47 F 41–51 M	35 !↓	
Hematology, Manual Diff			
Neutrophil (%)	40–70	61	
Lymphocyte (%)	22–44	53 !↑	
Monocyte (%)	0–7	6	
Eosinophil (%)	0–5	0	
Basophil (%)	0–2	0	
Blasts (%)	3–10	5	
Segs (%)	0–60	83 !↑	
Bands (%)	0–10	3	
Arterial Blood Gases (ABGs)			
pH	7.35–7.45	7.35	7.37
pCO$_2$ (mm Hg)	35–45	47 !↑	40.1
SO$_2$ (%)	≥95	92	90.2
CO$_2$ content (mmol/L)	25–30	32 !↑	29.8
O$_2$ content (%)	15–22	12 !↓	18
pO$_2$ (mm Hg)	≥80	85	87
HCO$_3^-$ (mEq/L)	21–28	29 !↑	27

Note: Values and units of measurement listed in these tables are derived from several resources. Substantial variation exists in the ranges quoted as "normal" and these may vary depending on the assay used by different laboratories.

Case Questions

I.   Understanding the Diagnosis and Pathophysiology

1.   COPD includes two distinct diagnoses. Outline the similarities and differences between emphysema and chronic bronchitis.

2.   What risk factors does Mrs. Hoffman have for this disease?

3.   Identify at least four signs and symptoms described in the physician's history and physical that are consistent with Mrs. Hoffman's diagnosis. Then describe the pathophysiology that may be responsible for each symptom.

4.   Mrs. Hoffman's medical record indicates previous pulmonary function tests as follows: baseline FEV[1] 50.7 L, FVC 51.5 L, FEV/FVC 46%. Define FEV, FVC, and FEV/FVC, and indicate how they are used in the diagnosis of COPD. How can these measurements be used in treating COPD?

5.   Look at Mrs. Hoffman's arterial blood gas values from the day she was admitted.

   a.   Why would arterial blood gases (ABGs) be drawn for this patient?

   b.   Define each of the following and interpret Mrs. Hoffman's values:

      pH:

      pCO_2:

      SO_2:

      HCO_3^-

    c.   Mrs. Hoffman was placed on oxygen therapy. What lab values tell you the therapy is working?

6.   Mrs. Hoffman has quit smoking. Shouldn't her condition now improve? Explain.

7.   What is a respiratory quotient? How is this figure related to nutritional intake and respiratory status?

II.   Understanding Nutrition Therapy

8.   What are the most common nutritional concerns for someone with COPD? Why is the patient diagnosed with COPD at higher risk for malnutrition?

III.   Nutrition Assessment

9.   Calculate Mrs. Hoffman's %UBW and BMI. Does either of these values indicate she is at nutritional risk? How would her 1+ bilateral pitting edema affect evaluation of her weight?

10.   Calculate Mrs. Hoffman's energy and protein requirements. What is your rationale?

11.   Using Mrs. Hoffman's nutrition history and 24-hour recall as a reference, do you think she has an adequate oral intake? Explain.

12.   Evaluate Mrs. Hoffman's laboratory values. Identify those that are abnormal. Which of these may be used to assess her nutritional status?

13.   Why may Mrs. Hoffman be at risk for anemia? Do her laboratory values indicate that she is anemic?

14.   What factors can you identify from her nutrition interview that contribute to her difficulty in eating?

IV. Nutrition Diagnosis

15. Select two high-priority nutrition problems and complete the PES statement for each.

V. Nutrition Intervention

16. For each of the PES statements you have written, establish an ideal goal (based on the signs and symptoms) and an appropriate intervention (based on the etiology).

17. What goals might you set for Mrs. Hoffman as she is discharged and beginning pulmonary rehabilitation?

VI. Nutrition Monitoring and Evaluation

18. You are now seeing Mrs. Hoffman at her second visit to pulmonary rehabilitation. She provides you with the following information from her food record. Her weight is now 116 lbs. She explains adjustment to her medications and oxygen at home has been difficult, so she hasn't felt like eating very much. When you talk with her, you find she is hungriest in the morning, and often by evening she is too tired to eat. She is having no specific intolerances, but she does tell you she hasn't consumed any milk products because she thought they would cause more sputum to be produced.

Monday
Breakfast: Coffee, 1 c with 2 tbsp nondairy creamer; orange juice 1 c; 1 poached egg; ½ slice toast

Lunch: ¼ tuna salad sandwich (made with 3 tbsp tuna salad on 1 slice wheat bread); coffee, 1 c with 2 tbsp nondairy creamer

Supper: Cream of tomato soup, 1 c; ½ slice toast; ½ banana; Pepsi—approx 36 oz

Tuesday
Breakfast: Coffee, 1 c with 2 tbsp nondairy creamer; ½ c orange juice; ½ c oatmeal with 2 tbsp brown sugar

Lunch: 1 chicken leg from Kentucky Fried Chicken; ½ c mashed potatoes; 2 tbsp gravy; coffee, 1 c with 2 tbsp nondairy creamer

Supper: Cheese, 2 oz; 8 saltine crackers; 1 can V8 juice (6 oz); Pepsi, approx. 36 oz

a. Is she meeting her calorie and protein goals?

b. What would you tell her regarding the use of supplements and/or milk and sputum production?

c. Using information from her food diary as a teaching tool, identify three interventions you would propose for Mrs. Hoffman to increase her calorie and protein intakes.

Bibliography

Academy of Nutrition and Dietetics. Evidence Analysis Library. Chronic Obstructive Pulmonary Disease Guideline. http://www.andeal.org/topic .cfm?menu=5301. Accessed on 03/24/15.

Academy of Nutrition and Dietetics. Nutrition Care Manual. Chronic Obstructive Pulmonary Disease (COPD). https://www.nutritioncaremanual.org /topic.cfm?ncm_category_id=1&lv1=5538&lv2 =22249&ncm_toc_id=22249&ncm_heading =Nutrition%20Care. Accessed on 03/24/15.

Bergman EA, Hawk SN. Diseases of the respiratory system. In: Nelms M, Sucher K, Lacey K. *Nutrition Therapy and Pathophysiology.* 3rd ed. Belmont, CA: Wadsworth, Cengage Learning; 2016:635–664.

Berthon BS, Wood LG. Nutrition and respiratory health—feature review. *Nutrients.* 2015;7:1618–1643.

Choudhury G, Rabinovich R, Macnee W. Comorbidities and systemic effects of chronic obstructive pulmonary disease. *Clinics in Chest Medicine.* 2014;35:101–130.

Collins PF, Elia M, Stratton RJ. Nutritional support and functional capacity in chronic obstructive pulmonary disease: A systematic review and meta-analysis. *Respirology.* 2013;18:616–629.

Grönberg AM, Slinde F, Engström CP, Hulthén L, Larsson S. Dietary problems in patients with severe chronic obstructive pulmonary disease. *J Hum Nutr Diet.* 2005;18(6):445–452.

Gologanu D, Ionita D, Gartonea T, Stanescu C, Bogdan MA. Body composition in patients with chronic obstructive pulmonary disease. *Maedica* (Buchar). 2014;9(1):25–32.

Hallin R, Koivisto-Hursti UK, Lindberg E, Janson C. Nutritional status, dietary energy intake and the risk of exacerbations in patients with chronic obstructive pulmonary disease (COPD). *Respir Med.* 2006;100:561–567.

Koehler F, Doehner W, Hoernig S, Witt C, Anker SD, John M. Anorexia in chronic obstructive pulmonary disease—Association to cachexia and hormonal derangement. *Int J Cardiol.* 2007;119:83–89.

National Guideline Clearinghouse (NGC). Guideline summary NGC-7966: Chronic obstructive pulmonary disease. In: National Guideline Clearinghouse (NGC). Rockville (MD): Agency for Healthcare Research and Quality (AHRQ); 2010 Oct. Available: http://www .guideline.gov. Accessed 02/07/15.

National Guideline Clearinghouse (NGC). Guideline synthesis: Chronic obstructive pulmonary disease (COPD): Diagnosis and management of acute exacerbations. In: National Guideline Clearinghouse (NGC). Rockville (MD): Agency for Healthcare Research and Quality (AHRQ); 2001 Dec (revised 2011 Oct). Available: http://www.guideline.gov. Accessed 02/07/15.

Nordén J, Grönberg AM, Bosaeus I, et al. Nutrition impact symptoms and body composition in patients with COPD. *Eur J Clin Nutr.* 2015;69(2):256–261.

Odencrants S, Ehnfors M, Grobe SJ. Living with chronic obstructive pulmonary disease: Part I. Struggling with meal-related situations: experiences among persons with COPD. *Scand J Caring Sci.* 2005;19:230–239.

Reeves A, White H, Sosnowski K, Tran K, Jones M, Palmer M. Energy and protein intakes of hospitalised patients with acute respiratory failure receiving non-invasive ventilation. *Clin Nutr.* 2014;33:1068–1073.

Schols AM. Nutrition as a metabolic modulator in COPD. *Chest.* 2013;144:1340–1345.

Schols AM, Ferreira IM, Franssen FM, et al. Nutritional assessment and therapy in COPD: A European Respiratory Society statement. *Eur Respir J.* 2014;44:1504–1520.

Internet Resources

American Lung Association: http://www.lung.org /lung-disease/copd/

Centers for Disease Control and Prevention: http://www .cdc.gov/copd/

COPD International: http://www.copd-international.com/

National Heart Lung and Blood Institute/ Learn More Breathe Better: http://www.nhlbi.nih.gov/health /educational/copd/

USDA Nutrient Data Laboratory: http://ndb.nal.usda.gov/

COPD with Respiratory Failure

Georgianna Sergakis, PhD, RRT, RCP
The Ohio State University

Objectives

After completing this case, the student will be able to:

1. Describe the pathophysiology of chronic obstructive pulmonary disease and its relationship to acute respiratory failure.
2. Describe the role of nutrition support in treatment of patients on mechanical ventilation.
3. Outline the metabolic implications of acute respiratory failure.
4. Interpret biochemical indices for assessment of respiratory function.
5. Interpret biochemical indices for assessment of nutritional status.
6. Plan, interpret, and evaluate nutrition support for mechanically ventilated patients.

Daishi Hayoto, a 65-year-old male, is brought to the University Hospital emergency department by his wife because he has been experiencing severe shortness of breath. Mr. Hayoto has a long-standing history of COPD.

Hayato, Daishi, Male, 65 y.o.

Allergies: Penicillin	**Code:** FULL	**Isolation:** None
Pt. Location: RM 405	**Physician:** M. McFarland	**Admit Date:** 3/26

Patient Summary: Acute respiratory distress, COPD, peripheral vascular disease with intermittent claudication

History:

Onset of disease: Patient was diagnosed with COPD 10 years ago, and notes a history of chronic tobacco use, 2 PPD for 50 years. He woke up in his usual state of health today with marked limitation of his exercise capacity due to dyspnea on exertion. He also notes two-pillow orthopnea, swelling in both lower extremities. Today while performing some yardwork he noted sudden onset of marked dyspnea beyond his usual shortness of breath with ADLs. His wife brought him to the emergency department right away. There, a chest radiograph showed a pneumothorax involving the left lung. Patient also states he gets cramping in his right calf when he walks. *[handwritten: lung collapse]*

Medical history: Cholecystectomy 20 years ago. Total dental extraction 5 years ago. Intermittent claudication. Claims to be allergic to penicillin. Diagnosed with emphysema more than 10 years ago; $FEV_1/FVC = 69\%$ and $FEV_1 = 60\%$ of predicted. Has been treated successfully with Combivent (Respimat® inhaler)—2 inhalations QID (each inhalation delivers 20 mcg ipratropium bromide; 100 mcg albuterol) and tiotropium DPI.

Surgical history: Cholecystectomy 20 years ago

Medications at home: Combivent inhaler, tiotropium bromide DPI, Lasix, O_2 2 L/hour via nasal cannula; wife notes that he is noncompliant. *[handwritten: K depleting]*

Tobacco use: Yes; 2 PPD for 50 years

Alcohol use: Yes; 1–2 drinks 1–2 ×/week

Family history: Father died of non-small cell lung cancer. Maternal grandfather also

[handwritten margin notes: d.f./labored breathing; discomf. breath lieing flt]

Demographics:

Marital status: Married, lives with wife, age 62, who is well; four adult children not living in the area

Years education: Bachelor's degree

Language: English and Japanese

Occupation: Retired manager of local grocery chain

Hours of work: N/A

Ethnicity: Nisei

Religious affiliation: Methodist

Admitting History/Physical:

Chief complaint: "My husband has had emphysema for many years. He was working in the yard today and got really short of breath. I called our doctor and she said to go straight to emergency."

Vital Signs: Temp: 98°F   Pulse: 118   Resp rate: 36
BP: 110/80   Height: 5'4"   Weight: 122 lbs

Heart: Normal heart sounds; no murmurs or gallops

HEENT: Within normal limits; fundoscopic exam reveals AV nicking

   Eyes: Pupil reflex normal

   Ears: Slight neurosensory deficit acoustically

Hayato, Daishi, Male, 65 y.o.
Allergies: Penicillin   **Code:** FULL   **Isolation:** None
Pt. Location: RM 405   **Physician:** M. McFarland   **Admit Date:** 3/26

Nose: Unremarkable

Throat: Jugular veins appear distended. Trachea is shifted to the right. Carotids are full, symmetrical, and without bruits.

Genitalia: Unremarkable

Rectal: Prostate normal; stool hematest negative

Neurologic: DTR full and symmetric; alert and oriented × 3

Extremities: Nails have tar stains, Cyanosis, 1+ pitting edema

Skin: Warm, dry to touch

Chest/lungs: Hyperresonance to percussion over the left chest anteriorly and posteriorly. Diminished breath sounds are noted over right chest with absent sounds on the left. Using accessory muscles at rest.

Abdomen: Old surgical scar RUQ. No organomegaly or masses. BS reduced.

Circulation: R femoral bruit present. Right PT and DP pulses were absent.

Nursing Assessment	3/26
Abdominal appearance (concave, flat, rounded, obese, distended)	rounded
Palpation of abdomen (soft, rigid, firm, masses, tense)	soft
Bowel function (continent, incontinent, flatulence, no stool)	continent
Bowel sounds (P=present, AB=absent, hypo, hyper)	
RUQ	P
LUQ	P
RLQ	P
LLQ	P
Stool color	brown
Stool consistency	soft
Tubes/ostomies	N/A
Genitourinary	
Urinary continence	catheter
Urine source	catheter
Appearance (clear, cloudy, yellow, amber, fluorescent, hematuria, orange, blue, tea)	clear, yellow
Integumentary	
Skin color	pale
Skin temperature (DI=diaphoretic, W=warm, dry, CL=cool, CLM=clammy, CD1=cold, M=moist, H=hot)	W
Skin turgor (good, fair, poor, TENT=tenting)	fair

(Continued)

Hayato, Daishi, Male, 65 y.o.
Allergies: Penicillin   **Code:** FULL   **Isolation:** None
Pt. Location: RM 405   **Physician:** M. McFarland   **Admit Date:** 3/26

Nursing Assessment *(Continued)*

Nursing Assessment	**3/26**
Skin condition (intact, EC=ecchymosis, A=abrasions, P=petechiae, R=rash, W=weeping, S=sloughing, D=dryness, EX=excoriated, T=tears, SE=subcutaneous emphysema, B=blisters, V=vesicles, N=necrosis)	SE at site of pneumothorax
Mucous membranes (intact, EC=ecchymosis, A=abrasions, P=petechiae, R=rash, W=weeping, S=sloughing, D=dryness, EX=excoriated, T=tears, SE=subcutaneous emphysema, B=blisters, V=vesicles, N=necrosis)	intact
Other components of Braden score: special bed, sensory pressure, moisture, activity, friction/shear (>18=no risk, 15–16=low risk, 13–14=moderate risk, ≤12=high risk)	activity, 18

CXR: increased AP diameter, flattened diaphragms, bullae noted in bilateral apices, and significant pneumothorax of the left upper lobe. There is a chest tube on the left side.

Orders:
Oxygen (titrate to keep SpO_2 >88%), ABG, continuous pulse oximetry, CBC, chemistry panel, UA repeat Chest X-ray, ECG, albuterol (2.5 mg) and ipratropium bromide (0.5mg) nebulizers Q4; albuterol (2.5mg) prn.
IVF D_5 ½ NS at TKO Solumedrol 10–40 mg q 4–6 hr; high dose = 30 mg/kg q 4–6 hr (2 days max)
NPO

Nutrition:
General: Wife relates general appetite is only fair. Usually breakfast is the largest meal. Appetite has been decreased for past several weeks. She states his highest weight was 135 lbs, but feels he weighs much less than that now.
Usual dietary intake:
AM: Egg, hot cereal, bread or muffin, hot tea (with milk and sugar)
Lunch: Soup, sandwich, hot tea (with milk and sugar)
Dinner: Small amount of meat, rice, 2–3 kinds of vegetables, hot tea (with milk and sugar)

24-hr recall: 2 scrambled eggs, few bites of Cream of Wheat, sips of hot tea, bite of toast; ate nothing rest of day—sips of hot tea

Food allergies/intolerances/aversions: NKA
Previous nutrition therapy? No
Food purchase/preparation: Wife
Vit/min intake: None

Anthropometric data: Ht 5'4", Wt 122 lbs, UBW 135 lbs

Hayato, Daishi, Male, 65 y.o.
Allergies: Penicillin
Pt. Location: RM 405

Code: FULL
Physician: M. McFarland

Isolation: None
Admit Date: 3/26

Laboratory Results

	Ref. Range	3/26 1405	3/27 0600
Chemistry			
Sodium (mEq/L)	136–145	138	
Potassium (mEq/L)	3.5–5.1	3.9	
Chloride (mEq/L)	98–107	101	
Carbon dioxide (CO_2, mEq/L)	23–29	45 !↑	
Bicarbonate (mEq/L)	23–28	38 !↑	
BUN (mg/dL)	0–20	11	
Creatinine serum (mg/dL)	0.6–1.1 F 0.9–1.3 M	0.7	
BUN/Crea ratio	10.0–20.0	15	
Uric acid (mg/dL)	2.8–8.8 F 4.0–9.0 M	7.1	
Est GFR, non-Afr Amer (mL/min/1.73 m^2)	>60	99	
Glucose (mg/dL)	70–99	108 !↑	
Phosphate, inorganic (mg/dL)	2.2–4.6	3.2	
Magnesium (mg/dL)	1.5–2.4	1.9	
Calcium (mg/dL)	8.6–10.2	9.1	
Anion gap (mmol/L)	10–20	2.9 !↓	
Osmolality (mmol/kg/H_2O)	275–295	285	
Bilirubin total (mg/dL)	≤1.2	1.3 !↑	
Bilirubin, direct (mg/dL)	<0.3	0.8 !↑	
Protein, total (g/dL)	6–7.8	6.1	
Albumin (g/dL)	3.5–5.5	3.4 !↓	
Prealbumin (mg/dL)	18–35	16 !↓	
Ammonia (NH_3, µg/L)	6–47	9	
Alkaline phosphatase (U/L)	30–120	114	
ALT (U/L)	4–36	15	
AST (U/L)	0–35	22	
CPK (U/L)	30–135 F 55–170 M	152	
Lactate dehydrogenase (U/L)	208–378	210	

(Continued)

Hayato, Daishi, Male, 65 y.o.
Allergies: Penicillin
Pt. Location: RM 405

Code: FULL
Physician: M. McFarland

Isolation: None
Admit Date: 3/26

Laboratory Results *(Continued)*

	Ref. Range	3/26 1405	3/27 0600
Cholesterol (mg/dL)	<200	155	
HDL-C (mg/dL)	>59 F, >50 M	32 !↓	
VLDL (mg/dL)	7–32	31	
LDL (mg/dL)	<130	142 !↑	
LDL/HDL ratio	<3.22 F <3.55 M	4.44 !↑	
Triglycerides (mg/dL)	35–135 F 40–160 M	155	
Coagulation (Coag)			
PT (sec)	11–13	12.7	
INR	0.9–1.1	0.97	
PTT (sec)	24–34	26	
Hematology			
WBC (× 10^3/mm³)	3.9–10.7	5.6	
RBC (× 10^6/mm³)	4.2–5.4 F 4.5–6.2 M	6.9 !↑	
Hemoglobin (Hgb, g/dL)	12–16 F 14–17 M	17.5 !↑	
Hematocrit (Hct, %)	37–47 F 41–51 M	54 !↑	
Hematology, Manual Diff			
Neutrophil (%)	40–70	52	
Lymphocyte (%)	22–44	10 !↓	
Monocyte (%)	0–7	3	
Eosinophil (%)	0–5	0	
Basophil (%)	0–2	0	
Blasts (%)	3–10	7	
Segs (%)	0–60	83 !↑	
Bands (%)	0–10	9	
Arterial Blood Gases (ABGs)			
pH	7.35–7.45	7.2 !↓	7.30 !↓
pCO₂ (mm Hg)	35–45	76 !↑	59 !↑
SaO₂ (%)	≥95	78 !↓	88 !↓

Hayato, Daishi, Male, 65 y.o.
Allergies: Penicillin
Pt. Location: RM 405

Code: FULL
Physician: M. McFarland

Isolation: None
Admit Date: 3/26

Laboratory Results *(Continued)*

	Ref. Range	3/26 1405	3/27 0600
O_2 content (%)	15–22	14 !↓	17
pO_2 (mm Hg)	≥80	56 !↓	88
Base excess (mEq/L)	+/–2	1	1
Base deficit (mEq/L)	+/–2	NA	NA
HCO_3^- (mEq/L)	21–28	38 !↑	30 !↑

Note: Values and units of measurement listed in these tables are derived from several resources. Substantial variation exists in the ranges quoted as "normal" and these may vary depending on the assay used by different laboratories.

Intake/Output

Date		3/27 0701–3/28 0700			
Time		0701–1500	1501–2300	2301–0700	Daily total
IN	Formula	200	200	Withheld due to high residuals	400
	Flush (mL/kg/hr)	50 (0.56)	50 (0.56)		100 (0.37)
	I.V. (mL/kg/hr)	400 (0.90)	400 (0.90)	800 (1.80)	1600 (1.20)
	I.V. piggyback				
	TPN				
	Total intake (mL/kg)	650 (11.7)	650 (11.7)	800 (14.4)	2100 (37.9)
OUT	Urine (mL/kg/hr)	325 (0.73)	575 (1.30)	765 (1.72)	1665 (1.25)
	Emesis output				
	Other				
	Stool	200	100		300
	Total output (mL/kg)	525 (9.5)	675 (12.2)	765 (13.8)	1965 (35.4)
Net I/O		+125	−25	+35	+135
Net since admission (3/26)		+125	+100	+135	+135

Case Questions

I.   Understanding the Disease and Pathophysiology

1.   Mr. Hayato was diagnosed with emphysema more than 10 years ago. Define *emphysema* and explain its underlying pathophysiology.

2.   In the emergency room, a chest tube was inserted into the left thorax with drainage under suction. Subsequently the oropharynx was cleared. A resuscitation bag and mask were used to ventilate the patient with high-flow oxygen. Endotracheal intubation was then performed using a laryngoscope so the trachea could be directly visualized to place a 8.0 endotracheal tube. The patient was then ventilated with the help of a volume-cycled ventilator. Initial ventilator settings are Assist-Control mode, frequency= 12 breaths/min, with a FiO_2 of 100%, a positive end-expiratory pressure (PEEP) of 6 cm H_2O, and a tidal volume of 400 mL (8 cc/kg of his IBW). Daily chest radiographs and ABGs were used each AM to adjust the ventilator settings. Define the following terms found in the history and physical for Mr. Hayato:

   a.   Dyspnea

   b.   Orthopnea

   c.   Pneumothorax

   d.   Endotracheal intubation

   e.   Cyanosis

3.   Identify features of the physician's physical examination consistent with his admitting diagnosis. Describe the pathophysiology that might be responsible for each physical finding.

II.   Understanding the Nutrition Therapy

4.   What is the relationship between nutritional status and respiratory function? Define *respiratory quotient* (RQ). What dietary factors affect RQ?

5. Do nutrition support and nutritional status play a role in enabling a patient to be weaned from a respiratory ventilator? Explain.

III. Nutrition Assessment

6. Evaluate Mr. Hayato's admitting anthropometric data.

7. Determine Mr. Hayato's energy and protein requirements. Justify your answer.

8. Determine Mr. Hayato's fluid requirements.

9. Evaluate Mr. Hayato's biochemical indices relevant to nutritional status on 3/26.

IV. Nutrition Diagnosis

10. Select two high-priority nutrition problems and complete the PES statement for each.

V. Nutrition Intervention

11. A nutrition consult was completed on 3/27, and enteral feedings were initiated. Mr. Hayato was started on Isosource HN @ 25 cc/hr continuously over 24 hours.

   a. At this rate, how many kcal and grams of protein should he receive per day?

   b. Calculate his nutrition prescription utilizing this enteral formula. Include the goal rate, free water requirements, and the appropriate progression of the rate.

12. What type of formula is Isosource HN? What are the percentages of kilocalories from carbohydrate, protein, and lipid? Is there a specific nutrient composition that should be considered in respiratory failure or the mechanically ventilated patient?

VI.   Nutrition Monitoring and Evaluation

13. Examine the intake/output record. How much enteral feeding (kcal, protein) did the patient receive?

14. You read in the physician's orders that the patient experienced high gastric residual volume (GRV) and the enteral feeding was discontinued. Define *high GRV*. Using evidence-based guidelines, what recommendations are given regarding definition of high GRV? What recommendations would you make?

15. Were any additional signs of EN intolerance documented? Do you agree with the decision to discontinue the feeding? Why or why not?

16. What options are available to improve tolerance of the tube feeding?

17. On 3/27, the enteral feeding was restarted at 25 mL/hr and then increased to 50 mL/hr after 12 hours. What were Mr. Hayato's energy and protein intakes for 3/27?

18. Examine the values documented for arterial blood gases (ABGs).

    a. On the day Mr. Hayato was intubated, his ABGs were as follows: pH 7.2, pCO_2 65, CO_2 35, pO_2 56, HCO_3^- 38. What can you determine from each of these values?

    b. On 3/28, while Mr. Hayato was on the ventilator, his ABGs were as follows: pH 7.36, pCO_2 63, pO_2 60, HCO_3^- 32. What can you determine from each of these values?

    c. On 3/30, after the enteral feeding was resumed, his ABGs were as follows: pH 7.22, pCO_2 66, pO_2 57, HCO_3^- 37. In addition, indirect calorimetry indicated an RQ of 0.95 and his measured energy intake was 1350 kcal. How does the patient's measured energy intake compare to your previous calculations? What does the RQ indicate?

19. The patient was weaned from the ventilator on 4/2 and discharged to home on 4/5. As Mr. Hayato is prepared for discharge, what nutritional goals might you set with him and his wife to improve his overall nutritional status?

Bibliography

Academy of Nutrition and Dietetics. Evidence Analysis Library. Chronic Obstructive Pulmonary Disease Guideline. http://www.andeal.org/topic .cfm?menu=5301&cat=3707. Accessed 3/30/15.

Academy of Nutrition and Dietetics. Evidence Analysis Library. Recommendations Summary. CI: Enteral Nutrition Energy Delivery. http://www.andeal.org /topic.cfm?menu=5302&cat=4888. Accessed 03/30/15.

Academy of Nutrition and Dietetics. Nutrition Care Manual. Chronic Obstructive Pulmonary Disease (COPD). https://www.nutritioncaremanual.org /topic.cfm?ncm_category_id=1&lv1=5538&lv2 =22249&ncm_toc_id=22249&ncm_heading =Nutrition%20Care. Accessed on 03/30/15.

Altintas ND, AydinK, Turkoglu MA, Abbasoglu O, Topeli A. Effect of enteral versus parenteral nutrition on outcome of medical patients requiring mechanical ventilation. *Nutr Clin Pract.* 2011;26:322–329.

Bergman EA, Hawk SN. Diseases of the respiratory system. In: Nelms M, Sucher K, Lacey K, Roth SL. *Nutrition Therapy and Pathophysiology.* 2nd ed. Belmont, CA: Wadsworth, Cengage Learning; 2011:648–681.

Brisard L, Le Gouge A, Lascarrou JB, et al. Impact of early enteral versus parenteral nutrition on mortality in patients requiring mechanical ventilation and catecholamines: Study protocol for a randomized controlled trial (NUTRIREA-2). *Trials.* 2014;15:507.

Choudhury G, Rabinovich R, Macnee W. Comorbidities and systemic effects of chronic obstructive pulmonary disease. *Clinics in Chest Medicine.* 2014;35(1):101–130.

Collins EG, Bauldoff G, Carlin B, et al. Clinical competency guidelines for pulmonary rehabilitation professionals: Position statement of the American Association of Cardiovascular and Pulmonary Rehabilitation. *J Cardiopulm Rehabil Prev.* 2014;34(5):291–302.

Decramer M, De Benedetto F, Del Ponte A, Marinari S. Systemic effects of COPD. *Respir Med.* 2005;99 Suppl B:S3–S10.

Demiling RH, DeSanti L. Effect of a catabolic state with involuntary weight loss on acute and chronic respiratory disease. Available from: http://www.med-scape .com/viewprogram/1816_pnt. Accessed 03/04/15.

Doley J, Mallampalli A, Sandberg M. Nutrition management for the patient requiring prolonged mechanical ventilation. *Nutr Clin Pract.* 2011;26:232–241.

National Guideline Clearinghouse (NGC). Guideline summary NGC-7966: Chronic obstructive pulmonary disease. In: National Guideline Clearinghouse (NGC). British Colombia: Medical Services Commission; 2011 Jan. Available: http://www .guideline.gov. Accessed 03/04/15.

National Guideline Clearinghouse (NGC). Guideline synthesis: Chronic obstructive pulmonary disease (COPD): Diagnosis and management of acute exacerbations. In: National Guideline Clearinghouse (NGC). Rockville, MD: Agency for Healthcare Research and Quality (AHRQ); 2001 Dec (revised 2011 Oct). Available: http://www.guideline.gov. Accessed 03/04/15.

Nelms MN, Habash D. Nutrition assessment: Foundation of the nutrition care process. In: Nelms M, Sucher K, Lacey K. *Nutrition Therapy and Pathophysiology.* 3rd ed. Belmont, CA: Wadsworth, Cengage Learning; 2016:36–71.

Nelms MN. Enteral and parenteral nutrition support. In: Nelms M, Sucher K, Lacey K. *Nutrition Therapy and Pathophysiology.* 3rd ed. Belmont, CA: Wadsworth, Cengage Learning; 2016:88–114.

Nelms MN. Metabolic stress and the critically ill. In: Nelms M, Sucher K, Lacey L. *Nutrition Therapy and Pathophysiology.* 3rd ed. Belmont, CA: Wadsworth, Cengage Learning; 2016:665–685.

Nici L, Donner C, Wouters E, et al. American Thoracic Society/European Respiratory Society statement on pulmonary rehabilitation. *Am J Respir Crit Care Med.* 2006;173(12):1390–413.

Patel V, Romano M, Corkins MR, et al. Nutrition Screening and Assessment in Hospitalized Patients: A survey of current practice in the United States. *Nutr Clin Pract.* 2014;29(4):483–490.

Schols AM. Nutritional advances in patients with respiratory diseases. *Eur Respir Rev.* 2015;24(135):17–22.

Ukleja A, Freeman KL, Gilbert K, et al. Standards for nutrition support: Adult hospitalized patients. *Nutr Clin Pract.* 2010;25:403–414.

🌐 Internet Resources

American Lung Association: http://www.lung.org /lung-disease/copd/

Centers for Disease Control and Prevention: http://www .cdc.gov/copd/

COPD International: http://www.copd-international.com/

National Heart Lung and Blood Institute—Learn More Breathe Better: http://www.nhlbi.nih.gov/health /public/lung/copd/index.htm

USDA Nutrient Data Laboratory: http://www.ars.usda .gov/main/site_main.htm?modecode=80-40-05-25.

Unit Ten

NUTRITION THERAPY FOR METABOLIC STRESS AND CRITICAL ILLNESS

The physiological response to stress, trauma, and infection has been an important area of nutrition research for the past several decades. This metabolic response is characterized by catabolism of stored nutrients to meet the increased energy requirements.

Unlike other situations in which the body faces increased energy requirements, the stress response demands a preferential use of glucose for fuel. Because glycogen stores are quickly depleted, the body turns to lean body mass for glucose produced via gluconeogenesis.

Under the influence of counterregulatory hormones such as glucagon, epinephrine, norepinephrine, and cortisol, as well as cytokines such as interleukin and tumor necrosis factor, the body shifts from its normal balanced state or anabolism to catabolism. All sources of fuel metabolism are affected by the stress response and the subsequent control of counterregulatory hormones. Despite increased lipolysis, the efficiency for the use of fatty acids and glycerol as sources of fuel is reduced.

The body's inability to keep up with the rate of protein catabolism results in loss of skeletal muscle and high urinary losses of nitrogen. The liver's rate of gluconeogenesis is increased, and hyperglycemia is common. In addition, many tissues—especially skeletal tissue—develop insulin resistance, which contributes to the hyperglycemic state.

Cases 28, 29, and 30 focus on the application of evidenced-based guidelines to guide the decision making for nutrition support. Nutrition support can serve as an integral component of the medical care and can impact the metabolic response. With increasing rates of obesity in the United States, the necessity of providing nutrition support in the morbidly obese patient (as in Case 30) is an increasingly common challenge for the registered dietitian.

Case 29 allows you to assess a patient with a burn injury. Burn injuries are an excellent example of the posttraumatic, hypermetabolic state. Determining nutritional needs, prescribing appropriate nutrition support, and monitoring daily progress are all addressed in this case. Other conditions resulting in metabolic stress include trauma, open wounds, and sepsis. These situations also demand close attention to nutrition support to minimize complications of protein-calorie malnutrition and to optimize recovery assisted by medical nutrition therapy. You can easily transfer the same concepts for nutrition assessment and support to other individual cases you may encounter.

Metabolic Stress and Trauma: Open Abdomen

Deborah Cohen, DCN, RD
University of New Mexico

Objectives

After completing the case, the student will be able to:

1. Apply the knowledge of the pathophysiology of trauma and metabolic stress in order to provide nutrition support for the critically ill patient.
2. Identify the basic components of indirect calorimetry.
3. State specific indications for the use of indirect calorimetry in critically ill patients.
4. Interpret the respiratory quotient.
5. Compare different predictive equations that are appropriate for use in the critically ill population.

6. Use current evidence-based guidelines to evaluate and plan nutrition support for the critically ill.

Juan Perez is a 29-year-old male admitted to the surgical intensive care unit with a gunshot wound to the abdomen. He experienced gastric, duodenal, and jejunal injuries, liver laceration, and a left pleural effusion.

Perez, Juan, Male, 29 y.o.
Allergies: NKA
Pt. Location: Bed #2 SICU

Code: FULL
Physician: D. Kuhls, MD

Isolation: Contact
Admit Date: 3/22

Patient Summary: The patient was brought into the emergency department by a friend after he was shot in the abdomen. He was vomiting blood, and complained of severe back and "stomach" pain. He was able to respond to a few questions initially but stated, "The pain is too bad for me to think." He denied being allergic to any medications or having any chronic medical problems.

History:
Medical history: Unremarkable
Surgical history: Unknown
Medications at home: Unknown
Tobacco use: Yes
Alcohol use: Unknown

Demographics:
Marital status: Single; lives with his brother, his brother's wife, and their two children, ages 2 and 4
Language: Spanish/English
Occupation: Convenience store clerk
Ethnicity: Hispanic
Religious affiliation: Catholic

Admitting History/Physical:
General appearance: Mildly obese 29-year-old Hispanic male on mechanical ventilation

Vital Signs: Temp: 102.5   Pulse: 135   Resp rate: 20
                    BP: 115/65   Height: 70"   Weight: 102.7 kg

Heart: Noncontributory
HEENT: NG tube in place for decompression
Genitalia: Deferred
Neurologic: Sedated
Extremities: 4+ bilateral edema
Skin: Warm, moist
Chest/lungs: Lungs clear to auscultation and percussion
Peripheral vascular: Pulses full—no bruits
Abdomen: Abdominal distention, wound VAC in place, three tubes draining peritoneal fluid, hypoactive BS present in all regions. Liver percusses 8 cm at the midclavicular line, one fingerbreadth below the right costal margin.

Dx: Abdominal GSW

Tx plan: Emergent OR

MD Progress Note:
Hospital Day #7
3/29 0840

Perez, Juan, Male, 29 y.o.
Allergies: NKA
Pt. Location: Bed #2 SICU

Code: FULL
Physician: D. Kuhls, MD

Isolation: Contact
Admit Date: 3/22

<u>Admission History</u>: Juan Perez is a 29-yo male who suffered a GSW to the abdomen. In the ED a FAST (focused assessment with sonography for trauma) scan was performed and found to be positive in the ED and he was transferred emergently to the OR. In the OR, he underwent exploratory laparotomy, gastric repair, control of liver hemorrhage, and resection of proximal jejunum, leaving his GI tract in discontinuity. Following the OR, he was transferred to the SICU intubated and hemodynamically stable.

Hospital Day #2 (3/24): Returned to surgery to remove packs and to reestablish bowel continuity. An abdominal vacuum-assisted closure (VAC) device was placed. Three Jackson Pratt drains left in place.

Hospital Day #3 (3/25): Returned to surgery for anastomotic leak—gastrojejunostomy tube inserted through the patient's stomach, with the jejunal limb shortened in order to provide antegrade intraluminal drainage, as well as retrograde jejunostomy tube for drainage.

Hospital Day #7 (3/29): Returned to surgery for abdominal washout, insertion of a distally placed jejunostomy tube for feeding, and a VAC change.

Subjective: Juan Perez previous 24 hours reviewed.

Vitals: Temp: 99.1 Pulse: 82 Resp rate: 15 BP: 122/78 Wt.: 109 kg
O_2 Sat (%): 93%

I/O last 3 completed shifts: *In:* 5472 (IV 1800, TPN 3312, IV Piggyback 360)
                                  Out: 4584 (Urine 2889, Other 1695)

<u>Physical Exam</u>
General/Constitutional: NAD, lying in bed, sedated
HEENT: Normocephalic, PERRL
Cardiac: RRR
Pulmonary/Chest: No wheezes or crackles
Abdominal: VAC in place, jejunostomy feeding tube in place, moderate distention with appropriate tenderness
Extremities: WNL
Periperal Vascular Exam: Peripheral pulses throughout
Neurological: Moves all extremities spontaneously—sedated
Skin: Warm, dry
IV Fluid: D5 0.45 @75 mL/h–KVO
Nutrition: NPO, TPN
Glycemic Control: Insulin drip as per institution protocol
Mobility: As tolerates per PT treatment plan

.... T. Franks, MD—Surgical Resident
.... D. Kuhls, MD—Trauma Attending

Nutrition Consult—Follow-up: 3/29 Hospital Day #7
<u>A</u>: 29-yo male s/p GSW to the abdomen with emergent exploratory laparatomy; s/p gastric repair, control of liver hemorrhage and resection of proximal jejunum—jejunostomy feeding tube in place. Ht.: 70" Adm Wt: 102.7 kg Current wt: 109 kg IBW: 75.45 kg

Perez, Juan, Male, 29 y.o.
Allergies: NKA
Pt. Location: Bed #2 SICU

Code: FULL
Physician: D. Kuhls, MD

Isolation: Contact
Admit Date: 3/22

Metabolic cart measurement: REE 3657 kcal RQ 0.76
Current nutrition support: Dextrose: 140 CAA: 60 FAT/L:20 Goal Rate: 135 mL/hr
Propofol @35 mL/hr providing additional 924 kcal for total of:
3888 kcal (51 kcal/kg IBW/day) and 194 g protein (2.6 g/kg IBW/day)
Labs and medications reviewed.
D: Increased energy expenditure related to open abdomen and posttrauma status as evidenced by metabolic cart measurement of 3657 kcal expenditure.
Altered GI function related to open abdomen and GSW with subsequent surgery as evidenced by lack of bowel sounds, no stool output, and continued wound VAC for open abdomen.
I: Current metabolic cart measurement does not indicate overfeeding so will recommend to continue current TPN. Recommend to initiate trickle feeds of Pivot at 5 mL/hr.
M/E: Will continue to monitor electrolytes, nutritional parameters, and metabolic tolerance of nutrition support daily. Would recommend to delay nitrogen balance study as it will most likely be inaccurate due to large amounts of protein losses via abdominal wounds.

.... L. Hall, MS, RD, CNSC

Nursing Assessment	3/29
Abdominal appearance (concave, flat, rounded, obese, distended)	distended—wound VAC in place
Palpation of abdomen (soft, rigid, firm, masses, tense)	NA
Bowel function (continent, incontinent, flatulence, no stool)	no stool
Bowel sounds (P=present, AB=absent, hypo, hyper)	
RUQ	AB
LUQ	AB
RLQ	AB
LLQ	AB
Stool color	N/A
Stool consistency	N/A
Tubes/ostomies	J-P drains—wound VAC
Genitourinary	
Urinary continence	catheter
Urine source	catheter
Appearance (clear, cloudy, yellow, amber, fluorescent, hematuria, orange, blue, tea)	cloudy, pale yellow
Integumentary	
Skin color	light brown

Perez, Juan, Male, 29 y.o.
Allergies: NKA   **Code:** FULL   **Isolation:** Contact
Pt. Location: Bed #2 SICU   **Physician:** D. Kuhls, MD   **Admit Date:** 3/22

Nursing Assessment *(Continued)*

Nursing Assessment	3/29
Skin temperature (DI=diaphoretic, W=warm, dry, CL=cool, CLM=clammy, CD+=cold, M=moist, H=hot)	DI
Skin turgor (good, fair, poor, TENT=tenting)	fair
Skin condition (intact, EC=ecchymosis, A=abrasions, P=petechiae, R=rash, W=weeping, S=sloughing, D=dryness, EX=excoriated, T=tears, SE=subcutaneous emphysema, B=blisters, V=vesicles, N=necrosis)	A, D
Mucous membranes (intact, EC=ecchymosis, A=abrasions, P=petechiae, R=rash, W=weeping, S=sloughing, D=dryness, EX=excoriated, T=tears, SE=subcutaneous emphysema, B=blisters, V=vesicles, N=necrosis)	intact
Other components of Braden score: special bed, sensory pressure, moisture, activity, friction/shear (>18 = no risk, 15–16 = low risk, 13–14 = moderate risk, ≤ 12 = high risk)	10

Intake/Output

Date	3/29 0701–3/30 0700			
Time	0701–1500	1501–2300	2301–0700	Daily total
IN P.O.	0	0	0	0
I.V.	600	600	600	1800
(mL/kg/hr)	(0.69)	(0.69)	(0.69)	(0.69)
I.V. piggyback	120	120	120	360
TPN	1104	1104	1104	3312
Total intake	1824	1824	1824	5472
(mL/kg)	(16.7)	(16.7)	(16.7)	(50.2)
OUT Urine	868	790	1231	2889
(mL/kg/hr)	(0.99)	(0.90)	(1.41)	(1.10)
Emesis output				
Other (JP drains)	525	555	615	1695
Stool				
Total output	1393	1345	1846	4584
(mL/kg)	(12.78)	(12.34)	(16.93)	(42.05)
Net I/O	+431	+479	−22	+888
Net since admission (3/22)	+3264	+3743	+3721	+3721

Perez, Juan, Male, 29 y.o.
Allergies: NKA
Pt. Location: Bed #2 SICU

Code: FULL
Physician: D. Kuhls, MD

Isolation: Contact
Admit Date: 3/22

Laboratory Results

	Ref. Range	3/29 1522	4/1 1809
Chemistry			
Sodium (mEq/L)	136–145	146 !↑	140
Potassium (mEq/L)	3.5–5.1	4.0	3.7
Chloride (mEq/L)	98–107	99	99
Carbon dioxide (CO_2, mEq/L)	23–29	25	26
BUN (mg/dL)	6–20	23 !↑	25 !↑
Creatinine serum (mg/dL)	0.6–1.1 F 0.9–1.3 M	1.4 !↑	1.6 !↑
BUN/Crea ratio	10.0–20.0	16.42	15.6
Uric acid (mg/dL)	2.8–8.8 F 4.0–9.0 M	8.9	
Glucose (mg/dL)	70–99	164 !↑	140 !↑
Phosphate, inorganic (mg/dL)	2.2–4.6	2.0 !↓	2.1 !↓
Magnesium (mg/dL)	1.5–2.4	1.9	1.5
Calcium (mg/dL)	8.6–10.2	7.1 !↓	
Osmolality (mmol/kg/H_2O)	275–295	309.3 !↑	296.7 !↑
Bilirubin total (mg/dL)	≤1.2	0.9	
Bilirubin, direct (mg/dL)	<0.3	0.15	
Protein, total (g/dL)	6–7.8	5.2 !↓	5.1 !↓
Albumin (g/dL)	3.5–5.5	1.4 !↓	1.9 !↓
Prealbumin (mg/dL)	18–35	3.0 !↓	5.0 !↓
Ammonia (NH_3, µg/L)	6–47	11	
Alkaline phosphatase (U/L)	30–120	540 !↑	
ALT (U/L)	4–36	435 !↑	
AST (U/L)	0–35	190 !↑	
CPK (U/L)	30–135 F 55–170 M	182 !↑	
Lactate dehydrogenase (U/L)	208–378	750 !↑	
C-reactive protein (mg/dL)	<1.0	245 !↑	220 !↑
Cholesterol (mg/dL)	<200	180	
HDL–C (mg/dL)	>59 F, >50 M	40 !↓	
VLDL (mg/dL)	7–32	110 !↑	
LDL (mg/dL)	<130	140 !↑	

Perez, Juan, Male, 29 y.o.
Allergies: NKA
Pt. Location: Bed #2 SICU

Code: FULL
Physician: D. Kuhls, MD

Isolation: Contact
Admit Date: 3/22

Laboratory Results *(Continued)*

	Ref. Range	3/29 1522	4/1 1809
LDL/HDL ratio	<3.22 F <3.55 M	3.5	
Triglycerides (mg/dL)	35–135 F 40–160 M	274 !↑	265 !↑
HbA$_{1C}$ (%)	<5.7	7.1 !↑	
Coagulation (Coag)			
PT (sec)	11–13	9 !↓	
INR	0.9–1.1	0.6 !↓	
PTT (sec)	24–34	21 !↓	
Hematology			
WBC (×10^3/mm^3)	3.9–10.7	15.2 !↑	
RBC (×10^6/mm^3)	4.2–5.4 F 4.5–6.2 M	3.2 !↓	
Hemoglobin (Hgb, g/dL)	12–16 F 14–17 M	14	
Hematocrit (Hct, %)	37–47 F 41–51 M	35 !↓	
Mean cell volume (µm^3)	80–96	82	
Mean cell Hgb (pg)	28–32	27 !↓	
Mean cell Hgb content (g/dL)	32–36	33	
RBC distribution (%)	11.6–16.5	12	
Platelet count (×10^3/mm^3)	150–350	180	
Urinalysis			
Collection method	—	catheter	
Color	—	pale yellow	
Appearance	—	cloudy	
Specific gravity	1.001–1.035	1.045 !↑	
pH	5–7	5.1	
Protein (mg/dL)	Neg	+ !↑	
Glucose (mg/dL)	Neg	+ !↑	
Ketones	Neg	+ !↑	
Blood	Neg	Neg	
Bilirubin	Neg	Neg	

(Continued)

Perez, Juan, Male, 29 y.o.
Allergies: NKA
Pt. Location: Bed #2 SICU

Code: FULL
Physician: D. Kuhls, MD

Isolation: Contact
Admit Date: 3/22

Laboratory Results *(Continued)*

	Ref. Range	3/29 1522	4/1 1809
Nitrites	Neg	Neg	
Urobilinogen (EU/dL)	<1.1	<0.1	
Leukocyte esterase	Neg	Neg	
Prot chk	Neg	Neg	
WBCs (/HPF)	0–5	0	
RBCs (/HPF)	0–2	0	
Bact	0	5 !↑	
Mucus	0	5 !↑	
Crys	0	0	
Casts (/LPF)	0	0	
Yeast	0	2 !↑	

Note: Values and units of measurement listed in these tables are derived from several resources. Substantial variation exists in the ranges quoted as "normal" and these may vary depending on the assay used by different laboratories.

Case Questions

I. Understanding the Disease and Pathophysiology

1. The patient has suffered a gunshot wound to the abdomen. This has resulted in an open abdomen. Define *open abdomen*. The medical record describes the use of a wound "VAC." Describe this procedure and its connection to the diagnosis for open abdomen.

2. The patient underwent gastric resection and repair, control of liver hemorrhage, and resection of the proximal jejunum, leaving his GI tract in discontinuity. Describe the potential effects of surgery on this patient's ability to meet his nutritional needs.

3. The metabolic stress response to trauma has been described as a progression through three phases: the ebb phase, the flow phase, and finally the recovery or resolution. Define each of these and determine how they may correspond to this patient's hospital course.

4. Acute-phase proteins are often used as a marker of the stress response. What is an acute-phase protein? What is the role of C-reactive protein in the nutritional assessment of critically ill trauma patients? What other acute-phase proteins may be followed to assess the inflammatory stress response?

II. Understanding the Nutrition Therapy

5. Metabolic stress and trauma significantly affect nutritional requirements. Describe the changes in nutrient metabolism that occur in metabolic stress. Specifically address energy requirements and changes in carbohydrate, protein, and lipid metabolism.

6. Are there specific nutrients that should be considered when designing nutrition support for a trauma patient? Explain the rationale and current recommendations regarding glutamine, arginine, and omega-3 fatty acids for this patient population.

7. Using current evidence-based guidelines, explain the decision-making process that would be applied in determining the route for nutrition support for the trauma patient.

III. Nutrition Assessment

8. Calculate and interpret the patient's BMI.

9. What factors make assessing his actual weight difficult on a daily basis?

10. Calculate energy and protein requirements for Mr. Perez. Use at least two methods (including the Penn State) to estimate his energy needs. Explain your rationale for using each one. For the Penn State calculation, the minute ventilation is 3.5 L/minute and the maximum temperature is 39.2.

11. What does indirect calorimetry measure?

12. Compare the estimated energy needs calculated using the predictive equations with each other and with those obtained by indirect calorimetry measurements.

13. Interpret the RQ value. What does it indicate?

14. What factors contribute to the elevated energy expenditure in this patient?

15. Mr. Perez was prescribed parenteral nutrition. Determine how many kilocalories and grams of protein are provided with his prescription. Read the nutrition consult follow-up and the I/O record. What was the total volume of PN provided that day?

16. Compare this nutrition support to his measured energy requirements obtained by the metabolic cart on 3/26. Based on the metabolic cart results, what changes would you recommend be made to the TPN regimen, if any? What are the limitations that prevent the health care team from making significant changes to the nutrition support regimen?

17. The patient was also receiving propofol. What is this, and why should it be included in an assessment of his nutritional intake? How much energy (total kcal, % kcal from fat) did it provide?

18. The RD recommended that trickle feeds be initiated. What is this and what is the rationale? The RD recommended the formula Pivot 1.5 for these trickle feeds. What type of formula is this, and what would be the rationale for choosing this formula?

19. List abnormal biochemical values for 3/29, describe why they might be abnormal, and explain any nutrition-related implications.

20. Current guidelines recommend using a nitrogen balance study to assess the adequacy of nutrition support.

    a. According to the Powell (2012) article (see bibliography below), what adjustments should be made to assess for nitrogen losses through fistulas, drains, or wound output?

    b. A 24-hour nitrogen collection is completed for Mr. Perez with results of UUN 42 g. Calculate his nitrogen balance.

IV.   Nutrition Diagnosis
21. Identify the nutrition diagnosis you would use in your follow-up note. Complete the PES statement.

V.   Nutrition Intervention
22. For the PES statement that you have written, establish an ideal goal (based on the signs and symptoms) and an appropriate intervention (based on the etiology).

VI.   Nutrition Monitoring and Evaluation
23. What are the standard recommendations for monitoring the nutritional status of a patient receiving nutrition support?

24. Hyperglycemia was noted in the laboratory results. Why is hyperglycemia of concern in the critically ill patient? How was this handled for this patient? What are the current recommendations for glycemic control in critically ill patients?

25. What would be the standard guidelines and subsequent recommendations to begin weaning TPN and increasing enteral feeds?

Bibliography

Bankhead R, Boullata J, Brantley S, et al. Enteral nutrition practice recommendations. *J Parenter Enteral Nutr.* 2009;33(2):122–167.

Byrnes MC, Reicks P, Irwin E. Early enteral nutrition can be successfully implemented in trauma patients with an "open abdomen." *Am J Surg.* 2010;199:359–363.

Carr JA. Abdominal compartment syndrome: A decade of progress. *J Am Coll Surgeons.* 2013;216:135–146.

Cohen D, Kuhls D. Energy expenditure and open abdomen following trauma. *Top Clin Nutr.* 2009;24:122–129.

Diaz JJ, et al. The management of the open abdomen in trauma and emergency general surgery: Part 1— damage control. *J Trauma.* 2010;68:1425–1438.

Friese RS. The open abdomen: Definitions, management principles and nutrition support considerations. *Nutr Clin Prac.* 2012;27:492–498.

McClave SA, Martindale RG, Vanek VW, et al. Guidelines for the provision and assessment of nutrition support therapy in the adult critically ill patient: Society of Critical Care Medicine and American Society for Parenteral and Enteral Nutrition. *J Parenter Enteral Nutr.* 2009;33:277–316.

McDonnell M, Umpierrez G. Insulin therapy for the management of hyperglycemia in hospitalized patients. *Endocrinology & Metabolism Clinics of North America* [serial online]. March 2012;41(1):175–201. Available from: CINAHL Plus with Full Text, Ipswich, MA. Accessed 10/26/15.

Nahikian-Nelms ML. Metabolic stress and the critically ill. In: Nelms M, Sucher K, Lacey K. *Nutrition Therapy and Pathophysiology.* 3rd ed. Belmont, CA: Cengage Learning; 2016:665–685.

Nahikian-Nelms ML, Habash D. Nutrition assessment: Foundation of the nutrition care process. In: Nelms M, Sucher K, Lacey K. *Nutrition Therapy and Pathophysiology.* 3rd ed. Belmont, CA: Cengage Learning, 2016:36–71.

Powell NJ, Collier B. Nutrition and the open abdomen. *Nutr Clin Pract.* 2012;27:499–506.

Preiser JC, van Zanten AR, Berger MM, et al. Metabolic and nutritional support in critically ill patients: Consensus and controversies. *Critical Care.* 2015;19(1):35.

Internet Resources

AND Evidence Analysis Library: http://www.andeal.org/

Nutrition Care Manual: http://www.nutritioncaremanual.org

Case 29

Nutrition Support for Burn Injury

Sheela Thomas, MS, RD, LD, CNSC
The Ohio State University Wexner Medical Center

Objectives

After completing this case, the student will be able to:

1. Understand the metabolic response to burn injury and the related nutritional considerations.
2. Understand the nutritional implications of the following: total body surface area burn; inhalation injury; circumferential burns; fluid resuscitation; age and comorbid conditions in burn injury.
3. Demonstrate the ability to assess the nutritional needs of patients with burn injury.
4. Evaluate the current literature regarding nutrition support for patients with burn injury.

5. Apply evidence-based guidelines for nutrition support in the critically ill burn patient.
6. Develop a nutrition care plan—with appropriate measurable goals, interventions, and strategies for monitoring and evaluation—that addresses the nutrition diagnoses for this case.

Mr. Angelo is a 65-year-old male who has been admitted to the surgical intensive care unit for treatment of serious burns estimated to cover 40% of his body, as well as suspected smoke inhalation injury.

Angelo, Joe, male, 65 y.o.

Allergies: NKA	**Code:** FULL	**Isolation:** None
Pt. Location: SICU Bed 36	**Physician:** L. Martin	**Admit Date:** 9/9

Patient Summary: Mr. Angelo is a 65-year-old male admitted as a level 2 trauma with 40% total body surface area burns after being involved in a trailer fire. He is admitted to the surgical intensive care unit for management of burn injury.

History:

Onset of disease: Patient is unclear about what occurred, and his story changed several times during assessment. Patient lost his job recently and was coming from Atlanta to move in with his parents. He was driving behind an RV in a caravan when the RV caught fire. Apparently he was in the front cab of the RV trying to put out an engine fire when his clothes caught on fire. He jumped out of the car and rolled on the ground to put out the flames. At one time he stated that he jumped into a ravine, but later he stated this was not the case. He received 1650 cc of normal saline en route to hospital. The burn involves the face, bilateral upper extremity, bilateral lower extremity circumferentially, scrotum, back, and buttocks. The ENT service evaluated the patient and performed a nasopharyngolaryngoscopy. Findings included laryngeal edema and soot on the vocal cords bilaterally. Recommendation is to intubate for airway protection due to edema and soot on the vocal cords. Patient does have occasional wheezing and some patchy infiltrates on chest X-ray that could be related to smoke inhalation. Pt was started on fluid resuscitation per Parkland formula using lactated Ringer's (LR) @ 610 mL/hr.

Medical history: Diabetes, HTN, GERD

Surgical history: s/p cholecystectomy 30 years ago

Medications at home: None

Tobacco use: Smokes 1 PPD for >30 yrs

Alcohol use: 2–3 beers daily and a case on Saturday and Sunday

Family history: Father: HTN; mother: anxiety disorder, HTN; brother: healthy

Demographics:

Years education: 11

Language: English only

Occupation: Unemployed

Household members: Lives alone

Ethnicity: Caucasian

Religious affiliation: Unknown

Primary Assessment per EMS:

Airway: Intact

Breathing: Clear

Circulation 2+ carotid and radial pulses, 2+ femoral, 1+ DP pulses diminished

Glasgow coma score: 14

Admitting History/Physical:

General appearance: Alert, cooperative, mild distress, appears stated age. The wounds appear to have ruptured blisters and devitalized skin. The patient's ROM to affected area is diminished in range with pain.

Angelo, Joe, male, 65 y.o.
Allergies: NKA
Pt. Location: SICU Bed 36

Code: FULL
Physician: L. Martin

Isolation: None
Admit Date: 9/9

Vital Signs: Temp: 100   Pulse: 120   Resp rate: 22
                   BP: 140/93   Height: 72"   Weight: 71.2 kg   SpO$_2$: 98%

HEENT: Head/Face: Non-rebreather mask in place. Burns involving entire face, singed eyebrows, hair, and facial hair.
Eyes: PERRLA
Ears: Clear
Nose: Soot noted in nares and oropharynx
Throat: Dry mucous membranes

Neck: C-collar in place
Lungs: Clear to auscultation bilaterally
Heart: Tachycardia, regular rhythm; S1, S2 normal, no murmur, click, rub, or gallop
Abdomen: Soft, skin tender. Bowel sounds normal. No masses, no organomegaly, partial thickness and 1st degree burns near umbilicus.
Upper extremities: Burns noted R bicep, forearm, hand, left bicep and hand, mostly second degree. Skin sloughing and devitalized tissue.
Lower extremities: Mostly full thickness burns noted to bilateral lower extremities circumferentially
Back: Second degree burns in mid and left back
Genitourinary: Erythema and blistering at head of penis and scrotum
Peripheral vascular: Pulses:
Right pulses: FEM: present 2+, POP: present 2+, DP: present 1+, PT: present 1+
Left pulses: FEM: present 2+, POP: present 2+, DP: present 1+, PT present 1+

Nursing Assessment	9/9
Abdominal appearance (concave, flat, rounded, obese, distended)	distended
Palpation of abdomen (soft, rigid, firm, masses, tense)	soft
Bowel function (continent, incontinent, flatulence, no stool)	continent
Bowel sounds (P=present, AB=absent, hypo, hyper)	
RUQ	P, hypo
LUQ	P, hypo
RLQ	P, hypo
LLQ	P, hypo
Stool color	none
Stool consistency	
Tubes/ostomies	N/A
Genitourinary	
Urinary continence	catheter
Urine source	catheter
Appearance (clear, cloudy, yellow, amber, fluorescent, hematuria, orange, blue, tea)	yellow

(Continued)

Angelo, Joe, male, 65 y.o.
Allergies: NKA   **Code:** FULL   **Isolation:** None
Pt. Location: SICU Bed 36   **Physician:** L. Martin   **Admit Date:** 9/9

Nursing Assessment *(Continued)*

Nursing Assessment	9/9
Integumentary	
Skin color	beefy red to pale
Skin temperature (DI=diaphoretic, W=warm, dry, CL=cool, CLM=clammy, CD1=cold, M=moist, H=hot)	CL, M
Skin turgor (good, fair, poor, TENT=tenting)	poor
Skin condition (intact, EC=ecchymosis, A=abrasions, P=petechiae, R=rash, W=weeping, S=sloughing, D=dryness, EX=excoriated, T=tears, SE=subcutaneous emphysema, B=blisters, V=vesicles, N=necrosis)	W, S, B, N
Mucous membranes (intact, EC=ecchymosis, A=abrasions, P=petechiae, R=rash, W=weeping, S=sloughing, D=dryness, EX=excoriated, T=tears, SE=subcutaneous emphysema, B=blisters, V=vesicles, N=necrosis)	B, D
Other components of Braden score: special bed, sensory pressure, moisture, activity, friction/shear (>18=no risk, 15–16=low risk, 13–14=moderate risk, >12=high risk)	10

Admission Orders:

Laboratory: C-reactive protein now and routine every Monday morning
CBC, EDIF, platelet routine every morning
Chem 7, IP, Mg, Ca routine every morning
Hemoglobin A_{1C} routine one time
Hepatic function panel routine, every Monday morning
Prealbumin now and routine every Monday morning
Ionized calcium routine every morning
PT, IR, PTT routine every morning
ABGs routine every morning

Radiology:

CT head, neck, abdomen
KUB—NG placement and enteral feeding tube placement verification
Chest X-ray for CVC placement and ET tube

Vital Signs: Routine, every 1 hour
I & O recorded every hour
NG tube to low intermittent suction
Oral care per ventilator protocol: Oral mouth swab every 4 hours and PRN. Teeth and gum brushing every 12 hours. Supraglottic oral suctioning every 8 hours and prior to manipulation of the ETT.

Notify burn MD during first 48 hours: If urinary output is less than 0.5 mL/kg/hr or greater than 1.0 mL/kg/hr. Notify for any fluid bolus orders for urinary output.

Angelo, Joe, male, 65 y.o.
Allergies: NKA   **Code:** FULL   **Isolation:** None
Pt. Location: SICU Bed 36   **Physician:** L. Martin   **Admit Date:** 9/9

Notify house officer:
If urinary output is less than 0.5 mL/kg/hr or greater than 1.0 mL/kg/hr.
Systolic blood pressure greater than 180, less than 90.
Diastolic blood pressure greater than 110, less than 60.
Heart rate greater than 120, less than 60.
Temperature greater than 102.
Respiratory rate greater than 28, less than 10.
Oxygen saturation less than 92%.
Absent peripheral pulses or decreased in Q1H circ checks.
If repleted with any electrolyte more than twice per day.

Diet: NPO with EN. Impact with Glutamine @ 20 mL/hr, advance 20 mL/hr every 4 hours to 60 mL/hr. Final goal rate per RD.

Activity:
Position any burned extremity elevated
Position HOB 30 degrees or greater
Position with no pillow under head if neck burns present

Scheduled and PRN Medications:
Ascorbic acid 500 mg every 12 hours
Chlorhexidine 0.12% oral solution 15 mL every 12 hours
Famotidine tablet 20 mg every 12 hours
Heparin injection 5,000 units every 8 hours
Insulin regular injection every 6 hours
Multivitamin tablet 1 tab daily
Zinc sulfate 220 mg daily
Methadone 5 mg every 8 hours
Oxandrolone 10 mg every 12 hours
Senna tablet 8.6 mg daily
Docusate oral liquid 100 mg every 12 hours
Silver sulfadiazine 1% cream topical application daily
Midazolam HCl (Versed) 100 mg in sodium chloride 0.9% 100 mL IV infusion, initiate infusion at 1 mg/hr
Hydromorphone (Dilaudid) injection 0.5–1 mg, intravenous every 3 hours as needed
Fentanyl (Sublimaze) injection 50–100 mcg intravenous every 15 minutes as needed
Propofol (Diprivan) 10 mg/mL premix infusion, start at 25 mcg/kg/min intravenous continuous
Thiamin 100 mg × 3 days
Folate 1 mg × 3 days

Dressing change:
Hydromorphone (Dilaudid) injection 0.5–1.5 mg, IV give 10 min prior to dressing change and every 15 min prn if pain score is greater than 4 out of 10 during dressing change.

Angelo, Joe, male, 65 y.o.
Allergies: NKA
Pt. Location: SICU Bed 36

Code: FULL
Physician: L. Martin

Isolation: None
Admit Date: 9/9

Ketamine 50 mg injection, administer as slow IV push over greater than 1 minute immediately prior to dressing change. If needed, may administer 50 mg IV push every 15 minutes for prn pain score greater than 4 out of 10 during dressing change up to 200 mg maximum.
Midazolam (Versed) 2–5 mg, intravenous. Administer as directed, for anxiety, pre- and intraprocedure pain management. Give 10 minutes prior to dressing change and may repeat prn during dressing change if duration greater than 60 minutes.
Oxycodone (Roxicodone) 5–10 mg, per NG tube every 4 hours as needed for moderate pain.

IVF: LR @ 610 mL/hr × first 8 hours and decrease to 305 mL/hr × 16 hours

Nutrition: NPO with TF Impact with Glutamine @ 60 mL/hr.
History: Not following any specific diet. Stable weight for past 6 months. Has not been monitoring blood glucose levels for about a year.

MD Progress Note:
9/11 0500
Subjective: 65-yo male who presented as level 1 trauma with 40% total body surface area burns. Intubated on arrival to SICU for airway protection. Plan per burn team to do bronchoscopy at 11:30 today. Patient with significant respiratory acidosis. S/P escharotomy of bilateral lower extremities overnight per trauma team. Hypotensive overnight. Received 4 L of fluids.

Principal Problem:
Burn involving 40% body surface area
Active problems:
Respiratory failure
Acute pain due to injury
Oliguria
Malnutrition
Vitals: Temp: 100.2 Pulse: 104 Resp. rate: 18 BP: 87/59 O_2 Sat (%) 100%

Hemodynamic/Invasive Device Data (24 hours):
Arterial Line (1) Monitoring
Arterial Line (1) BP: 87/59 mm Hg
Arterial Line (1) MAP: 71 mm Hg

Ventilation/Oxygen Therapy (24 hours):
Oxygen therapy
O_2 Sat (%): 100%
Oxygen therapy O_2 device: Ventilator (mechanical ventilation)
FIO_2%: 40%
Ventilator settings and monitoring (adult)

Angelo, Joe, male, 65 y.o.
Allergies: NKA   **Code:** FULL   **Isolation:** None
Pt. Location: SICU Bed 36   **Physician:** L. Martin   **Admit Date:** 9/9

Ventilator type: 840
Adult/Pediatric Modes SIMV-BiPhasic: SIMV VC
Set/target tidal volume: 550
Set rate: 18
RR total (breaths/min): 18
PEEP: 5
Pressure support: 10
Peak inspiratory pressure (cmH$_2$O): 18
I:E ratio: 1:2.30

Fluid Management (24 hours):
I/O last 3 completed shifts
In: 16425 mL
Out: 1696 mL
Urine output: 1295 mL (18 mL/kg)

Physical Exam:
General appearance: Intubated, sedated
Head: Burns involving entire face, singed eyebrows, hair, and facial hair
Back: Partial thickness burns over lower back and buttocks
Lungs: Clear to auscultation bilaterally
Heart: Tachycardia, regular rhythm; S1, S2 normal, no murmur, click, rub, or gallop
Abdomen: Soft, non-tender. Bowel sounds normal. No masses, no organomegaly, partial thickness
and 1st degree burns near umbilicus.
Male genitalia: Abnormal findings: blistering over scrotum and head of penis
Extremities: Partial thickness burns to bilateral upper extremities and full thickness circumferential
burns to lower extremities. S/P escharotomy of bilateral lower extremities.

Assessment/Plan:
40% TBSA burn: Managed per burn team. Continue daily dressing changes. OR today for debride-
ment and split thickness skin grafting.
Respiratory failure: Intubated 9/9 for airway protection. Bronchoscopy at 11:30 today.
Pain: Versed gtt, increase methadone to 10 mg every 8 hours. Dilaudid and fentanyl pm. Wean
propofol to off possibly by the end of the day. Currently at 25 mL/hr.
Hyperkalemia: Secondary to metabolic, respiratory acidosis. Improving. Last K$^+$5.9. Continue to
resuscitate with LR.
Protein-calorie malnutrition: Advance TF to goal rate per nutrition.
Acute kidney injury: Continue fluid resuscitation.

.... L. Martin MD

Angelo, Joe, male, 65 y.o.
Allergies: NKA   **Code:** FULL   **Isolation:** None
Pt. Location: SICU Bed 36   **Physician:** L. Martin   **Admit Date:** 9/9

Intake/Output

Date		9/09 0700–9/10 0659			
Time		0700–1459	1500–2259	2300–0659	Daily total
IN	P.O.	**0**	**0**	**0**	**0**
	I.V.	**4880**	**2440**	**2440**	**9760**
	(mL/kg/hr)	(8.6)	(4.3)	(4.3)	(5.71)
	IV bolus	**1000**	**1000**	**4000**	**6000**
	Enteral feeding	**0**	**228**	**337**	**565**
	IV piggyback	**0**	**100**	**0**	**100**
	Total intake	**5880**	**3768**	**6777**	**16425**
	(mL/kg)	(82.6)	(52.9)	(95.2)	(230.7)
OUT	Urine	**665**	**325**	**305**	**1295**
	(mL/kg/hr)	(1.2)	(0.6)	(0.5)	(0.76)
	Emesis output				
	NG Tube	**0**	**300**	**100**	**400**
	Stool	**0**	**0**	**31**	**31**
	Total output	**665**	**625**	**405**	**1695**
	(mL/kg)	(9.3)	(8.8)	(5.7)	(23.8)
Net I/O		**+5215**	**+3143**	**+6372**	**+14730**
Net since admission (9/09)		**+5215**	**+8358**	**+14730**	**+14730**

Laboratory Results

	Ref. Range	9/9 0200
Chemistry		
Sodium (mEq/L)	136–145	137
Potassium (mEq/L)	3.5–5.1	5.9 !↑
Chloride (mEq/L)	98–107	113 !↑
Carbon dioxide (CO_2, mEq/L)	23–29	20 !↓
Bicarbonate (mEq/L)	23–28	19 !↓
BUN (mg/dL)	6–20	13
Creatinine serum (mg/dL)	0.6–1.1 F 0.9–1.3 M	1.36 !↑
BUN/Crea ratio	10.0–20.0	10.3
Uric acid (mg/dL)	2.8–8.8 F 4.0–9.0 M	8.1
Est GFR, non-Afr Amer (mL/min/1.73 m^2)	>60	54 !↓

Angelo, Joe, male, 65 y.o.
Allergies: NKA   **Code:** FULL   **Isolation:** None
Pt. Location: SICU Bed 36   **Physician:** L. Martin   **Admit Date:** 9/9

Laboratory Results *(Continued)*

	Ref. Range	**9/9 0200**
Glucose (mg/dL)	70–99	211 !↑
Phosphate, inorganic (mg/dL)	2.2–4.6	3.4
Magnesium (mg/dL)	1.5–2.4	1.4 !↓
Calcium (mg/dL)	8.6–10.2	6.9 !↓
Anion gap (mmol/L)	10–20	5.0 !↓
Osmolality (mmol/kg/H_2O)	275–295	295
Bilirubin total (mg/dL)	≤1.2	1.2
Bilirubin, direct (mg/dL)	<0.3	0.2
Protein, total (g/dL)	6–7.8	4.7 !↓
Albumin (g/dL)	3.5–5.5	2.1 !↓
Prealbumin (mg/dL)	18–35	12 !↓
Ammonia (NH_3, μg/L)	6–47	16
Alkaline phosphatase (U/L)	30–120	70
ALT (U/L)	4–36	21
AST (U/L)	0–35	44 !↑
C-reactive protein (mg/dL)	<1.0	12 !↑
Coagulation (Coag)		
PT (sec)	11–13	12.7
INR	0.9–1.1	0.98
PTT (sec)	24–34	26
Hematology		
WBC ($\times 10^3$/mm^3)	3.9–10.7	18.1 !↑
RBC ($\times 10^6$/mm^3)	4.2–5.4 F 4.5–6.2 M	5.97
Hemoglobin (Hgb, g/dL)	12–16 F 14–17 M	18.7 !↑
Hematocrit (Hct, %)	37–47 F 41–51 M	54.4 !↑
Arterial Blood Gases (ABGs)		
pH	7.35–7.45	7.31 !↓
pCO_2 (mm Hg)	35–45	39.8
SO_2 (%)	≥95	99.8
CO_2 content (mmol/L)	25–30	27
O_2 content (%)	15–22	21

(Continued)

Angelo, Joe, male, 65 y.o.
Allergies: NKA
Pt. Location: SICU Bed 36

Code: FULL
Physician: L. Martin

Isolation: None
Admit Date: 9/9

Laboratory Results *(Continued)*

	Ref. Range	**9/9 0200**
pO$_2$ (mm Hg)	≥80	106.5
HCO$_3^-$ (mEq/L)	21–28	19.6 !↓
COHb (%)	<2	0.9

Note: Values and units of measurement listed in these tables are derived from several resources. Substantial variation exists in the ranges quoted as "normal" and these may vary depending on the assay used by different laboratories.

Case Questions

I.   Understanding the Diagnosis and Pathophysiology

1.   Describe how burn wounds are classified. Identify and describe Mr. Angelo's burn injuries.

2.   Explain the "rule of nines" used in assessment of burn injury.

3.   Mr. Angelo's fluid resuscitation order was: *LR @ 610 mL/hr × first 8 hours and decrease to 305 mL/hr × 16 hours.* What is the primary goal of fluid resuscitation? Briefly explain the Parkland formula. What common intravenous fluid is used in burn patients for fluid resuscitation? What are the components of this solution?

4.   What is inhalation injury? How can it affect patient management?

5.   Burns are often described as one of the most metabolically stressful injuries. Discuss the effects of a burn on metabolism and how this will affect nutritional requirements.

6.   List all medications that Mr. Angelo is receiving. Identify the action of each medication and any drug–nutrient interactions that you should monitor.

II.   Understanding the Nutrition Therapy

7.   Using evidence-based guidelines, describe the potential benefits of early enteral nutrition in burn patients.

8.   What are the common criteria used to assess readiness for the initiation of enteral nutrition in burn patients?

9.   What are the specialized nutrient recommendations for the enteral nutrition formula administered to burn and trauma patients per ASPEN/SCCM guidelines?

What additional micronutrients will need supplementation in burn therapy?

What dosages are recommended?

III. Nutrition Assessment

10. Using Mr. Angelo's height and admit weight, calculate IBW, %IBW, BMI, and BSA.

11. Energy requirements can be estimated using a variety of equations. The Xie and Zawacki equations are frequently used. Estimate Mr. Angelo's energy needs using these equations. How many kcal/kg does he require based on these equations?

12. Determine Mr. Angelo's protein requirements. Provide the rationale for your estimate.

13. The MD's progress note indicates that the patient is experiencing acute kidney injury. What is this? If the patient's renal function continues to deteriorate and he needs continuous renal replacement therapy, what changes will you make to your current nutritional regimen and why?

14. This patient is receiving the medication propofol. Using the information that you listed in question #6 and #11, what changes will you make to your nutritional regimen and how will you assess tolerance to this medication?

IV. Nutrition Diagnosis

15. Identify at least two of the most pertinent nutrition problems and the corresponding nutrition diagnoses.

16. Write your PES statement for each nutrition problem.

V. Nutrition Intervention

17. The patient is receiving enteral feeding using Impact with Glutamine @ 60 mL/hr. Determine the energy and protein provided by this prescription. Provide guidelines to meet the patient's calculated needs using the Xie equation.

18. By using the information on the intake/output record, determine the energy and protein provided during this time period. Compare the energy and protein provided by the enteral feeding to your estimation of Mr. Angelo's needs.

19. One of the residents on the medical team asks you if he should stop the enteral feeding because the patient's blood pressure has been unstable. What recommendations can you make to the patient's critical care team regarding enteral feeding and hemodynamic status?

VI. Nutrition Monitoring and Evaluation

20. List factors that you would monitor to assess the tolerance to and adequacy of nutrition support.

21. What is the best method to assess calorie needs in critically ill patients? What are the factors that need to be considered before the test is ordered?

22. Write an ADIME note that provides your nutrition assessment and enteral feeding recommendations and/or evaluation of the current enteral feeding orders.

Bibliography

Abdullahi A, Jeschke MG. Nutrition and Anabolic Pharmacotherapies in the Care of Burn Patients. *Nutr Clin Pract*. 2014;29:621–630.

Bankhead R, Boullata J, Brantley S, et al. Enteral nutrition practice recommendations. *JParenter Enteral Nutr*. 2009;33:122–167.

Bittner EA, Shank E, Woodson L, Martyn JA. Acute and perioperative care of the burn-injured patient. *Anesthesiology*. 2015;122:448–464.

Chan MM, Chan GM. Nutritional therapy for burns in children and adults. *Nutrition*. 2009;25:261–269.

Coen JR, Carpenter AM, Shupp JW, et al. The results of a national survey regarding nutritional care of obese burn patients. *J Burn Care & Res*. 2011;32:561–565.

Collier BR, Cherry-Bukowiec JR, Mills Mary E. Trauma, Surgery and Burns. In: ASPEN Adult Nutrition Support Core Curriculum. 2nd ed. 2012;392–411.

Diaz C, Herndon DN, Porter C, et al. Effects of pharmacological interventions on muscle protein synthesis and breakdown in recovery from burns. *Burns*. 2015;41:649–657.

Endorf FW, Ahrenholz D. Burn management. *Curr Op in Crit Care*. 2011;17:601–605.

Foster K. Clinical guidelines in the management of burn injury: A review and recommendations from the organization and delivery of burn care committee. *J Burn Care Res*. 2014;35:271–283.

Graves C, Saffle J, Cochran A. Actual burn nutrition care practices: An update. *J Burn Care Res*. 2009;30:77–82.

Hall B. Care for the patient with burns in the trauma rehabilitation setting. *Critical Care Nursing Quarterly*. 2012;3:272–280.

Holt B, Graves C, Faraklas I, Cochran A. Compliance with nutrition support guidelines in acutely burned patients. *Burns*. 2012;38:645–649.

Kurmis R, Heath K, Ooi S, et al. A Prospective Multi-Center Audit of Nutrition Support Parameters Following Burn Injury. *J Burn Care & Res*. 2015;36:471–477.

Kurmis R, Parker A, Greenwood J. The use of immunonutrition in burn injury care: Where are we? *J Burn Care & Res*. 2010;31:677–691.

Latenser BA. Critical care of the burn patient: The first 48 hours. *Crit Care Med*. 2009;37:2819–2826.

Legrand M, Guttormsen AB, Berger MM. Ten tips for managing critically ill burn patients: Follow the RASTAFARI! *Intensive Care Med*. 2015;41:1107–1109.

Mahanna E, Crimi E, White P, Mann DS, Fahy BG. Nutrition and metabolic support for critically ill patients. *Curr Opin Anaesthesiol*. 2015;28:131–138.

Masters B, Aarabi S, Sidhwa F, Wood F. High-carbohydrate, high-protein, low-fat versus low-carbohydrate, high-protein, high-fat enteral feeds for burns. *Cochrane Database of Systematic Reviews*. 2012;1:Article No.: CD006122.DOI:10.1002/14651858. CD006122.pub3.

McClave SA, et al. Guidelines for the provision and assessment of nutrition support therapy in the adult critically ill patient: Society of Critical Care Medicine (SCCM) and American Society for Parenteral and Enteral Nutrition (ASPEN). *J Parenter Enteral Nutr*. 2009;33:277–316.

Moore CL, Schmidt PM. A burn progressive care unit: Customized care from admission through discharge. *Perioperative Nursing Clinics*. 2012;7:99–105.

Mendonfa MN, Gragnani A, Masako F. Burns, metabolism and nutritional requirements. *Nutr Hosp*. 2011;26:692–700.

Nahikian-Nelms ML. Metabolic stress and the critically ill. In: Nelms M, Sucher K, Lacey K. *Nutrition Therapy and Pathophysiology*. 3rd ed. Belmont, CA: Wadsworth, Cengage Learning; 2016:665–685.

Nahikian-Nelms ML, Habash D. Nutrition assessment: Foundation of the nutrition care process. In: Nelms M, Sucher K, Lacey K. *Nutrition Therapy and Pathophysiology*. 3rd ed. Belmont, CA: Wadsworth, Cengage Learning; 2016:36–71.

Nordlund MJ, Pham TN, Gibran NS. Micronutrients after burn injury: A review. *J Burn Care & Res*. 2014;35:121–133.

Ridley E, Gantner D, Pellegrino V. Nutrition therapy in critically ill patients—A review of current evidence for clinicians. *Clin Nutr*. 2015;34:565–571.

Rodriguez NA, Jeschke MG, Williams FN, Kamolz LP, Herndon DN. Nutrition in burns: Galveston contributions. *JPEN*. 2011;35:704–14.

Shields BA, Pidcoke HF, Chung KK, et al. Are visceral proteins valid markers for nutritional status in burn intensive care unit? *J Burn Care Res*. 2015;36:375–380.

Sudenis T, Hall K, Carlotto R. Enteral nutrition: What the dietitian prescribes is not what the burn patient gets! *J Burn Care Res*. 2015;36:297–305.

Sullivan J. Nutrition and metabolic support in severe burn injury. *Support Line*. 2010;32:3–13.

Vanek VW, et al. A.S.P.E.N. Position Paper: Parenteral Nutrition Glutamine Supplementation. *Nutrition in Clinical Practice*. 2011;26:479–494.

Internet Resources

AND Evidence Analysis Library: http://www.andeal .org
American Burn Association: http://www.ameriburn.org

Nutrition Care Manual: http://www.nutritioncaremanual.org
UpToDate: http://www.uptodate.com/contents/overview -of-nutritional-support-for-moderate-to-severe-burn -patients

Nutrition Support in Sepsis and Morbid Obesity

Objectives

After completing this case, the student will be able to:

1. Identify the current surgical procedures used for bariatric surgery.
2. Identify the physiological consequences of bariatric surgery.
3. Describe the pathophysiology of sepsis.
4. Apply evidence-based guidelines for provision of nutrition support in the morbidly obese patient.
5. Identify specific nutrients that may assist with treatment of sepsis.

6. Describe refeeding syndrome and the current recommendations for its prevention.
7. Interpret nutrition assessment data to assist with the design of measurable goals, interventions, and strategies for monitoring and evaluation that address the nutrition diagnoses for the patient.

Chris McKinley is a 37-year-old obese male admitted to the MICU from the ED with probable sepsis 4 months after undergoing a Roux-en-Y gastric bypass.

McKinley, Chris, Male, 37 y.o.
Allergies: NKA
Pt. Location: MICU Bed #5

Code: FULL
Physician: P Walker

Isolation: None
Admit Date: 2/23

Patient Summary: Mr. McKinley has suffered from type 2 diabetes mellitus, hyperlipidemia, hypertension, and osteoarthritis over the previous 10 years. Mr. McKinley has weighed over 250 lbs since age 15 with steady weight gain since that time. He had attempted to lose weight numerous times but the most weight he ever lost was 75 lbs, which he regained over the following two-year period. He had recently reached his highest weight of 425 lbs, lost 24 lbs prior to his planned bariatric surgery through the preoperative nutrition education program, and then had the Roux-en-Y gastric bypass surgery 4 months ago. He has done well at home with a total weight loss of approximately 100 lbs to date. Now, however, he is admitted to the MICU from the ER with probable sepsis.

History:

Onset of disease: Experienced flu-like symptoms over previous 48 hours and then became acutely short of breath—brought to ER at that time.
Medical history: Type 2 diabetes mellitus, hypertension, hyperlipidemia, osteoarthritis
Surgical history: s/p Roux-en-Y gastric bypass surgery November 1; R total knee replacement 3 years previous
Medications at home: Lovastatin 60 mg/day (previously on Lantus and metformin—off diabetes medications for 2 months)
Tobacco use: None
Alcohol use: Socially, 2–3 beers per week—has not had alcohol since surgery
Family history: Father: Type 2 DM, CAD, Htn, COPD; Mother: Type 2 DM, CAD, osteoporosis

Demographics:

Marital status: Single
Number of children: 0
Years education: Associate's degree
Language: English only
Occupation: Office manager for real estate office
Hours of work: 8–5 daily—sometimes on weekends
Household members: Lives with roommate
Ethnicity: Caucasian
Religious affiliation: None stated

Admitting History/Physical:

Chief complaint: On mechanical ventilation
General appearance: Obese white male

Vital Signs: Temp: 102.5   Pulse: 98   Resp rate: 23
                    BP: 135/90   Height: 5'10"   Weight: 325 lbs

Heart: Elevated rate, regular rhythm, normal heart; diminished distal pulses. Exam reveals no gallop and no friction rub.

McKinley, Chris, Male, 37 y.o.
Allergies: NKA   **Code:** FULL   **Isolation:** None
Pt. Location: MICU Bed #5   **Physician:** P Walker   **Admit Date:** 2/23

HEENT: Head: WNL
                  Eyes: PERRLA
                  Ears: Clear
                  Nose: WNL
                  Throat: Dry mucous membranes without exudates or lesions
Genitalia: Normally developed 37-year-old male
Extremities: Ecchymosis, abrasions, petechiae on lower extremities, 2≦ pitting edema
Skin: Warm, dry to touch
Chest/lungs: Respirations rapid with rales
Peripheral vascular: Diminished pulses bilaterally
Abdomen: Obese, rash present under skinfolds

Nursing Assessment	2/23
Abdominal appearance (concave, flat, rounded, obese, distended)	obese
Palpation of abdomen (soft, rigid, firm, masses, tense)	soft
Bowel function (continent, incontinent, flatulence, no stool)	continent
Bowel sounds (P=present, AB=absent, hypo, hyper)	
RUQ	P
LUQ	P
RLQ	P
LLQ	P
Stool color	light brown
Stool consistency	formed
Tubes/ostomies	NA
Genitourinary	
Urinary continence	NA
Urine source	catheter
Appearance (clear, cloudy, yellow, amber, fluorescent, hematuria, orange, blue, tea)	clear, yellow
Integumentary	
Skin color	pale
Skin temperature (DI=diaphoretic, W=warm, dry, CL=cool, CLM=clammy, CD1=cold, M=moist, H=hot)	W, M
Skin turgor (good, fair, poor, TENT=tenting)	good
Skin condition (intact, EC=ecchymosis, A=abrasions, P=petechiae, R=rash, W=weeping, S=sloughing, D=dryness, EX=excoriated, T=tears, SE=subcutaneous emphysema, B=blisters, V=vesicles, N=necrosis)	EC, A, R

(Continued)

McKinley, Chris, Male, 37 y.o.
Allergies: NKA   **Code:** FULL   **Isolation:** None
Pt. Location: MICU Bed #5   **Physician:** P Walker   **Admit Date:** 2/23

Nursing Assessment *(Continued)*

Nursing Assessment	2/23
Mucous membranes (intact, EC=ecchymosis, A=abrasions, P=petechiae, R=rash, W=weeping, S=sloughing, D=dryness, EX=excoriated, T=tears, SE=subcutaneous emphysema, B=blisters, V=vesicles, N=necrosis)	intact
Other components of Braden score: special bed, sensory pressure, moisture, activity, friction/shear (>18 = no risk, 15–16 = low risk, 13–14 = moderate risk, ≤12 = high risk)	13

Orders:

Initiate Sepsis Bundle Orders: Central line placement; arterial line placement—arterial line care per protocol
If SBP <90 or MAP <65: norepinephrine 4 mcg/min; dopamine 5 mcg/kg/min; epinephrine 1 mcg/min
Normal Saline 500 mL bolus until CVP 8–12, then continue at 150 mL/hr
ECG, urine culture, U/A with microscopic; blood culture 1st and 2nd peripheral site
Serum lactate
Basic metabolic panel
Hepatic function panel, CBC, EDIF, platelets.
Insert peripheral IV and maintain venous access
Vancomycin 2 g in sodium chloride IVPB
Piperacillin-tazobactam (Zosyn) 4.5 g in dextrose 100 mL IVPB
Height, Weight, Intake/Output
Insert feeding tube—nutrition consult

Nutrition:

Meal type: NPO
Fluid requirement: 1800–2000 mL

MD Progress Note:

2/24
Subjective: Chris McKinley's previous 24 hours reviewed
Vitals: Temp: 102.4, Pulse: 88, Resp rate: 30, BP: 108/58
Urine Output: 3270 mL, Glu 220

Physical Exam:
HEENT: Obese neck, no adenopathy, no JVD appreciated, RIJ CVC in place
Neck: WNL
Heart: Regular rate, regular rhythm, no M/R/G appreciated
Lungs: Coarse breath sounds bilaterally with scattered rhonchi R>L; no wheezes or crackles
Abdomen: Morbidly obese, soft, non-distended, no organomegaly, bowel sounds present

McKinley, Chris, Male, 37 y.o.
Allergies: NKA
Pt. Location: MICU Bed #5

Code: FULL
Physician: P Walker

Isolation: None
Admit Date: 2/23

Extremities: Good radial pulses bilaterally. Ecchymosis, abrasions, petechiae on lower extremities, 2+ pitting edema.
Skin: WNL
Neurologic: Intubated, sedated, pupils equal and reactive to light

Assessment/Plan: 37-yo male transferred from ED with severe sepsis, pneumonia. Maintain current mechanical ventilation; cultures pending but will continue vancomycin and Zosyn. Sedation with Versed and fentanyl. Initiate enteral feeding per nutrition consult.

.... P. Walker, MD

Intake/Output

Date		2/23 0701–2/24 0700			
Time		0701–1500	1501–2300	2301–0700	Daily total
IN	P.O.	0	0	0	0
	I.V.	1550	1200	1200	3950
	(mL/kg/hr)	(1.31)	(1.01)	(1.01)	(1.11)
	I.V. piggyback	250	250	250	750
	TPN	0	0	0	0
	Total intake	1800	1450	1450	4700
	(mL/kg)	(12.2)	(9.81)	(9.81)	(31.8)
OUT	Urine	1320	1000	950	3270
	(mL/kg/hr)	(1.12)	(0.85)	(0.80)	(0.92)
	Emesis output				
	Other				
	Stool				
	Total output	1320	1000	950	3270
	(mL/kg)	(8.93)	(6.77)	(6.43)	(22.1)
Net I/O		+480	+450	+500	+1430
Net since admission (2/23)		+480	+930	+1430	+1430

McKinley, Chris, Male, 37 y.o.
Allergies: NKA
Pt. Location: MICU Bed #5

Code: FULL
Physician: P Walker

Isolation: None
Admit Date: 2/23

Laboratory Results

	Ref. Range	2/23 0600
Chemistry		
Sodium (mEq/L)	136–145	136
Potassium (mEq/L)	3.5–5.1	5.8 !↑
Chloride (mEq/L)	98–107	99
Carbon dioxide (CO_2, mEq/L)	23–29	31 !↑
Bicarbonate (mEq/L)	23–28	24
BUN (mg/dL)	6–20	15
Creatinine serum (mg/dL)	0.6–1.1 F 0.9–1.3 M	0.9
BUN/Crea ratio	10.0–20.0	16.7
Uric acid (mg/dL)	2.8–8.8 F 4.0–9.0 M	5.1
Est GFR, non-Afr Amer (mL/min/1.73 m²)	>60	109
Glucose (mg/dL)	70–99	385 !↑
Phosphate, inorganic (mg/dL)	2.2–4.6	2.1 !↓
Magnesium (mg/dL)	1.5–2.4	1.8
Calcium (mg/dL)	8.6–10.2	9.5
Anion gap (mmol/L)	10–20	13
Osmolality (mmol/kg/H_2O)	275–295	289
Bilirubin total (mg/dL)	≤1.2	1.3 !↑
Bilirubin, direct (mg/dL)	<0.3	0.7 !↑
Protein, total (g/dL)	6–7.8	5.8 !↓
Albumin (g/dL)	3.5–5.5	1.9 !↓
Prealbumin (mg/dL)	18–35	11 !↓
Ammonia (NH_3, µg/L)	6–47	35
Alkaline phosphatase (U/L)	30–120	118
ALT (U/L)	4–36	39 !↑
AST (U/L)	0–35	41 !↑
CPK (U/L)	30–135 F 55–170 M	220 !↑
Lactate dehydrogenase (U/L)	208–378	401 !↑
C-reactive protein (mg/dL)	<1.00	110 !↑

McKinley, Chris, Male, 37 y.o.
Allergies: NKA
Pt. Location: MICU Bed #5

Code: FULL
Physician: P Walker

Isolation: None
Admit Date: 2/23

Laboratory Results (Continued)

	Ref. Range	2/23 0600
Fibrinogen (mg/dL)	160–450	525 !↑
Lactate (mEq/L)	0.3–2.3	4.2 !↑
Cholesterol (mg/dL)	<200	320 !↑
HDL-C (mg/dL)	>59 F, >50 M	32 !↓
VLDL (mg/dL)	7–32	45 !↑
LDL (mg/dL)	<130	232 !↑
LDL/HDL ratio	<3.22 F <3.55 M	7.5 !↑
Triglycerides (mg/dL)	35–135 F 40–160 M	245 !↑
HbA$_{1C}$ (%)	<5.7	6.8 !↑
Coagulation (Coag)		
PT (sec)	11–13	14.5 !↑
INR	0.9–1.1	1.4 !↑
PTT (sec)	24–34	37 !↑
Hematology		
WBC ($\times 10^3$/mm^3)	3.9–10.7	23.5 !↑
RBC ($\times 10^6$/mm^3)	4.2–5.4 F 4.5–6.2 M	5.5
Hemoglobin (Hgb, g/dL)	12–16 F 14–17 M	12.5 !↓
Hematocrit (Hct, %)	37–47 F 41–51 M	38 !↓
Platelet count ($\times 10^3$/mm^3)	150–350	210
Transferrin (mg/dL)	250–380 F 215–365 M	385 !↑
Ferritin (mg/mL)	20–120 F 20–300 M	14 !↓
Vitamin B$_{12}$ (ng/dL)	24.4–100	25
Folate (ng/dL)	5–25	15
Urinalysis		
Collection method	—	catheter
Color	—	yellow

(Continued)

McKinley, Chris, Male, 37 y.o.
Allergies: NKA
Pt. Location: MICU Bed #5

Code: FULL
Physician: P Walker

Isolation: None
Admit Date: 2/23

Laboratory Results *(Continued)*

	Ref. Range	2/23 0600
Appearance	—	Clear
Specific gravity	1.001–1.035	1.004
pH	5–7	6.9
Protein (mg/dL)	Neg	+ !↑
Glucose (mg/dL)	Neg	+ !↑
Ketones	Neg	+ !↑
Blood	Neg	Neg
Bilirubin	Neg	Neg
Nitrites	Neg	Neg
Urobilinogen (EU/dL)	<1.0	0.3
Leukocyte esterase	Neg	Neg
Prot chk	Neg	Neg
WBCs (/HPF)	0–5	2
RBCs (/HPF)	0–2	1
Bact	0	+ !↑
Mucus	0	0
Crys	0	0
Casts (/LPF)	0	0
Yeast	0	0

Note: Values and units of measurement listed in these tables are derived from several resources. Substantial variation exists in the ranges quoted as "normal" and these may vary depending on the assay used by different laboratories.

Case Questions

I.   Understanding the Pathophysiology

1.   Mr. McKinley's admission orders indicate he is being treated for probable sepsis and SIRS. Define these conditions.

2.   Describe the metabolic alterations that occur as a result of sepsis and the systemic inflammatory response. Using the medical record information, identify the specific criteria that are consistent with the diagnosis of sepsis.

3.   Mr. McKinley had a Roux-en-Y gastric bypass 4 months ago and has lost approximately 100 lbs. Describe this procedure. Identify the most probable nutritional concerns associated with this rapid weight loss/surgical procedure.

II.   Understanding the Nutrition Therapy

4.   Using evidenced-based guidelines and the research literature, determine whether Mr. McKinley should receive nutrition support. Address the pros/cons of PN versus EN; early enteral feeding; and full versus trophic feeding. Use this discussion to provide a rationale for your decisions.

5.   How will Mr. McKinley's bariatric surgery affect your recommendations for nutrition support?

6.   Discuss the current literature recommendations for supplementation of omega-3-fatty acids, glutamine, arginine and antioxidants in nutrition support during sepsis.

7.   Define *refeeding syndrome*. How will Mr. McKinley's recent 100-lb weight loss affect your nutrition support recommendations regarding risk of refeeding syndrome?

III.   Nutrition Assessment

8.   Assess Mr. McKinley's height and weight. Calculate his BMI and % usual body weight.

9.   After reading the physician's history and physical, identify any signs or symptoms that are most likely a consequence of Mr. McKinley's admitting critical illness.

10. Identify any abnormal biochemical indices and discuss the probable underlying etiology.

11. Which laboratory measurements are consistent with sepsis and metabolic stress?

12. Assess Mr. McKinley's current hydration status using the first 24 hours of I/O and the nursing assessment.

13. Determine Mr. McKinley's energy and protein requirements. Explain the rationale for the method you used to calculate these requirements.

IV.   Nutrition Diagnosis

14. Identify the pertinent nutrition problems and the corresponding nutrition diagnoses.

15. Are you able to diagnose Mr. McKinley using the proposed ASPEN/AND criteria for malnutrition? If so, describe the information you used to make this diagnosis.

V.   Nutrition Intervention

16. Outline the nutrition support regimen you would recommend for Mr. McKinley. This should include formula choice (and rationale) and rate initiation and advancement.

VI.   Nutrition Monitoring and Evaluation

17. Identify the steps you would take to monitor Mr. McKinley's nutritional status in the intensive care unit.

18. What factors may affect his tolerance to enteral feeding?

19. Write a note for your initial inpatient nutrition assessment with nutrition support recommendations.

Bibliography

Academy of Nutrition and Dietetics Nutrition Care Manual. Bariatric Surgery. Available at: https://www.nutritioncaremanual.org/topic.cfm?ncm_category_id=1&lv1=5545&lv2=16927&ncm_toc_id=16927&ncm_heading=Nutrition%20Care. Accessed 07/06/15.

Arabi YM, Tamim HM, Dhar GS, et al. Permissive underfeeding and intensive insulin therapy in critically ill patients: A randomized controlled trial. *Am J Clin Nutr.* 2011;93:569–577.

Bastarache JA, Ware LB, Girard TD, Wheeler AP, Rice W. Markers of inflammation and coagulation may be modulated by enteral feeding strategy. *J Parenter Enteral Nutr.* 2012;36:732–740.

Davis CJ, Sowa D, Keim KS, et al. The use of prealbumin and C-reactive protein for monitoring nutrition support in adult patients receiving enteral nutrition in an urban medical center. *J Parenter Enteral Nutr.* 2012;36:197–204.

Dellinger RP, Levy MM, Rhodes A, et al: Surviving Sepsis Campaign: International guidelines for management of severe sepsis and septic shock: 2012. *Crit Care Med.* 2013;41:580–637.

Desai SV, Mcclave SA, Rice TW. Nutrition in the ICU: An evidence-based approach. *Chest.* 2014;145:1148–1157.

Dickerson RN. Hypocaloric, high protein nutrition therapy for critically ill patients with obesity. *Nutr Clin Pract.* 2014;29:48–54.

Elke G, Heyland DK. Enteral nutrition in critically ill septic patients-less or more? *J Parenter Enteral Nutr.* 2015;39:786–791.

Elke G, Wang M, Weiler N, Day AG, Heyland DK. Close to recommended caloric and protein intake by enteral nutrition is associated with better clinical outcome of critically ill septic patients: Secondary analysis of a large international nutrition database. *Crit Care.* 2014;18:R29.

Fraipoint V, Preiser JC. Energy estimation and measurement in critically ill patients. *JPEN.* 2013;37:705–713.

Fremont RD and Rice TW. Pros and cons of feeding the septic intensive care patient. *Nutr Clin Pract.* 2015; 30:344–350.

Gariballa S. Refeeding syndrome: A potentially fatal condition but remains underdiagnosed and undertreated. *Nutrition.* 2008;24:604–606.

Hurt RT and Frazier TH. Obesity. In: ASPEN Adult Nutrition Support Core Curriculum. 2nd ed. 2012:603–619.

Jeejeebhoy KN. Permissive underfeeding of the critically ill patient. *Nutr Clin Pract.* 2004;19:477–480.

Kastrup M, Spies C. Less is more? Is permissive underfeeding in crtically ill patients necessary? *Am J Clin Nutr.* 2011;94:957–958.

Kushner RF, Drover JW. Current strategies of critical care assessment and therapy of the obese patient (hypocaloric feeding): What are we doing and what do we need to do? *J Parenter Enteral Nutr.* 2011;35(5 Suppl):36S–43S.

Kwon Y, Kim HJ, Lo menzo E, Park S, Szomstein S, Rosenthal RJ. Anemia, iron and vitamin B12 deficiencies after sleeve gastrectomy compared to Roux-en-Y gastric bypass: A meta-analysis. *Surg Obes Relat Dis.* 2014;10:589–597.

Laferrère B. Diabetes remission after bariatric surgery: Is it just the incretins? *International Journal of Obesity.* 2011;35:S22–S25.

McClave SA, Martindale G, Rice TW, Heland DK. Feeding the critically ill patient. *Critical Care Medicine.* 2014;42:2600–2610.

Miller KR, Kiraly L, Martindale RG. Critical Care Sepsis. In: ASPEN Adult Nutrition Support Core Curriculum. 2nd ed. 2012:377–391.

Mogensen KM, Andrew BY, Corona JC, Robinson ML. Validation of the Society of Critical Care Medicine and American Society for Parenteral and Enteral Nutrition recommendations for caloric provision to critically ill obese patients: A pilot study. *J Parenter Enteral Nutrition.* 2015; DOI: 10.1177/0148607115584001. Accessed: July 6, 2015.

Nelms M. Metabolic stress and the critically ill. In: Nelms M, Sucher K, Lacey K. *Nutrition Therapy and Pathophysiology.* 3rd ed. Belmont, CA: Cengage Learning; 2016:665–685.

Owais AR, Bumby RF, MacFie J. Review article: Permissive underfeeding in short-term nutritional support. *Aliment Pharmacol Ther.* 2010;32:628–636.

Owers EL, Reeves AI, Ko SY, et al. Rates of adult acute inpatients documented as at risk of refeeding syndrome by dietitians. *Clin Nutr.* 2015;34:134–139.

Preiser JC, Van zanten AR, Berger MM, et al. Metabolic and nutritional support of critically ill patients: Consensus and controversies. *Crit Care.* 2015;19:737.

Rice TW. Immunonutrition in critical illness: Limited benefit, potential harm. *JAMA.* 2014; 312: 490–491.

Tresley J, Sheean PM. Refeeding syndrome: Recognition is the key to prevention and management. *J Am Diet Assoc.* 2008;108:2105–2108.

Ukleja A, Freeman KL, Gilbert K, et al. Standards for nutrition support: Adult hospitalized patients. *Nutr Clin Pract.* 2010;25:403–414.

Wichansawakun S, Kim DW, Young L, Apovian C. Metabolic support of the obese Intensive Care Unit patient. In: Mullin GE, Cheskin LJ, Matarese LE. *Integrative Weight Management, A Guide for Clinicians.* New York: Humana Press. 2014:215–224.

Young Choi E, Park DA, Park J. Calorie intake of enteral nutrition and clinical outcomes in acutely critically ill patients: A meta-analysis of randomized controlled trials. *J Parenter Enteral Nutr.* 2015;39:291–300.

Internet Resources

American Society for Metabolic and Bariatric Surgery: http://ASMBS.org

Nutrition Care Manual: http://www.nutritioncaremanual.org

Sepsis Alliance: http://www.sepsisalliance.org/

Surviving Sepsis Campaign: http://www.survivingsepsis.org/Pages/default.aspx

U.S. National Library of Medicine: http://www.ncbi.nlm.nih.gov/pubmedhealth/PMH0001687/

Unit Eleven

NUTRITION THERAPY FOR NEOPLASTIC DISEASE

The layperson often uses *cancer* as a name for one disease. The term *cancer*, or *neoplasm*, actually describes any condition in which cells proliferate at a rapid rate and in an unrestrained manner. Each type of cancer is a different disease with different origins and responses to therapy. It is difficult to generalize about the role of nutrition in cancer treatment, because each diagnosis is truly an individual case. However, it is obvious to any clinician participating in the care of cancer patients that nutrition problems are common.

More than 80 percent of patients with cancer experience some degree of malnutrition. Nutrition problems may be some of the first symptoms the patient recognizes. Unexplained weight loss, changes in ability to taste, or a decrease in appetite are often present at diagnosis. The malignancy itself may affect not only energy requirements, but also the metabolism of nutrients.

As the patient begins therapy for a malignancy—surgery, radiation therapy, chemotherapy, immuno-therapy, or bone marrow transplant—treatment side effects occur that can affect nutritional status. And, as with many medical conditions, cancer patients also face significant psychosocial issues. Can nutrition make a difference? Adequate nutrition helps prevent surgical complications, meet increased energy and protein requirements, and repair and rebuild tissues, which cancer therapies often damage. Furthermore, good nutrition allows increased tolerance of therapy and helps maintain the patient's quality of life.

Case 31 is set after therapy has been completed and the patient is in a recovery phase. Nutrition recommendations change at this stage to focus on improvement in overall health and cancer prevention. Using the National Cancer Institute guidelines, you will be able to help this patient focus on key nutrients that have been linked to cancer prevention. Case 32 allows you to plan nutritional care for some of the most common problems during cancer diagnosis and therapy.

Nutrition and Breast Cancer

Colleen Spees, PhD, RDN, LD, FAND
The Ohio State University

Objectives

After completing this case, the student will be able to:

1. Explain the staging for diagnosis of breast cancer.
2. Understand the current medical treatments used for breast cancer and the nutritional consequences of each treatment.
3. Interpret nutrition assessment data to assist with the design of measurable survivorship goals, nutrition and physical activity interventions, and strategies for monitoring and evaluation that address the nutrition diagnoses for the survivor.
4. Apply evidence-based guidelines for provision of nutritional care for the breast cancer survivor.
5. Identify dietary patterns that may assist with prevention of cancer using evidence-based resources.
6. Provide evidence-based recommendations for use of supplements and complementary and alternative medicine for the cancer survivor.

Jennifer Smith is a 61-year-old female referred to the outpatient Registered Dietitian Nutritionist at the university oncology clinic during her regular clinic visit.

Smith, Jennifer, Female, 61 y.o.

Allergies: NKFA	**Code:** FULL	**Isolation:** None
Pt. Location: Outpatient Oncology Clinic	**Physician:** M. Johnson	**Admit Date:** 7/8

Patient Summary: Jennifer Smith is a 61-year-old female who was diagnosed with breast cancer—Stage IIB Invasive Ductal Carcinoma T2N1miM0 18 months previously. She was treated with R mastectomy followed by radiation and chemotherapy. She received chemotherapy with Docetaxel, doxorubicin, and cyclophosphamide every three weeks for six cycles. This was followed with radiation therapy to the chest wall. She has completed treatment and most recently completed reconstructive surgery.

History:

Onset of disease: Dx: Stage IIB Invasive Ductal Carcinoma T2N1miM0
Medical history: Type 2 DM
Surgical history: s/p Hysterectomy, s/p R mastectomy, s/p deep inferior epigastric perforator flap reconstructive surgery 6 weeks ago
Medications at home: metformin
Tobacco use: none
Alcohol use: 1–2 × per week—white and red wine
Family history: Mother and sister—breast cancer; father—diabetes, CHD

Demographics:

Marital status: Married
Number of children: 4 children—ages 32, 30, 27, 24
Education: 4 years college
Language: English only
Occupation: Sales manager for national cosmetic company
Hours of work: Currently not working but plans to return in the next few weeks
Household members: Husband—youngest child home for summer
Ethnicity: Caucasian
Religious affiliation: Methodist

History/Physical:

Chief complaint: Here for follow-up 3 months. Last treatment
General appearance: Pleasant, overweight woman

Vital Signs:

Temp: 98.6	Pulse: 73	Resp rate: 15
BP: 127/78	Height: 5'5"	Weight: 175 lbs

Heart: Regular rate and rhythm, normal heart sounds—no clicks, murmurs, or gallops
HEENT: Head: WNL
    Eyes: PERRLA
    Ears: Clear
    Nose: WNL
    Throat: Moist mucous membranes without exudates or lesions
Genitalia: Normal female

Smith, Jennifer, Female, 61 y.o.
Allergies: NKFA   **Code:** FULL   **Isolation:** None
Pt. Location: Outpatient Oncology Clinic   **Physician:** M. Johnson   **Admit Date:** 7/8

Neurologic: Alert and oriented × 3
Extremities: Noncontributory
Skin: Smooth, warm, dry, excellent turgor, no edema
Chest/lungs: Lungs clear
Peripheral vascular: Pulse 4+ bilaterally, warm, no edema
Abdomen: Healing postsurgical wounds

Nutrition:

General: Patient reports that her usual weight prior to breast cancer diagnosis was 195 lbs. She experienced loss of appetite, nausea, vomiting, diarrhea, and mucositis during chemo treatments. She also states that she had extreme fatigue throughout both chemo and radiation. She states that she is feeling much better and appetite "unfortunately" has returned to normal. She admits that she is glad she has lost weight and would like to continue to lose weight—"I know that this will keep me healthier". Mrs. Smith is interested in changing her diet to try and keep her cancer from coming back and wants advice on how to do this. She has considered becoming a vegetarian and wonders if this will be a good thing for her. She is not exercising yet due to the recent reconstructive surgery but would like to start something besides just walking—which she does every day with her dogs. She walks her golden retrievers twice a day for about ½ mile each time.

24 hour recall:

AM:	1 c coffee (brewed black)
	Cheerios—1 c with ½ c fresh strawberries
	Almond milk —1 c
Snack:	2 c coffee (brewed black)
	Granola bar
Lunch:	Tuna salad—made with egg and mayonnaise—¾ c in a fresh tomato
	20 wheat thins eaten with tuna salad
	1 can diet cola
PM:	8 oz filet mignon grilled
	1 large baked potato with 2 tbsp butter, salt, and pepper
	Dinner salad with ranch-style dressing (3 tbsp)—lettuce, spinach, croutons, sliced cucumber
	1 glass of Riesling white wine (~ 6 oz)
HS snack:	1 glass of Riesling white wine (~ 6 oz)—3 oz cheese and ~ 10 wheat thin crackers

Food allergies/intolerances/aversions: No known
Previous nutrition therapy? Yes. If yes, when: several years ago Where? Local diabetes association— attended diabetes classes.
Food purchase/preparation: Self and husband
Vit/min intake: Multivitamin/mineral daily

Smith, Jennifer, Female, 61 y.o.
Allergies: NKFA   **Code:** FULL   **Isolation:** None
Pt. Location: Outpatient Oncology Clinic   **Physician:** M. Johnson   **Admit Date:** 7/8

Laboratory Results

	Ref. Range	7/1 0600 (fasting)
Chemistry		
Sodium (mEq/L)	136–145	138
Potassium (mEq/L)	3.5–5.1	3.7
Chloride (mEq/L)	98–107	101
Carbon dioxide (CO_2, mEq/L)	23–29	25
Bicarbonate (mEq/L)	23–28	24
BUN (mg/dL)	6–20	11
Creatinine serum (mg/dL)	0.6–1.1 F 0.9–1.3 M	0.8
BUN/Crea ratio	10.0–20.0	13.75
Uric acid (mg/dL)	2.8–8.8 F 4.0–9.0 M	3.1
Est GFR, non-Afr Amer (mL/min/1.73 m²)	>60	82
Glucose (mg/dL)	70–99	137 !↑
Phosphate, inorganic (mg/dL)	2.2–4.6	3.8
Magnesium (mg/dL)	1.5–2.4	1.9
Calcium (mg/dL)	8.6–10.2	9.1
Anion gap (mmol/L)	10–20	13
Osmolality (mmol/kg/H_2O)	275–295	288
Bilirubin total (mg/dL)	≤1.2	0.7
Bilirubin, direct (mg/dL)	<0.3	0.1
Protein, total (g/dL)	6–7.8	6.9
Albumin (g/dL)	3.5–5.5	3.8
Prealbumin (mg/dL)	18–35	30
Ammonia (NH_3, µg/L)	6–47	8
Alkaline phosphatase (U/L)	30–120	42
ALT (U/L)	4–36	11
AST (U/L)	0–35	17
CPK (U/L)	30–135 F 55–170 M	44
Lactate dehydrogenase (U/L)	208–378	210
C-reactive protein (mg/dL)	<1.00	1.1 !↑
Cholesterol (mg/dL)	<200	210 !↑

Smith, Jennifer, Female, 61 y.o.
Allergies: NKFA
Pt. Location: Outpatient Oncology Clinic

Code: FULL
Physician: M. Johnson

Isolation: None
Admit Date: 7/8

Laboratory Results *(Continued)*

	Ref. Range	7/1 0600 (fasting)
HDL-C (mg/dL)	>59 F, >50 M	72
VLDL (mg/dL)	7–32	31
LDL (mg/dL)	<130	107
LDL/HDL ratio	<3.22 F <3.55 M	1.48
Triglycerides (mg/dL)	35–135 F 40–160 M	155 !↑
HbA$_{1c}$ (%)	<5.7	6.8 !↑
Hematology		
WBC (×10^3/mm^3)	3.9–10.7	5.2
RBC (×10^6/mm^3)	4.2–5.4 F 4.5–6.2 M	4.3
Hemoglobin (Hgb, g/dL)	12–16 F 14–17 M	11.9 !↓
Hematocrit (Hct, %)	37–47 F 41–51 M	36 !↓
Platelet count (×10^3/mm^3)	150–350	201
Transferrin (mg/dL)	250–380 F 215–365 M	385 !↑
Ferritin (mg/mL)	20–120 F 20–300 M	55
Urinalysis		
Collection method	—	Clean catch
Color	—	yellow
Appearance	—	clear
Specific gravity	1.001–1.035	1.005
pH	5–7	5.9
Protein (mg/dL)	Neg	Neg
Glucose (mg/dL)	Neg	Neg
Ketones	Neg	Neg
Blood	Neg	Neg
Bilirubin	Neg	Neg
Nitrites	Neg	Neg
Urobilinogen (EU/dL)	<1.0	Neg

(Continued)

Smith, Jennifer, Female, 61 y.o.
Allergies: NKFA   **Code:** FULL   **Isolation:** None
Pt. Location: Outpatient Oncology Clinic   **Physician:** M. Johnson   **Admit Date:** 7/8

Laboratory Results (Continued)

	Ref. Range	**7/1 0600 (fasting)**
Leukocyte esterase	Neg	Neg
Prot chk	Neg	Neg
WBCs (/HPF)	0–5	2
RBCs (/HPF)	0–2	1
Bact	0	0
Mucus	0	0
Crys	0	0
Casts (/LPF)	0	0
Yeast	0	0

Note: Values and units of measurement listed in these tables are derived from several resources. Substantial variation exists in the ranges quoted as "normal" and these may vary depending on the assay used by different laboratories.

Case Questions

I.   **Understanding the Pathophysiology**

1.   Describe the incidence and prevalence of breast cancer in the United States. How has this changed over the previous decade?

2.   What are the risk factors for developing breast cancer? Explain potential genetic and environmental risk factors. Does Mrs. Smith have any of these in her history?

3.   Explain Mrs. Smith's diagnosis: Stage IIB Invasive Ductal Carcinoma T2N1miM0. Specifically discuss the type of breast cancer and the staging of her diagnosis.

4.   She was treated with Docetaxel, Doxorubicin, and Cyclophosphamide chemotherapy regimen. What are these medications and how do they work?

5.   Mrs. Smith was also treated with radiation therapy. What is the basic mechanism of using radiation therapy as a component of treatment for breast cancer?

6.   What are the major side effects of her chemotherapy and radiation therapy?

7.   Mrs. Smith recently underwent reconstructive surgery. She had the deep inferior epigastric perforator (DIEP) flap reconstructive procedure. Describe this procedure.

II.   **Understanding the Nutrition Therapy**

8.   What are the general principles of nutrition therapy for a patient undergoing treatment for a malignancy?

9.   Now that Mrs. Smith has completed treatment for her breast cancer, what general nutrition recommendations can be made for prevention of cancer and specifically for breast cancer?

10.   Are there specific vitamin, mineral, or herbal supplements that are recommended for prevention of the recurrence of breast cancer?

11. What are the general nutrition therapy recommendations for Type 2 diabetes?

III. Nutrition Assessment

12. Assess Mrs. Smith's height and weight. Calculate her BMI and % usual body weight.

13. Identify any abnormal biochemical indices and discuss the probable underlying etiology.

14. Determine Mrs. Smith's energy and protein requirements. Explain the rationale for the method you used to calculate these requirements.

15. Mrs. Smith is taking Metformin. What is this medication and what is the mechanism of action?

16. Will recommendations for Type 2 DM impact the cancer prevention and survivorship recommendations that you have discussed in question #9?

IV. Nutrition Diagnosis

17. Identify at least 2 pertinent nutrition problems and the corresponding nutrition diagnoses.

18. Write two PES statements for each nutrition diagnosis you have identified.

V. Nutrition Intervention

19. Identify three major changes in Mrs. Smith's dietary intake that would be consistent with cancer prevention and survivorship guidelines, allow for continued weight loss and support the care of her Type 2 Diabetes.

20. Mrs. Smith has asked about becoming a vegetarian. Describe your response to this question and provide an evidence-based rationale for your recommendation.

21. For each PES statement and the responses to #19, establish an ideal goal (based on the signs and symptoms) and appropriate intervention (based on the etiology).

22. Mrs. Smith is interested in specific supplements that may help in cancer prevention. What would you tell her based upon the evidence? Provide suggestions for resources for Mrs. Smith that would support her decision making in regards to complementary and alternative medicine.

23. Mrs. Smith has asked about recommendations for physical activity. Provide credible resources and recommendations to her about physical activity. Determine at least three recommendations for increasing her physical activity.

VI. Nutrition Monitoring and Evaluation
24. Write a note for your initial outpatient nutrition assessment and nutrition recommendations.

Bibliography

American Cancer Society: ACS Guidelines on Nutrition and Physical Activity for Cancer Prevention. Available from: http://www.cancer.org/healthy/eathealthygetactive/acsguidelinesonnutritionphysicalactivityforcancer-prevention/nupa-guidelines-toc. Accessed 07/07/15.

American Institute for Cancer Research. Recommendations for Cancer Prevention. Available from: http://www.aicr.org/reduce-your-cancer-risk/recommendations-for-cancer-prevention/. Accessed 07/07/15.

Bradbury KE, Appleby PN, Key TJ. Fruit, vegetable, and fiber intake in relation to cancer risk: Findings from the European Prospective Investigation into Cancer and Nutrition (EPIC). *Am J Clin Nutr*. 2014;100:394S–398S.

Chages V, Romieu I. Nutrition and breast cancer. *Maturitas*. 2014;77:7–11.

Cohen D. Neoplastic Disease. In: Nelms M, Sucher K, Lacey K. *Nutrition Therapy and Pathophysiology* 3rd ed. Belmont, CA: Cengage Learning; 2016:702–734.

Dennis Parker EA, Sheppard VB, Adams-Campbell L. Compliance with national nutrition recommendations among breast cancer survivors in "Stepping Stone". *Integr Cancer Ther*. 2014;13:114–120.

Goff DC, Lloyd-Jones DM, Bennett G, et al. 2013 ACC/AHA Guideline on the Assessment of Cardiovascular Risk: A report of the American College of Cardiology/American Heart Association Task Force on practice guidelines. *J Am Coll Cardiol*. 2014;63:2935–2959.

Hebuterne X, Lemaire E, Michallet M, et al. Prevalence of malnutrition and current use of nutrition support in patients with cancer. *J Parenter Enteral Nutr*. 2014;38:196–204.

Izano MA, Fung TT, Chiuve SS, Hu FB, Homes MD. Are diet quality scores after breast cancer diagnosis associated with improved breast cancer survival? *Nutr Cancer*. 2013;65:820–826.

Kwok A, Palermo C, Boitong A. Dietary experiences and support needs of women who gain weight following chemotherapy for breast cancer. *Support Care Cancer*. 2015;23:1561–1568.

McDonald C, Bauer J, Capra S, Coll J. The muscle mass, omega-3-diet, exercise and lifestyle (MODEL) study – A randomized controlled trial for women who have completed breast cancer treatment. *BMC Cancer*. 2014;14:264–287.

Rossi RE, Pericleous M, Mandair D, et al. The role of dietary factors in prevention of breast cancer. *Anticancer Res*. 2014;34:6861–6875.

Schiavon CC, Vieira FG, Ceccatto V, et al. Nutrition education intervention for women with breast cancer: Effect on nutritional factors and oxidative stress. *J Nut Educ Behav*. 2015;47:2–9.

Vance V, Campbell S, McCargar L, et al. Dietary changes and food intake in the first year after breast cancer treatment. *Appl Physio Nutr Metab*. 2014;39:707–714.

Internet Resources

National Cancer Institute: www.cancer.gov

Nutrition in Cancer Care - for Health Professionals. http://www.cancer.gov/about-cancer/treatment/side-effects/appetite-loss/nutrition-hp-pdq

American Cancer Society: ACS Guidelines on Nutrition and Physical Activity for Cancer Prevention. Available from: http://www.cancer.org/healthy/eathealthygetactive/acsguidelinesonnutritionphysicalactivityforcancerpre-vention/nupa-guidelines-toc. Accessed: July 7, 2015.

American Institute for Cancer Research. http://www.aicr.org/reduce-your-cancer-risk/recommendations-for-cancer-prevention/

Case 32

Tongue Cancer Treated with Surgery, Radiation, and Chemotherapy

Dena Champion, MS, RD, CNSC
Ohio State University Wexner Medical Center

Objectives

After completing this case, the student will be able to:

1. Identify and explain common metabolic and nutritional problems associated with malignancy.
2. Explain complications of medical treatment for cancer and the potential nutritional consequences.
3. Apply understanding of nutrition support in the treatment of and recovery from malignancy.
4. Analyze nutrition assessment data to evaluate nutritional status and identify specific nutrition problems.
5. Determine nutrition diagnoses and write appropriate PES statements.
6. Evaluate the adequacy of an enteral feeding regimen for a cancer patient.

Nick Seyer is a 58-year-old man who presents to his dentist for a routine cleaning. During examination, his dentist notices a small tongue mass, and Mr. Seyer admits to associated pain. His dentist refers him to an ear, nose, and throat (ENT) physician, who decides to biopsy the area.

Seyer, Nick, Male, 58 y.o.

Allergies: None	**Code:** FULL	**Isolation:** None
Pt. Location: RM 832	**Physician:** H. Brown	**Admit Date:** 9/5

Patient Summary: The biopsy revealed a stage IV T2 N2b, HPV (human papilloma virus) positive, squamous cell carcinoma (SCC) of the right anterior tongue.

History:

Onset of disease: Odynophagia × 5–6 months

Medical history: Hypertension, which he states is well controlled. Patient describes noticing a "pimple" on his tongue approximately 5–6 months ago. He noticed that this mass seemed to slowly get worse and he began having significant pain with eating. He states this is especially true with spicy or acidic foods like salsa, hot sauce, or orange juice. He has noted an approximately 30-pound weight loss over 5–6 months. He never expected that cancer could be the cause.

Medications at home: Metoprolol

Tobacco use: Yes, 2 ppd; wife also smokes.

Alcohol use: Yes, 1–2 drinks most nights of the week.

Family history: What? Liver cancer. Who? Mother—died age 58.

Demographics:

Marital status: Married

Household members: Wife, age 52; son, age 18; two other sons are away at college—ages 19 and 22

Years education: Some college

Language: English only

Occupation: Contractor

Hours of work: Variable but usually 5–6 days per week—starts as early as 6:30 and works often until after 6 pm

Ethnicity: Caucasian

Religious affiliation: Catholic

Admitting History/Physical:

Chief complaint: Tongue pain for several months that has progressively gotten worse. Weight loss due to pain with eating.

Vital Signs:	Temp: 98.3°F	Pulse: 88	Resp rate: 13
	BP: 132/92	Height: 6'3"	Weight: 198 lbs

Heart: Unremarkable

HEENT: Positive for hearing loss and sore throat. Negative for ear pain, nosebleeds, congestion, hoarse voice, rhinorrhea, and sinus pain. There is no tinnitus or ear discharge.

  Eyes: Sunken; sclera clear without evidence of tears

  Ears: Clear

  Nose: Dry mucous membranes

  Throat: Dry mucous membranes, no inflammation

Genitalia: Unremarkable

Rectal: Prostate normal; stool hematest negative

Neurologic: Alert, oriented × 3

Seyer, Nick, Male, 58 y.o.
Allergies: None
Pt. Location: RM 832

Code: FULL
Physician: H. Brown

Isolation: None
Admit Date: 9/5

Extremities: Joints appear prominent with evidence of some muscle wasting. No edema.
Skin: Warm, dry
Chest/lungs: Clear to auscultation and percussion
Abdomen: Negative for pain or tenderness.

Orders:

Surgery consult to evaluate for possible surgical resection.
Radiation oncologist and medical oncologists consulted to evaluate for postoperative external beam
radiation therapy and chemotherapy.

.... R. Brown MD

Nursing Assessment	9/5
Abdominal appearance (concave, flat, rounded, obese, distended)	rounded
Palpation of abdomen (soft, rigid, firm, masses, tense)	soft
Bowel function (continent, incontinent, flatulence, no stool)	continent
Bowel sounds (P=present, AB=absent, hypo, hyper)	
RUQ	P
LUQ	P
RLQ	P
LLQ	P
Stool color	brown
Stool consistency	soft
Tubes/ostomies	N/A
Genitourinary	
Urinary continence	yes
Urine source	clean catch
Appearance (clear, cloudy, yellow, amber, fluorescent, hematuria, orange, blue, tea)	clear, yellow
Integumentary	
Skin color	pale
Skin temperature (DI=diaphoretic, W=warm, dry, CL=cool, CLM=clammy, CD+=cold, M=moist, H=hot)	W
Skin turgor (good, fair, poor, TENT=tenting)	fair
Skin condition (intact, EC=ecchymosis, A=abrasions, P=petechiae, R=rash, W=weeping, S=sloughing, D=dryness, EX=excoriated, T=tears, SE=subcutaneous emphysema, B=blisters, V=vesicles, N=necrosis)	D
Mucous membranes (intact, EC=ecchymosis, A=abrasions, P=petechiae, R=rash, W=weeping, S=sloughing, D=dryness, EX=excoriated, T=tears, SE=subcutaneous emphysema, B=blisters, V=vesicles, N=necrosis)	D

(Continued)

Seyer, Nick, Male, 58 y.o.
Allergies: None   **Code:** FULL   **Isolation:** None
Pt. Location: RM 832   **Physician:** H. Brown   **Admit Date:** 9/5

Nursing Assessment *(Continued)*

Nursing Assessment	9/5
Other components of Braden score: special bed, sensory pressure, moisture, activity, friction/shear (>.18=no risk, 15–16=low risk, 13–14=moderate risk,≤12=high risk)	activity, 16

Nutrition:

General: Mr. Seyer noted decreased intake prior to admission. He states this is mainly related to tongue pain, but also thinks his appetite is poor, and he feels full quickly when eating. He does not have any problem swallowing. He is not having nausea or vomiting.

Usual dietary intake:
AM: Used to eat eggs, bacon, toast, and juice every morning, but for at least the past month he has eaten only eggs or oatmeal instead. He states that the toast is too dry and difficult to chew and the bacon isn't appealing. Juice causes significant discomfort.
Lunch: Previously, ate cold lunch packed for the work site. This included sandwich, cold meat or other leftovers from previous dinner, fruit, cookies, and tea. Lately he is drinking Ensure Active High Protein or a smoothie from McDonald's. He states drinking is easier than eating. Sometimes he doesn't eat lunch at all due to pain.
Dinner: He used to eat large portions of meat with a starch, vegetables, and salad. He usually drinks 2–3 beers after dinner. Lately he has found meat and salad difficult to eat. He prefers soups, mashed potatoes, etc. He is still drinking beer after dinner.

24-hour recall:
AM: 1 packet of instant oatmeal; sips of coffee
Lunch: 6 oz chicken noodle soup with 2–4 crackers
Dinner: Macaroni and cheese—homemade, ½ c
Bedtime: 1 scoop of chocolate ice cream

Food allergies/intolerances/aversions: None
Previous nutrition therapy? No
Food purchase/preparation: Wife
Vit/min intake: None. Used to take a multivitamin, but hasn't in years.

Laboratory Results

	Ref. Range	9/5 0832	9/11 0832
Chemistry			
Sodium (mEq/L)	136–145	137	136
Potassium (mEq/L)	3.5–5.1	3.8	3.6
Chloride (mEq/L)	98–107	101	99
Carbon dioxide (CO_2, mEq/L)	23–29	26	25
BUN (mg/dL)	6–20	9	10

Seyer, Nick, Male, 58 y.o.
Allergies: None
Pt. Location: RM 832

Code: FULL
Physician: H. Brown

Isolation: None
Admit Date: 9/5

	Ref. Range	9/5 0832	9/11 0832
Creatinine serum (mg/dL)	0.6–1.1 F 0.9–1.3 M	0.9	0.9
Glucose (mg/dL)	70–99	71	98
Phosphate, inorganic (mg/dL)	2.2–4.6	3.2	
Magnesium (mg/dL)	1.5–2.4	1.8	1.8
Calcium (mg/dL)	8.6–10.2	9.1	9.4
Bilirubin, direct (mg/dL)	<0.3	0.2	0.3 !↑
Protein, total (g/dL)	6–7.8	5.7 !↓	5.7 !↓
Albumin (g/dL)	3.5–5.5	3.1 !↓	3.0 !↓
Prealbumin (mg/dL)	18–35	15 !↓	12 !↓
Ammonia (NH_3, µg/L)	6–47	11	21
Alkaline phosphatase (U/L)	30–120	101	99
ALT (U/L)	4–36	21	33
AST (U/L)	0–35	32	27
CPK (IU/L)	30–135 F 55–170 M	162	145
Lactate dehydrogenase (U/L)	208–378	300	290
Cholesterol (mg/dL)	<200	180	170
HDL-C (mg/dL)	>59 F, >50 M	47 !↓	
LDL (mg/dL)	<130	129	
LDL/HDL ratio	<3.22 F <3.55 M	2.74	
Triglycerides (mg/dL)	35–135 F 40–160 M	158	
Coagulation (Coag)			
PT (sec)	11–13	12	12.8
Hematology			
WBC ($\times 10^3$/mm^3)	3.9–10.7	5.2	6.9
RBC ($\times 10^6$/mm^3)	4.2–5.4 F 4.5–6.2 M	4.2 !↓	4.3 !↓
Hemoglobin (Hgb, g/dL)	12–16 F 14–17 M	13.5 !↓	13.9 !↓
Hematocrit (Hct, %)	37–47 F 41–51 M	38 !↓	38 !↓
Mean cell volume (µm^3)	80–96	90	86
Mean cell Hgb (pg)	28–32	32.4 !↑	32.3 !↑

(Continued)

Seyer, Nick, Male, 58 y.o.
Allergies: None   **Code:** FULL   **Isolation:** None
Pt. Location: RM 832   **Physician:** H. Brown   **Admit Date:** 9/5

Laboratory Results *(Continued)*

	Ref. Range	9/5 0832	9/11 0832
Mean cell Hgb content (g/dL)	32–36	35.5	36.5 !↑
Platelet count (×10³/mm³)	150–350	250	232
Ferritin (mg/mL)	20–120 F 20–300 M	220	208
Hematology, Manual Diff			
Neutrophil (%)	40–70	55	65
Lymphocyte (%)	22–44	25	35
Monocyte (%)	0–7	4	5
Eosinophil (%)	0–5	0.5	0
Segs (%)	0–60	55	60
Bands (%)	0–10	4	3

Note: Values and units of measurement listed in these tables are derived from several resources. Substantial variation exists in the ranges quoted as "normal" and these may vary depending on the assay used by different laboratories.

Intake/Output

Date		9/11 0701–9/12 0700			
Time		0701–1500	1501–2300	2301–0700	Daily total
IN	tube feeding formula	**600**	**535**	**600**	**1735**
	tube feeding flush (mL/kg/hr)	**50** (0.90)	**50** (0.81)	**50** (0.90)	**150** (0.87)
	I.V. (mL/kg/hr)	**800** (1.11)	**800** (1.11)	**800** (1.11)	**2400** (1.11)
	I.V. piggyback				
	TPN				
	Total intake (mL/kg)	**1450** (16.11)	**1385** (15.39)	**1450** (16.11)	**4285** (47.61)
OUT	Urine (mL/kg/hr)	**1100** (1.53)	**1700** (2.36)	**900** (1.25)	**3700** (1.71)
	Emesis output				
	Other				
	Stool	0	0	300	300
	Total output (mL/kg)	**1100** (12.22)	**1700** (18.89)	**1200** (13.33)	**4000** (44.44)
Net I/O		+350	−315	+250	+285
Net since admission (9/5)		+400	+85	+335	+335

Case Questions

I.   Understanding the Disease and Pathophysiology

1.   Mr. Seyer has been diagnosed with cancer of the tongue, which is a type of head and neck cancer. Head and neck cancers are categorized by the area where they begin. Describe these primary areas.

2.   What are the major risk factors for development of head and neck cancer? Does Mr. Seyer's medical record indicate that he has any of these risk factors?

3.   Mr. Seyer's biopsy results indicated an HPV positive tumor. What is HPV? Does this imply a better or worse outcome?

4.   Mr. Seyer's cancer was described as Stage IV T2 N2b. Explain this terminology, which is used to describe staging for malignancies.

5.   Cancer is generally treated with a combination of therapies. These can include surgical resection, radiation therapy, chemotherapy, and immunotherapy. The type of malignancy and staging of the disease will, in part, determine the types of therapies that are prescribed. Define and describe each of these therapies. Briefly describe the mechanism for each. In general, how do they act to treat a malignancy?

6.   Mr. Seyer had a partial glossectomy and right neck dissection on 9/7. Describe these surgical procedures. How may these procedures affect him nutritionally?

II.   Understanding the Nutrition Therapy

7.   Many cancer patients experience changes in nutritional status. Briefly describe the potential effect of cancer on nutritional status.

8.   Surgery, radiation, and chemotherapy affect nutritional status. Describe potential nutritional and metabolic effects of these treatments.

III.   Nutrition Assessment

9. Calculate and evaluate Mr. Seyer's %UBW and BMI.

10. Summarize your findings regarding his weight status. Classify the severity of his weight loss. What factors may have contributed to his weight loss? Explain.

11. What does research tell us about the relationship between significant weight loss and prognosis in cancer patients?

12. Estimate Mr. Seyer's energy and protein requirements based on his current weight.

13. Estimate Mr. Seyer's fluid requirements based on his current weight.

14. What factors noted in Mr. Seyer's history and physical (as well as other medical/nutritional history) may indicate problems with eating prior to admission?

15. Mr. Seyer is currently receiving enteral nutrition, specifically Isosource HN at 75 mL/hr per PEG tube.

    a. Calculate the amount of energy and protein that will be provided at this rate.

    b. Next, by assessing the information in the intake/output record, determine the actual amount of enteral nutrition he received on September 11.

    c. Compare this to his estimated nutrient requirements.

    d. Compare fluids required to fluids received. Is he meeting his fluid requirements? How did you determine this? Why would you evaluate his output when assessing his fluid intake?

16. What type of formula is Isosource HN? One of the residents taking care of Mr. Seyer asks about a formula with a higher concentration of omega-3 fatty acids, antioxidants, arginine, and glutamine that could promote healing after surgery. What does the evidence indicate regarding nutritional needs for cancer patients and, in particular, nutrients to promote postoperative wound healing? What formulas may meet this profile? List them and discuss why you chose them.

17. Are any clinical signs of malnutrition noted in the patient's admission history and physical?

18. Review the patient's chemistries upon admission. Identify any that are abnormal and describe their clinical significance for this patient, including the likely reason for each abnormality and its nutritional implications.

19. Mr. Seyer has been diagnosed with a life-threatening illness. What is the definition of *terminal illness*?

20. The literature describes how a patient and his family may experience varying levels of emotional response to a terminal illness. These may include anger, denial, depression, and acceptance. How may this affect the patient's nutritional intake? How would you handle these components in your nutritional care? What questions might you have for Mr. Seyer or his family? List three.

IV. Nutrition Diagnosis

21. Select two high-priority nutrition problems after Mr. Seyer's surgery and complete the PES statement for each.

V. Nutrition Intervention

22. For each of the PES statements you have written, establish an ideal goal (based on the signs and symptoms) and an appropriate intervention (based on the etiology).

23. Does his current nutrition support meet his estimated nutritional needs? If not, determine the recommended changes. Discuss any areas of deficiency and ideas for implementing a new plan.

24. How may these interventions (from question #22) change as he progresses postoperatively? Discuss how Mr. Seyer may transition from enteral feeding to an oral diet.

VI. Nutrition Monitoring and Evaluation

25. List the factors you should monitor for Mr. Seyer while he is receiving enteral nutrition therapy.

26. Mr. Seyer will receive radiation therapy and chemotherapy as an outpatient. In question #8, you identified potential nutritional complications with both. Choose one of these nutritional complications and describe the nutrition intervention that would be appropriate for you to recommend.

27. Identify major assessment indices you would use to monitor his nutritional status once he begins therapy.

Bibliography

Academy of Nutrition and Dietetics Nutrition Care Manual. Head and Neck Cancer Nutrition Therapy. Available from: https://www.nutritioncaremanual.org/client_ed.cfm?ncm_client_ed_id=135&actionxm=ViewAll. Accessed 04/03/15.

Aiko S, Yoshizumi Y, Tsuwano S, Shimanouchi M, Sugiura Y, Maehara T. The effects of immediate enteral feeding with a formula containing high levels of omega-3 fatty acids in patients after surgery for esophageal cancer. *J Parenter Enteral Nutr.* 2005 May–Jun; 29(3):141–147.

Bossola, M. Interventions in head and neck cancer patients undergoing chemoradiotherapy: A narrative review. *Nutrients.* 2015;7:265–276.

Churma SA, Horrell CJ. Esophageal and gastric cancers. In: Kogut VJ and Luthringer SL. *Nutritional Issues in Cancer Care.* Pittsburgh, PA: Oncology Nursing Society; 2005:45–63.

Cohen DA, Sucher K. Neoplastic disease. In: Nelms M, Sucher K, Lacey K. *Nutrition Therapy and Pathophysiology.* 3rd ed. Belmont, CA: Cengage Learning; 2016:686–710.

Dalianis, T. Human papillomavirus and oropharyngeal cancer, the epidemics, and significance of additional clinical biomarkers for prediction of response to therapy (Review). *Int J Oncol.* 2014;44:1799–1805.

De Luis DA, Izaola O, Cuellar L, Terroba MC, Martin T, Aller R. High dose of arginine enhanced enteral nutrition in postsurgical head and neck cancer patients. A randomized clinical trial. *Eur Rev Med Pharmacol Sci.* 2009;13:279–283.

Fessler T, Havrilla C. Nutrition support for esophageal cancer patients—Strategies for meeting the challenges while improving patient care. *Today's Dietitian.* 2012;14:1–4.

Laskar SG, Swain M. HPV positive oropharyngeal cancer and treatment deintensification: How pertinent is it? *J Cancer Res Ther.* 2015;11:6–9.

National Cancer Institute. Grief, Bereavement, and Coping with Loss. Available from: http://www.cancer.gov/cancertopics/pdq/supportivecare/bereavement/HealthProfessional. Accessed 04/07/15.

Internet Resources

American Cancer Society: How are oral cavity and oropharyngeal cancers staged?: http://www.cancer.org/cancer/oralcavityandoropharyngealcancer/detailedguide/oral-cavity-and-oropharyngeal-cancer-staging

American Cancer Society: http://www.cancer.org/index

Academy of Nutrition and Dietetics Evidence Analysis Library: Fish Oil, Lean Body Mass and Weight in Adult Oncology Patients 2013. : http://www.andeal.org

Cancer Support Community: http://www.cancersupportcommunity.org/MainMenu/About-Cancer/Understanding-Cancer

Head and Neck Cancer Guide: Ablative Surgeries: http://www.headandneckcancerguide.org/adults/cancer-diagnosis-treatments/surgery-and-rehabilitation/cancer-removal-surgeries/

National Cancer Institute: Head and Neck Cancers: http://www.cancer.gov/cancertopics/types/head-and-neck/head_neck_fact_sheet

National Cancer Institute: HPV and Cancer: http://www.cancer.gov/cancertopics/causes-prevention/risk/infectious-agents/hpv-fact-sheet

National Cancer Institute: Radiation Therapy and Cancer: http://www.cancer.gov/cancertopics/treatment/types/radiation-therapy/radiation-fact-sheet

Appendix A

COMMON MEDICAL ABBREVIATIONS

AAL	anterior axillary line
ac	before meals
ACTH	adrenocorticotropic hormone
AD	Alzheimer's disease
ad lib	as desired (ad libitum)
ADA	American Diabetes Association
ADL	activities of daily living
AGA	antigliadin antibody
AIDS	acquired immunodeficiency syndrome
ALP (Alk phos)	alkaline phosphatase
ALS	amyotrophic lateral sclerosis
ALT	alanine aminotransferase
ANC	absolute neutrophil count
ANCA	antineutrophil cytoplasmic antibody
AND	Academy of Nutrition and Dietetics
AP	anterior posterior
ARDS	adult respiratory distress syndrome
ARF	acute renal failure, acute respiratory failure
ASA	acetylsalicylic acid, aspirin
ASCA	antisaccharomyces antibody
ASHD	arteriosclerotic heart disease
AST	aspartate aminotransferase
AV	arteriovenous
BANDS	neutrophils
BCAA	branched-chain amino acids
BE	barium enema
BEE	basal energy expenditure
BG	blood glucose
bid	twice a day (bis in die)
bili	bilirubin
BM	bowel movement
BMI	body mass index
BMR	basal metabolic rate
BMT	bone marrow transplant
BP (B/P)	blood pressure
BPD	bronchopulmonary dysplasia
BPH	benign prostate hypertrophy
bpm	beats per minute, breaths per minute
BS	bowel sounds, breath sounds, or blood sugar
BSA	body surface area
BUN	blood urea nitrogen
c	cup
c̄	with
C	centigrade

c/o	complains of
CA	cancer; carcinoma
CABG	coronary artery bypass graft
CAD	coronary artery disease
CAPD	continuous ambulatory peritoneal dialysis
cath	catheter, catheterize
CAVH	continuous arteriovenous hemofiltration
CBC	complete blood count
cc	cubic centimeter
C.C.E.	clubbing, cyanosis, or edema
CCK	cholecystokinin
CCU	coronary care unit
CDAI	Crohn's disease activity index
CDC	Centers for Disease Control and Prevention
CHD	coronary heart disease
CHF	congestive heart failure
CHI	closed head injury
CHO	carbohydrate
CHOL	cholesterol
CKD	chronic kidney disease
cm	centimeter
CNS	central nervous system
COPD	chronic obstructive pulmonary disease
CPK	creatinine phosphokinase
Cr	creatinine
CR	complete remission
CSF	cerebrospinal fluid
CT	computed tomography
CVA	cerebrovascular accident
CVD	cardiovascular disease
CVP	central venous pressure
CXR	chest X-ray
d/c	discharge
D/C	discontinue
D5NS	dextrose, 5% in normal saline
D5W	dextrose, 5% in water
DASH	Dietary Approaches to Stop Hypertension
DBW	desirable body weight
DCCT	Diabetes Control and Complications Trial
DKA	diabetic ketoacidosis
dL	deciliter
DM	diabetes mellitus
DRI	Dietary Reference Intake

DTR	deep tendon reflex		HS or h.s.	hours of sleep
DTs	delirium tremens		HTN	hypertension
DVT	deep vein thrombosis		Hx	history
Dx	diagnosis		I & O (I/O)	intake and output
ED	emergency department		i.e.	that is
e.g.	for example		IBD	inflammatory bowel disease
ECF	extracellular fluid		IBS	irritable bowel syndrome
ECG/EKG	electrocardiogram		IBW	ideal body weight
EEG	electroencephalogram		ICF	intracranial fluid
EGD	esophagogastroduodenoscopy		ICP	intracranial pressure
ELISA	enzyme-linked immunosorbent assay		ICS	intercostal space
EMA	antiendomysial antibody		ICU	intensive care unit
EMG	electromyography		IGT	impaired glucose tolerance
EOMI	extra-ocular muscles intact		IM	intramuscularly
ERT	estrogen replacement therapy		inc	incontinent
ESR	erythrocyte sedimentation rate		INR	international normalized ratio (in regard to prothrombin time)
F	Fahrenheit			
FBG	fasting blood glucose		IV	intravenous
FBS	fasting blood sugar		J	joule
FDA	Food and Drug Administration		K	potassium
FEF	forced mid-expiratory flow		kcal	kilocalorie
FEV	forced-expiratory volume		KCl	potassium chloride
FFA	free fatty acid		kg	kilogram
FH	family history		KS	Kaposi's sarcoma
FTT	failure to thrive		KUB	kidney, ureter, bladder
FUO	fever of unknown origin		L	liter
FVC	forced vital capacity		lb	pounds
FX	fracture		LBM	lean body mass
g	gram		LCT	long-chain triglyceride
g/dL	grams per deciliter		LDH	lactic dehydrogenase
GB	gallbladder		LES	lower esophageal sphincter
GERD	gastroesophageal reflux disease		LFT	liver function test
GFR	glomerular filtration rate		LIGS	low intermittent gastric suction
GI	gastrointestinal		LLD	left lateral decubitus position
GM-CSF	granulocyte/macrophage colony stimulating factor		LLQ	lower left quadrant
			LMP	last menstrual period
GTF	glucose tolerance factor		LOC	level of consciousness
GTT	glucose tolerance test		LP	lumbar puncture
GVHD	graft versus host disease		LUQ	left upper quadrant
h	hour		lytes	electrolytes
H & P (HPI)	history and physical		MAC	midarm circumference
HAV	hepatitis A virus		MAMC	midarm muscle circumference
HbA_{1c}	glycosylated hemoglobin		MAOI	monoamine oxidase inhibitor
HBV	hepatitis B virus		MCHC	mean corpuscular hemoglobin concentration
HC	head circumference			
Hct	hematocrit		MCL	midclavicular line
HCV	hepatitis C virus		MCT	medium-chain triglyceride
HDL	high-density lipoprotein		MCV	mean corpuscular volume
HEENT	head, eyes, ears, nose, throat		mEq	milliequivalent
Hg	mercury		mg	milligram
Hgb	hemoglobin		Mg	magnesium
HHNS	hyperosmolar hyperglycemic nonketotic (syndrome)		MI	myocardial infarction
			mm	millimeter
HIV	human immunodeficiency virus		mmHg	millimeters of mercury
HLA	human leukocyte antigen		MNT	medical nutrition therapy
HOB	head of bed		MOM	Milk of Magnesia
HR	heart rate		mOsm	milliosmol

MR	mitral regurgitation	R/O	rule out
MRI	magnetic resonance imaging	RA	rheumatoid arthritis
MVA	motor vehicle accident	RBC	red blood cell
MVI	multiple vitamin infusion	RBW	reference body weight
N	nitrogen	RD	registered dietitian
N/V	nausea and vomiting	RDA	Recommended Dietary Allowance
NG	nasogastric	RDS	respiratory distress syndrome
NH_3	ammonia	REE	resting energy expenditure
NICU	neurointensive care unit, neonatal intensive care unit	RLL	right lower lobe
		RLQ	right lower quadrant
NKA	no known allergies	ROM	range of motion
NKDA	no known drug allergies	ROS	review of systems
NPH	neutral protamine Hagedorn insulin	RQ	respiratory quotient
NPO	nothing by mouth	RR	respiratory rate
NSAID	nonsteroidal antiinflammatory drug	RUL	right upper lobe
NTG	nitroglycerin	RUQ	right upper quadrant
O_2	oxygen	Rx	take, prescribe, or treat
OA	osteoarthritis	$\bar{s}$	without
OC	oral contraceptive	S/P	status post
OHA	oral hypoglycemic agent	SBGM	self blood glucose monitoring
OR	operating room	SBO	small bowel obstruction
ORIF	open reduction internal fixation	SBS	short bowel syndrome
OT	occupational therapist	SGOT	serum glutamic oxaloacetic transaminase (now known as AST)
OTC	over the counter		
$paCO_2$	partial pressure of dissolved carbon dioxide in arterial blood	SGPT	serum glutamic pyruvic transaminase (now known as ALT)
paO_2	partial pressure of dissolved oxygen in arterial blood	SOB	shortness of breath
		SQ	subcutaneous
pc	after meals	stat	immediately
PCM	protein-calorie malnutrition	susp	suspension
PD	Parkinson's disease	T	temperature
PE	pulmonary embolus	T & A	tonsillectomy and adenoidectomy
PED	percutaneous endoscopic duodenostomy	T, tbsp	tablespoon
		t, tsp	teaspoon
PEEP	positive end-expiratory pressure	T_3	triiodothyronine
PEG	percutaneous endoscopic gastrostomy	T_4	thyroxine
PEM	protein-energy malnutrition	TB	tuberculosis
PERRLA	pupils equal, round, and reactive to light and accommodation	TEE	total energy expenditure
		TF	tube feeding
pH	hydrogen ion concentration	TG	triglyceride
PKU	phenylketonuria	TIA	transient ischemic attack
PMI	point of maximum impulse	TIBC	total iron binding capacity
PMN	polymorphonuclear	TKO	to keep open
PN	parenteral nutrition	TLC	total lymphocyte count
PO	by mouth (per os)	TNM	tumor, node, metastasis
PPD	packs per day	TPN	total parenteral nutrition
PPN	peripheral parenteral nutrition	TSF	triceps skinfold
prn	may be repeated as necessary (pro re nata)	TSH	thyroid stimulating hormone
		TURP	transurethral resection of the prostate
pt	patient		
PT	patient, physical therapy, prothrombin time	UA	urinalysis
		UBW	usual body weight
PTA	prior to admission	UL	Tolerable Upper Intake Level
PTT	partial thromboplastin time	URI	upper respiratory infection
PUD	peptic ulcer disease	UTI	urinary tract infection
PVC	premature ventricular contraction	UUN	urine urea nitrogen
PVD	peripheral vascular disease	VLCD	very-low-calorie diet

VOD	venous occlusive disease	WNL	within normal limits
VS	vital signs	wt	weight
w.a.	while awake	WW	whole wheat
WBC	white blood cell	yo	year old

Note: Abbreviations can vary from institution to institution. Although the student will find many of the accepted variations listed in this appendix, other references may be needed to supplement this list.

Notations that Should Not Be Used[a]

Inappropriate Abbreviation(s) or Figures	Best Practices
U, u	Write "unit"
IU	Write "International Unit"
Q.D., QD, q.d., qd	Write "daily"
Q.O.D., QOD, q.o.d., qod	Write "every other day"
Trailing zero (X.0 mg)	Write "1" (do not use a trailing zero with a whole number)
Lack of leading zero (.5)	Write "0.5" (use a leading zero when recording a value less than one)
MS, MSO_4	Write "morphine sulfate"
$MgSO_4$	Write "magnesium sulfate"

[a] Joint Commission (http://www.jointcommission.org/facts_about_do_not_use_list/. Accessed August 8, 2015.

NORMAL VALUES FOR PHYSICAL EXAMINATION

Vital Signs

Temperature

Rectal: C = 37.6°/F = 99.6°
Oral: C = 37°/F = 98.6° (± 1°)
Axilla: C = 37.4°/F = 97.6°

Blood Pressure: average 120/80 mmHg

Heart Rate (beats per minute)

Age	At Rest Awake	At Rest Asleep	Exercise or Fever
Newborn	100–180	80–160	≤220
1 week–3 months	100–220	80–200	≤220
3 months–2 years	80–150	70–120	≤200
2–10 years	70–110	60–90	≤200
11 years-adult	55–90	50–90	≤200

Respiratory Rate (breaths per minute)

Age	Respirations
Newborn	35
1–11 months	30
1–2 years	25
3–4 years	23
5–6 years	21
7–8 years	20
9–10 years	19
11–12 years	19
13–14 years	18
15–16 years	17
17–18 years	16–18
Adult	12–20

Cardiac Exam: carotid pulses equal in rate, rhythm, and strength; normal heart sounds; no murmurs present

HEENT Exam (head, eyes, ears, nose, throat)

Mouth: pink, moist, symmetrical; mucosa pink, soft, moist, smooth

Gums: pink, smooth, moist; may have patchy pigmentation

Teeth: smooth, white, shiny

Tongue: medium red or pink, smooth with free mobility, top surface slightly rough

Eyes: pupils equal, round, reactive to light and accommodation

Ears: tympanic membrane taut, translucent, pearly gray; auricle smooth without lesions; meatus not swollen or occluded; cerumen dry (tan/light yellow) or moist (dark yellow/brown)

Nose: external nose symmetrical, nontender without discharge; mucosa pink; septum at the midline

Pharynx: mucosa pink and smooth

Neck: thyroid gland, lymph nodes not easily palpable or enlarged

Lungs: chest contour symmetrical; spine straight without lateral deviation; no bulging or active movement within the intercostal spaces during breathing; respirations clear to auscultation and percussion

Peripheral Vascular: normal pulse graded at 3+, which indicates that pulse is easy to palpate and not easily obliterated; pulses equal bilaterally and symmetrically

Neurological: normal orientation to people, place, time, with appropriate response and concentration

Skin: warm and dry to touch; should lift easily and return back to original position, indicating normal turgor and elasticity

Abdomen: umbilicus flat or concave, positioned midway between xyphoid process and symphysis pubis; bowel motility notes normal air and fluid movement every 5–15 seconds; graded as normal, audible, absent, hyperactive, or hypoactive

ROUTINE LABORATORY TESTS WITH NUTRITIONAL IMPLICATIONS[1]

This table presents a partial listing of some uses of commonly performed lab tests that have implications for nutritional problems.

Laboratory Test	Acceptable Range	Description
Hematology		
Red blood cell (RBC) count ($\times 10^6$/mm³)	4.2–5.4 F 4.5–6.2 M	Number of RBC; aids evaluation of anemias.
Hemoglobin (Hgb, g/dL)	12–16 F 14–17 M	Hemoglobin content of RBC; aids evaluation of anemias.
Hematocrit (Hct, %)	37–47 F 41–51 M	Percentage RBC in total blood volume; aids evaluation of anemias.
Mean corpuscular volume (MCV µm³)	80–96	RBC size; helps to distinguish between microcytic and macrocytic anemias.
Mean corpuscular hemoglobin concentration (MCHC g/dL)	32–36	Hb concentration within RBCs; helps to distinguish iron-deficiency anemia.
White blood cell (WBC) count ($\times 10^3$/mm³)	3.9–10.7	Number of WBC; general assessment of immune function and/or presence of infection and inflammation.
Blood Chemistry		
Serum Proteins		
Total protein (g/dL)	6–7.8	Protein levels are not specific to disease or highly sensitive; they can reflect poor protein intake, illness or infections, changes in hydration or metabolism, pregnancy, or medications.
Albumin (g/dL)	3.5–5.5	May reflect chronic PEM; slow to respond to improvement or worsening of disease. Synthesis rate decreases during inflammation.
Transferrin (mg/dL)	250–380 F 215–365 M	May reflect illness, chronic PEM, or iron deficiency; slightly more sensitive to changes than albumin. Synthesis rate decreases during inflammation.
Prealbumin (mg/dL)	18–35	May reflect PEM; more responsive to health status changes than albumin or transferrin. Synthesis rate decreases during inflammation.
C-reactive protein (mg/dL)	<1.00	Acute-phase protein—indicator of inflammation or disease.
Fibrinogen (mg/dL)	160–450	Acute-phase protein—indicator of inflammation or disease.
Lactate (mEq/L)	0.3–2.3	Reflective of lactic acidosis—elevated during periods of critical illness.
Serum Enzymes		
Creatine kinase (CK, CPK) (U/L)	30–135 F 55–170 M	Different forms of CK are found in the muscle, brain, and heart. High blood levels may indicate heart attack, brain tissue damage, or skeletal muscle injury.

Lactate dehydrogenase (LDH) (IU/L)	208–378	LDH is found in many tissues. Specific types may be elevated after heart attack, lung damage, or liver disease.
Alkaline phosphatase (U/L)	30–120	Found in many tissues; often measured to evaluate liver function.
Aspartate aminotransferase (AST, formerly SGOT) (U/L)	0–35	Usually monitored to assess liver damage; elevated in most liver diseases. Levels are somewhat increased after tissue damage.
Alanine aminotransferase (ALT, formerly SGPT) (U/L)	4–36	Usually monitored to assess liver damage; elevated in most liver diseases. Levels are somewhat increased after tissue damage.
Serum Electrolytes		
Sodium (mEq/L)	136–145	Helps to evaluate hydration status or neuromuscular, kidney, and adrenal functions.
Potassium (mEq/L)	3.5–5.1	Helps to evaluate acid-base balance and kidney function; can detect potassium imbalances.
Chloride (mEq/L)	95–107	Helps to evaluate hydration status and detect acid-base and electrolyte imbalances.
Other		
Glucose (mg/dL)	70–99	Detects risk of glucose intolerance, diabetes mellitus, and hypoglycemia; helps to monitor diabetes treatment.
Glycosylated hemoglobin (HbA$_{1c}$) (%)	<5.7	Used to monitor long-term blood glucose control (average over previous 120 days).
Blood urea nitrogen (BUN) (mg/dL)	6–20	Primarily used to monitor renal function; value is altered by liver failure, dehydration, or shock.
Uric acid (mg/dL)	2.8–8.8 F 4.0–9.0 M	Used for detecting gout or changes in renal function; levels affected by age and diet; varies among different ethnic groups.
Creatinine (serum or plasma) (mg/dL)	0.6–1.1 F 0.9–1.3 M	Used to monitor renal function.

Note: μm = micrometer; dL = deciliter; pg = picogram; U/L = units per liter; mEq = milliequivalents

Note: Values and units of measurement listed in these tables are derived from several resources. Substantial variation exists in the ranges quoted as "normal" and these may vary depending on the assay used by different laboratories.

GROWTH CHARTS FOR CASE 25

Stature-for-Age and Weight-for-Age Percentiles: Girls, 2 to 20 Years

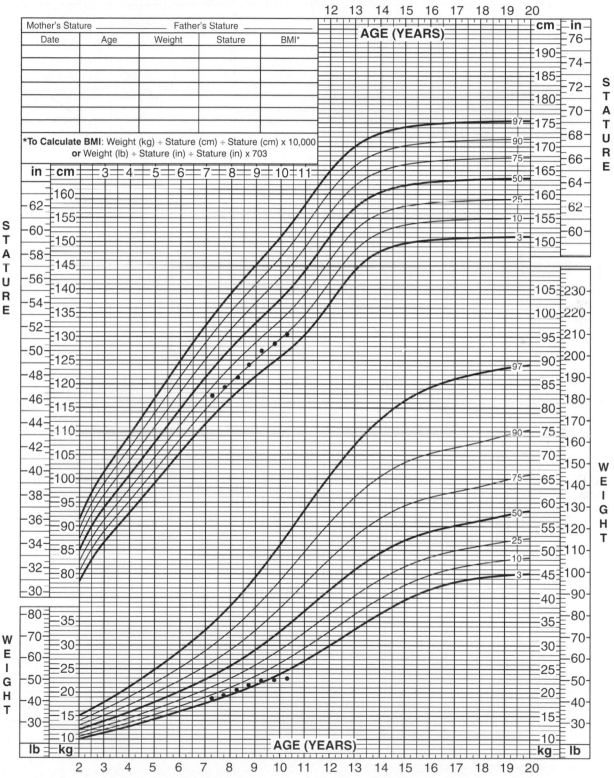

Mother's Stature _____		Father's Stature _____		
Date	Age	Weight	Stature	BMI*

*To Calculate BMI: Weight (kg) ÷ Stature (cm) ÷ Stature (cm) x 10,000
or Weight (lb) ÷ Stature (in) ÷ Stature (in) x 703

Source: Centers for Disease Control and Prevention. National Center for Health Statistics. 2000 CDC Growth Charts: United States. Available at http://www.cdc.gov/growthcharts. Accessed April 10, 2008.

Body Mass Index-for-Age Percentiles: Girls, 2 to 20 Years

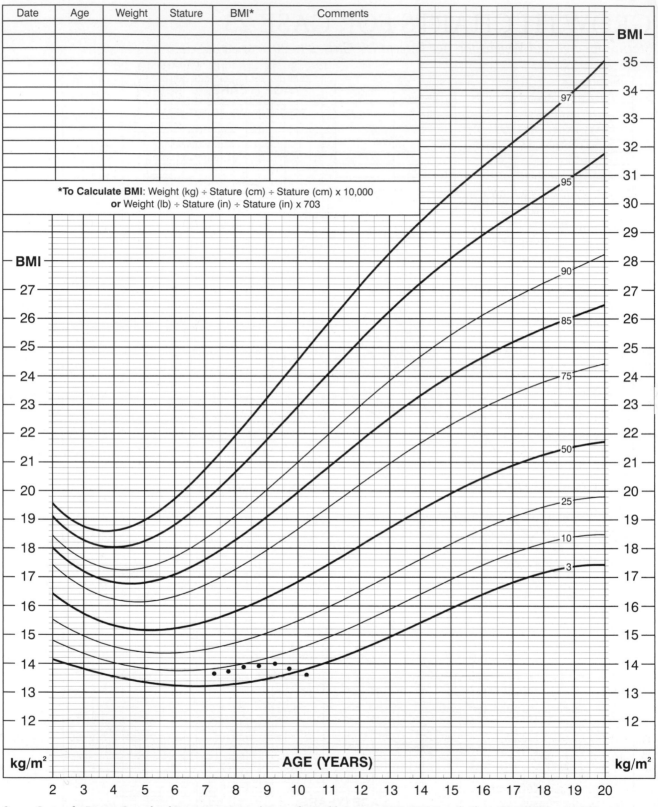

Source: Centers for Disease Control and Prevention. National Center for Health Statistics. 2000 CDC Growth Charts: United States. Available at http://www.cdc.gov/growthcharts. Accessed April 10, 2008.

INDEX